Emerging Technologies and Work-Integrated Learning Experiences in Allied Health Education

Indu Singh
Griffith University, Australia

Karun Raghuvanshi
Caterpillar of Australia Pty Ltd, Australia

A volume in the Advances in Educational Technologies and Instructional Design (AETID) Book Series

IGI Global
DISSEMINATOR OF KNOWLEDGE

Published in the United States of America by
IGI Global
Information Science Reference (an imprint of IGI Global)
701 E. Chocolate Avenue
Hershey PA, USA 17033
Tel: 717-533-8845
Fax: 717-533-8661
E-mail: cust@igi-global.com
Web site: http://www.igi-global.com

Library of Congress Cataloging-in-Publication Data

Names: Singh, Indu, 1961- editor. | Raghuvanshi, Karun, 1985- editor.
Title: Emerging technologies and work-integrated learning experiences in allied health education / Indu Singh and Karun Raghuvanshi, editors.
Description: Hershey, PA : Information Science Reference, [2018]
Identifiers: LCCN 2017023183| ISBN 9781522538509 (hardcover) | ISBN 9781522538516 (ebook)
Subjects: LCSH: Medical education--Technological innovations. | Medicine--Study and teaching (Continuing education)
Classification: LCC R735 .E45 2018 | DDC 610.71/1--dc23 LC record available at https://lccn.loc.gov/2017023183

This book is published in the IGI Global book series Advances in Educational Technologies and Instructional Design (AETID) (ISSN: 2326-8905; eISSN: 2326-8913)

British Cataloguing in Publication Data
A Cataloguing in Publication record for this book is available from the British Library.

All work contributed to this book is new, previously-unpublished material.
The views expressed in this book are those of the authors, but not necessarily of the publisher.

For electronic access to this publication, please contact: eresources@igi-global.com.

Advances in Educational Technologies and Instructional Design (AETID) Book Series

ISSN:2326-8905
EISSN:2326-8913

Editor-in-Chief: Lawrence A. Tomei, Robert Morris University, USA

MISSION

Education has undergone, and continues to undergo, immense changes in the way it is enacted and distributed to both child and adult learners. From distance education, Massive-Open-Online-Courses (MOOCs), and electronic tablets in the classroom, technology is now an integral part of the educational experience and is also affecting the way educators communicate information to students.

The **Advances in Educational Technologies & Instructional Design (AETID) Book Series** is a resource where researchers, students, administrators, and educators alike can find the most updated research and theories regarding technology's integration within education and its effect on teaching as a practice.

COVERAGE

- Hybrid Learning
- Curriculum Development
- Social Media Effects on Education
- Digital Divide in Education
- Classroom Response Systems
- Instructional Design
- E-Learning
- Higher Education Technologies
- Web 2.0 and Education
- Instructional Design Models

IGI Global is currently accepting manuscripts for publication within this series. To submit a proposal for a volume in this series, please contact our Acquisition Editors at Acquisitions@igi-global.com or visit: http://www.igi-global.com/publish/.

The Advances in Educational Technologies and Instructional Design (AETID) Book Series (ISSN 2326-8905) is published by IGI Global, 701 E. Chocolate Avenue, Hershey, PA 17033-1240, USA, www.igi-global.com. This series is composed of titles available for purchase individually; each title is edited to be contextually exclusive from any other title within the series. For pricing and ordering information please visit http://www.igi-global.com/book-series/advances-educational-technologies-instructional-design/73678. Postmaster: Send all address changes to above address.

Titles in this Series

For a list of additional titles in this series, please visit: https://www.igi-global.com/book-series/advances-educational-technologies-instructional-design/73678

Deviant Communication in Teacher-Student Interactions Emerging Research and Opportunities
Eletra Gilchrist-Petty (The University of Alabama in Huntsville, USA)
Information Science Reference • ©2018 • 133pp • H/C (ISBN: 9781522527794) • US $125.00

Culturally Engaging Service-Learning With Diverse Communities
Omobolade O. Delano-Oriaran (St. Norbert College, USA) Marguerite W. Penick-Parks (University of Wisconsin – Oshkosh, USA) and Suzanne Fondrie (University of Wisconsin – Oshkosh, USA)
Information Science Reference • ©2018 • 359pp • H/C (ISBN: 9781522529002) • US $225.00

Enhancing Education and Training Initiatives Through Serious Games
John Denholm (The University of Manchester, UK & University of Warwick, UK) and Linda Lee-Davies (The University of Manchester, UK & Wroxton College of Fairleigh Dickinson University, USA)
Information Science Reference • ©2018 • 311pp • H/C (ISBN: 9781522536895) • US $185.00

A Simplex Approach to Learning, Cognition, and Spatial Navigation Emerging Research ...
Pio Alfredo Di Tore (University of Salerno, Italy)
Information Science Reference • ©2018 • 116pp • H/C (ISBN: 9781522524557) • US $125.00

Digital Transformation and Innovation in Chinese Education
Hiller A. Spires (North Carolina State University, USA)
Information Science Reference • ©2018 • 362pp • H/C (ISBN: 9781522529248) • US $195.00

Applications of CALL Theory in ESL and EFL Environments
James Perren (Alliant International University, USA) Ken Kelch (Alliant International University, USA) Jin-suk Byun (Alliant International University, USA) Seth Cervantes (Alliant International University, USA) and Setareh Safavi (Alliant International University, USA)
Information Science Reference • ©2018 • 360pp • H/C (ISBN: 9781522529330) • US $195.00

For an enitre list of titles in this series, please visit: https://www.igi-global.com/book-series/advances-educational-technologies-instructional-design/73678

IGI Global
DISSEMINATOR OF KNOWLEDGE

701 East Chocolate Avenue, Hershey, PA 17033, USA
Tel: 717-533-8845 x100 • Fax: 717-533-8661
E-Mail: cust@igi-global.com • www.igi-global.com

Editorial Advisory Board

List of Reviewers

Table of Contents

Detailed Table of Contents

Allied healthcare professionals are an integral part of multidisciplinary healthcare teams requiring highly skilled and competent members from every discipline. Clinical and allied health education in Australia is challenged by increasing student numbers, changing healthcare practices, and service pressures impacting the clinical training of students. There is a need to optimise the effectiveness and efficiency of the way students develop their professional skills. New technological approaches deliver student-centered education involving work-integrated learning. This chapter covers different strategies developed and implemented over time, merging various technologies in an innovative manner providing better standardized skills and competencies to more students within limited resources to prepare them for a global inter-professional multidisciplinary healthcare team providing efficient service to society. It will also provide future directions to adapt technology from the non-healthcare industry to healthcare training and share some strategies of bringing the workplace to the classroom.

The scholarship of learning and teaching (SoLT) involves research into practices of teaching, learning, and curriculum. SoLT's main principle is that effective teachers in higher education should engage in scholarly teaching practices as a matter of course by staying in touch with the latest research developments in their discipline, integrating these developments into their curriculum, and routinely gathering and using student feedback to guide curriculum review and improvement. SoLT research focuses on understanding student learning in order to improve the teaching and learning experience for participants. SoLT principles are particularly important in pharmacology and chemistry education because they entail rich content that is rapidly changing. Over the years, the discipline of pharmacology has undergone rapid expansion and advancement: the number of United States Food and Drug Administration-approved drugs has increased exponentially, patients have become more educated, and our knowledge of the mechanisms underlying many adverse drug events and interactions has evolved.

Teaching anatomy has traditionally been restricted to didactic lectures and cadaveric dissection, where students are required to rote learn, without focus on analysis, conceptualisation, and clinical reasoning. A shift in pedagogical practices has occurred with rapidly developing online technologies now embedded within many university degree programs. Anatomy education has evolved to include new teaching modalities, such as computer-assisted learning including the use of 2D images or 3D models, web-based interactive games, virtual reality, augmented simulation, and haptics. Dissection courses have been found to be time-consuming and expensive, and in many universities, time committed to teaching is on the decline, there are increased costs associated with running body donation programs, and larger student numbers have led to fewer laboratory sessions available to students for learning. This chapter focuses on the use of digital atlases as a useful supplement to teaching anatomy in not only medical but all the allied health professions.

Nutritional genomics is a fast-growing area of precision medicine. It is expected that dietitians will be key players in this area. This chapter discusses the current state of industry, from research to the availability of commercial products, their regulation, and consumer perceptions. Current issues and controversies surrounding the readiness, availability, and delivery of this technology to consumers are examined, and finally, an education framework describing core competencies is presented. The framework aims to provide dietitians with the necessary tools to evaluate and make decisions on the potential for translation of this technology to clinical practice for disease prevention and management.

Adaptive learning platforms that individualize each learner's experience according to their input have only recently become widely accessible. This chapter illustrates some of the potential of adaptive learning platforms and describes a case study where this emerging technology has been used with physiotherapy students in a simulated clinical setting. Aspects of patient care scenarios presented with an adaptive learning platform were interleaved with live simulated patient interactions. Evaluation of the projects and the benefits and challenges of using adaptive learning platforms in biomedical education are discussed.

Distance learning is becoming increasingly common in the higher education sector. Student flexibility and inability of students to access education in remote regions are the main drivers of remote learning. There are many tools available that enable remote learning to reach geographically isolated and remote students as well as to provide extra flexibility to local students. This chapter explores current and emerging tools for flexible remote learning. Specifically, this chapter looks at current and new tools used in remote learning as effective tools for university students as well as

Design and manufacturing of dental restorations has evolved to embrace digital technology. So too has the paradigm of learning and teaching dental prosthetics. Once a didactic teacher-driven process, it has become student-focused, reliant on collaboration and directed toward employability. This chapter describes the stages, processes, and experiences of developing a collaborative partnership to "internationalize" dental technologist curricula which led to a model for developing shared digital resources and enhanced work-integrated learning. The discussion is supported by reflection of dental technology student learning experiences from Oslo and Akershus University College and Griffith University. Issues, controversies, and problems are explored through a descriptive analysis of experiences that aim to encourage other academics to rethink curriculum design, delivery, and assessment to create international partnerships. International collaboration in higher education can provide academics with a platform to share digital resources and create flexible, transferable qualifications.

Students commencing clinical placements often have difficulty applying their knowledge to produce meaningful clinical interactions. Patient-centred simulation can provide a bridge to clinical practice but can be expensive. This chapter describes the development and evaluation of a simulated environment integrating patient-centred simulation with an online adaptive learning platform to assist students to transition from classroom to placement. Student confidence increased significantly from pre- to post-simulation in all 12 areas that were surveyed from 3.4/6 (2.9–4.2) to 3.9/6 (3.7-4.5). Ninety-one percent of students felt better prepared for placement. The activity was not assessable and students rated this aspect highly for engagement and efficacy of learning. Student marks on their subsequent clinical placement were significantly higher for professional behavior, communication, and evidence-based practice compared with previous cohorts of students who had not undertaken a similar program.

In light of the changing landscape of workforce demand, digital technologies are becoming increasingly important to support students with their studies and professional preparation. As such, tertiary institutions are embedding curriculum approaches focused on the development of employability skills and drawing upon technology in order to prepare students for the real world of work in a manner that is scalable and transferable. Digital technologies such as ePortfolios have become an increasingly utilized platform for reflection, evidencing professional competencies and professional branding. Within this chapter, the authors discuss the benefits and limitations of these platforms from the perspectives of students, staff, professional, and institutional contexts. Case studies are utilzsed to demonstrate ePortfolios in practice across the allied health disciplines and key research questions and solutions for the future are discussed.

The fourth industrial revolution has seen significant national and international workplace change, with greater emphasis on innovation and digital adaptation. In response, universities across the sector are recognizing the importance of supporting the education of work-ready graduates and the continuing professional development of the existing professional workforce. Digital technologies have the potential to facilitate the development of employability skills such as digital literacy and reflection and foster continuing links to the profession and learning community. This chapter discusses the importance of embedding authentic, digitally enabled employability curriculum across the student and professional lifecycle, and showcases practice in the context of health professional education. A matrix for the selection of technologies that support the development of employability skills is also proposed and discussed.

Foreword

The changing landscape of higher education necessitates the use of digital technology in providing a flexible, learner-centred experience. This book focuses on learner-centred curriculum design across the student lifecycle and reports on different technological initiatives and measures for student engagement, learning, and outcomes. The aim is to inspire designers and educators to consider digital technologies as a tool for enhancing student experience and teaching and learning practices, to assist in the education of highly skilled and proficient Allied Health professionals.

As designers and educators, we are acutely aware that there isn't a systematic approach to the use of digital technologies within the teaching and learning context. This book serves as a useful reference as it provides guidelines and considerations for identifying and selecting digital technology that is fit-for-pedagogical-purpose - connecting what we do as designers and educators to learning practices and behaviour. It provides insights into learner behaviour and preferences, reflecting trends in learner-centred design, including frameworks that can be used to inform and enhance practice in support of student learning and success.

Case studies highlight the challenges and successes of digital technology initiatives implemented at different stages of the student lifecycle and as such, it serves as a roadmap and register of lessons learned. Authors give a practical view of how digital learning tools such as virtual reality and adaptive learning platforms, can assist with clinical skill development and work-integrated learning. The role and value of these technologies in providing opportunities for learners to engage with authentic professional practices and tools is also highlighted throughout.

The authors have a combined experience of many years across research, higher education and professional roles. The text is a valuable resource for educational designers, curriculum designers and educators navigating the pedagogical literature and the ever-expanding and diverse landscape of digital technologies within higher education. Each chapter provides insight into different approaches and levels of engagement with digital technology from the learner and educator perspective.

The book provides an evidence-base to inform how we select and use technology to support skill development and employability initiatives in health professional education. From project proposal, through design, implementation and evaluation, the embedded case studies serve as a useful reference for educators, offering insights into what we are likely to encounter in terms of technology enhanced education and in particular, future directions for Allied Health education.

The authors are commended for showcasing the value of collaboration between professional and academic roles in implementing technologies across curricula to support the education of highly skilled and work-ready health professionals.

Jenny Campagnolo
Griffith University, Australia

Preface

BACKGROUND

Allied health practices particularly laboratory medicine are ever evolving disciplines of health care. The rate of industrial automation as a result of global economic crisis has led to heavy duty high throughput product line commercialisation of health industry. The education industry though trying to keep up with the industry has in fragmented non-standardized ways incorporated various means of information and communication technologies (ICT). Besides the internet and ICT, web based learning, is advancing at a very fast rate. This has impacted on both the design and delivery of education to health science students with a strong focus on electronic learning (E-learning) and 3D virtual reality not only in modelling teaching resources but also by bringing a 360 degree panoramic view of an interactive industry layout into the classroom. Tertiary education faces a number of common challenges such as increasing class size, diverse cultural backgrounds, limited resources and teaching facilities as well as concerns around the alignment of course curriculum to graduate capabilities. This book aims to show various ways of embracing not only individual isolated digital interventions but mixed mode combinations of information science and technology with standardized education of health sciences, which is easy to incorporate within limited resources.

Industrial automation has had a global impact on clinical laboratories and the biopharmaceutical science industry. The adaptation of total laboratory automation (TLA) and advancing technology alongside innovative information software, has not only changed the working environment for technicians and scientists but has also transformed the way students are being trained and educated. This book, 'Emerging Technologies and Work-Integrated Learning Experiences in Allied Health Education', will discuss current implementation of technologies in health science education. It will then consider the future direction of the application of upcoming technologies in tertiary education.

Industry demand for universally adaptive multi-skilled work ready graduates has challenged the need to educate our future health professional to meet the demands of this global workforce. The recent advancements and applications of E-learning tools and 3D modelling in improving student engagement/accessibility and learning outcomes in foundation courses, such as anatomy, physiology and chemistry, as well as advanced courses of laboratory medicine, pharmacology, physiotherapy and genetics. Electronic body tissue and blood cell atlases (E-Atlas) demonstrate the link between pathology and the underlying anatomy, particularly when accessed through smart phone applications and other personal digital devices. Besides 24 hours access to class room material, the additional benefits include the support of undergraduate employability through the vertical and horizontal scaffolding and linking of courses across year levels. Web-based electronic learning (E-learning) tools such as simulated virtual labs, demonstration videos and mobile micro-computing (such as the Raspberry Pi) as well as the use of public databases of genetic and other information are increasingly becoming a part of modern educational systems that can break down many traditional access barriers to learning resources, such as access to current and expensive resources without the financial burden, as well as provide an interactive learning environment for students to gain a wide variety of practical experience.

The end product of the tertiary system is to produce highly employable graduates. Integrating technology based blended/E-learning approach into the various teaching modules can assist the students in meeting the growing demands of an industry, which seeks modern and work ready graduates in the field of ever increasing automation. This book shows how information science and technology has been trialled and can be used in standardizing tertiary health education to produce graduates who are; better prepared, require less on job training, are more globally aware and adaptable, and equipped to further their own carriers through self-directed life-long learning.

THE CHALLENGES

E-learning is being increasingly embraced in tertiary education at numerous institutions and has gained approval from both the students and the teachers. Currently most of the e-learning tools are fragmented, incorporating just one or other technologies in class rooms. The objective of this book is to demonstrate that standardised mix-mode of complementary various online learning tools is required to cater for student from different socio-economic and educational backgrounds and across the institutions and borders.

Modern technology in teaching institutions helps advance and incorporate the E-learning tools into educational facilities, which can have very positive impact. It can not only expand educational access and enhance exposure to real world learnings but it can also better prepare our graduates for future employability and success in all aspects of their social and educational means of life through everyday mediums.

To see the real value, it is important to pay attention to a significant shift that has not only caused a digital divide but also a cognitive divide between students based on their level of literacy within the IT medium. One of the many reasons for this divide can be the diversity in the rate by which technology is being incorporated into the early education system across different universities and countries. The paradigm shift from face-to face learning using mixed mode learning is heavily based on technology and its consistency in delivery and accessibility. These are still institutional barriers that can decelerate learning potential. This publication aims to bring those issues to the forefront and suggest ways of dealing with those issues by incorporating various technologies to complement each other as a flexible student directed life-long learning and continuous professional development as part of their long-term career path.

Modes of teaching and learning to be embedded in this book will include constructivist teaching methods and active learning strategies to enhance student knowledge and prepare them for the digital age. This mode of teaching can also enable students to develop skills such as critical analysis and personal interpretation of knowledge.

SEARCHING FOR A SOLUTION

About a decade ago there were multiple publications including books written about use of technology in teaching and flexible learning for students' convenience was the focus. As a result of that the upsurge in teaching and learning research led to distance learning, online learning, flip classrooms and use of electronic portfolios as innovative ideas in practice today in most institutions. The medical education and training changed face since then in last 4-5 years there have been some books and publications in use of smart phones, videos and modelling technology with 3D emerging as a winner.

However, there is no publication bringing various technologies together to scaffold the complex discipline divided teaching together into holistic multidisciplinary education system based on assessing the skills and competencies used for new employee training in the industry. This book is different from any other in the market as it encourages collaborating instead of competing within and with other institutes or teaching organisations and complement training with industry involvement.

This book will be useful for tertiary health educational institutions for both clinical and allied health teaching as well as secondary school teachers. Besides educational institutions this will also make a good reference material for health industry for training their new employees and upgrading the skills and professional development of their experienced and mature employees. The regional training organisations and professional exam bodies and training programs will be able to adopt or incorporate some of the suggestions made in this book as part of their professional body support system for fellowship and other registration exams in various disciplines of allied health, nursing, pharmacy, nutrition and dietetics to name a few.

ORGANIZATION OF THE BOOK

The book is organized into 14 chapters. A brief description of each of the chapters follows:

Chapter 1 identifies current challenges in learning and teaching of allied health care profession students due to increasing student numbers, changing health care practices and service pressures. These factors have an impact on the clinical placement training of students to complement their knowledge gained in classroom. A need was identified to optimise the effectiveness and efficiency of the way students develop their professional experience and thereafter expertise. Various technologies have been used as new approaches to delivering education which is student-centred involving work integrated active learning. It will introduce different strategies developed and implemented over time and merging of various technologies in an innovative manner to meet the challenge of providing better standardized skills and competencies to more students within limited resources to prepare them for global inter professional multidisciplinary health care team providing efficient service to society.

Chapter 2 reflects on the establishment and implementation of e-learning tools in higher education has been researched for at least two decades. There is plethora of commercial e-learning tools but the main question remains whether they have any impact on student performance and preference. This chapter is going to look at the history of e-learning tools, evaluate studies that examined the benefit of those tools and then provide a framework for designing successful e-learning tools that can benefit student learning and teaching. The results of three case studies will be discussed to support the framework design of the e-learning tools.

Chapter 3 shows the shift from traditional didactic lectures and cadaveric dissection in teaching anatomy to pedagogical practices has occurred with rapidly developing online technologies now embedded within many university degree programs. Anatomy education has evolved to include new teaching modalities such as computer-assisted learning including the use of 2D images or 3D models, web-based interactive games, virtual reality, augmented simulation and haptics. Dissection courses have been found to be time-consuming and expensive, and in many universities, time committed to teaching is on the decline, there are increased costs associated with running body donation programs and larger student numbers have led to fewer laboratory sessions available to students for learning. This chapter focuses on the use of digital atlases as a useful supplement to teaching anatomy in not only medical, but the allied health professions.

Chapter 4 examines emerging technologies in the field of nutritional genomics, the study of interaction between diet, the genome and health, and discuss the importance of evolving dietetics education in the context of dietitians being key players in the delivery of this technology to consumers. Although it has been argued that the evidence base for translating the outcomes of nutritional genomics research into personalized nutritional advice is immature, nutritional genomics tests are now available to the public and are being used in health care. Dietitians are well placed as leaders in the nutrition field to further the understanding of translation of the science into practice, and to provide guidance for the development and delivery of this technology in an evidence based way due to their expertise in nutrition and biomedical science. It is clear that in order for this to occur, dietetics education needs to evolve to enable dietitians to be competent and confident in all aspects of genetic driven nutrition care from ethical and legal considerations, interpreting complex genetic information contextualized within the nutrition care process, determining the clinical utility of various nutritional genetics tests for different clients, and effectively educating clients about the information that the data reveals.

Chapter 5 shares use of Adaptive learning platforms which individualize each learner's experience according to their input have only recently become widely accessible. This chapter illustrates some of the potential of adaptive learning platforms and describes a case study where this emerging technology has been used with Physiotherapy students in a simulated clinical setting. Aspects of patient care scenarios presented with an adaptive learning platform were interleaved with live simulated patient interactions. Evaluation of the projects and the benefits and challenges of using adaptive learning platforms in biomedical education are discussed.

Chapter 6 visits distance learning that has emerged as a popular conduit for the delivery of higher education. Student flexibility and inability of students in remote regions are the main drivers of remote learning. There are many tools available that enable remote learning to reach geographically isolated and remote students as well as providing extra flexibility to local students. This chapter explores current and emerging tools for flexible remote learning. Specifically this chapter will look at current and new tools used in remote learning as effective tools for university students as well as graduate continuing learning. The tools, benefits and models of remote learning will be discussed. The objective of the chapter is to discuss the current and emerging tools in remote learning and its importance in emerging technologies and work integrated learning in allied health.

Chapter 7 highlights utility and incorporation of increasing automation along with other recent advancements in the field of pathology into the classroom. It demonstrates importance of integrating e-learning technologies with the program Medical Laboratory Science (MLS). E-learning tools such as 3D virtual pathology laboratory, e-portfolio using pebble pad and Rasberry Pi (RPi) have been added to the Medical laboratory Science program at Griffith University, Gold Coast campus. Incorporation of these e-learning tools has the ability to potentially improve learning outcomes and increase the chances the employability by aiding in the production of work ready graduates. The aim of the following article is highlight the recent developments, issues and possible solutions along with future directions in the development and integration of these e-learning tools into the MLS.

Chapter 8 continues to explore work integrated learning in the classroom by presenting virtual microscopy as a method by which real-time microscopic illustrations get transmitted digitally via computer networks. There is increasing evidence suggest that these virtual microscopy combined with other didactic methods in teaching make significant improvements in student interaction and curiosity in histopathology and haematology teaching The introduction of virtual microscopy has broadened the field of e-learning in histopathology and haematology curriculum. Own and other case studies have proved the technological benefits of virtual microscopy in interacting off-campus students and educators. Recent technological advances have improved the use of virtual microscopy and enabled them for routine diagnostics. In this chapter, we have discussed the significance, usefulness and limitations of virtual microscopy in education. Also, the chapter has provided several technical considerations to develop a friendly web-based virtual microscopy tool in teaching.

Chapter 9 dwells into more clinical aspects of designing and manufacturing of dental restorations evolved to embrace digital technology. So too has the paradigm of learning and teaching dental prosthetics. Once a didactic teacher driven process, it has become student focused, reliant on collaboration and directed toward employability.

This chapter describes the stages, processes and experiences of developing a collaborative partnership to 'internationalize' dental technologist curricula which led to a model for developing shared digital resources, and enhance work integrated learning. The discussion is supported by the reflections of dental technology students learning experiences from Oslo and Akershus University College and Griffith University. Issues, controversies and problems are explored through a descriptive analysis of experiences that aims to encourage other academics to rethink curriculum design, delivery and assessment to create international partnerships. International collaboration in higher education can provide academics with a platform to share digital resources and create flexible, transferable qualifications.

Chapter 10 is the innovative case study describing trials to meet the challenge of Students commencing clinical placements, who often have difficulty applying their knowledge to produce meaningful clinical interactions. Patient-centred simulation can provide a bridge to clinical practice but can be expensive. This chapter will describe the development and evaluation of a simulated environment integrating patient-centred simulation with an online adaptive learning platform to assist students to transition from classroom to placement. Student confidence increased significantly from pre- to post-simulation in all 12 areas that were surveyed from 3.4/6 (2.9–4.2) to 3.9/6 (3.7-4.5). Ninety-one percent of students felt better prepared for placement. The activity was not assessable and students rated this aspect highly for engagement and efficacy of learning. Student marks on their subsequent clinical placement were significantly higher for professional behavior, communication and evidence-based practice compared with previous cohorts of students who had not undertaken a similar program.

Chapter 11 describes the real meaning of higher education and its outcome by embedding employability using digital approaches in curriculum of graduating students. It discusses the impact of industrial revolution not only on the work places but how to use these innovative, and digital adaptations for the benefit of ultimate aim of tertiary allied health care student's education that is employment at the end of graduation cycle. Universities across the sector are recognizing the importance of supporting the education of work-ready graduates and the continuing professional development of the existing professional workforce. Digital technologies have the potential to facilitate the development of employability skills such as digital literacy and reflection and foster continuing links to the profession and learning community. This chapter discusses the importance of embedding authentic, digitally–enabled employability curriculum across the student and professional lifecycle and showcases practice in the context of health professional education. A matrix for the selection of technologies that support the development of employability skills is also proposed and discussed.

Chapter 12 re-emphasises employability through use of ePortfolios and digital technologies as learning and teaching tool by embedding curriculum approaches focused on the development of employability skills and drawing upon technology to prepare students for the real world of work in a manner that is scalable and transferable. Digital technologies such as ePortfolios have become an increasingly utilised platform for reflection, evidencing professional competencies and professional branding. Within this chapter, the authors discuss the benefits and limitations of these platforms from the perspectives of students, staff, professional, and institutional contexts. Case studies will be utilised to demonstrate ePortfolios in practice across the Allied Health Disciplines and key research questions and solutions for the future are discussed.

Chapter 13 brings it all together by defining Digital technologies as integral component in the education of students in the allied health care curricula which includes dental technology, physiotherapy, pharmacy, nutrition and dietetics, nursing and medical laboratory science programs. This Chapter summarises the array of digital technologies that have implemented for the education of allied health care students as documented in the Chapters in this book.

The digital technologies have been used for curriculum design, to engage and facilitate the understanding of fundamental concepts in relevant to the disciplines, the development of active learning strategies as well as the design of critical thinking and clinical reasoning education. Online digital atlases and libraries are providing flexible resources for students to use as study tools or while on industry placement. Adaptive digital learning communication technologies are evolving as is the use of virtual reality for teaching. Communication technologies have become an essential component of the allied health care education as students are required to work with patients, other allied health care practitioners, clinical placement coordinators and academic staff.

As students are developing skills for their profession, the digital technologies have provided a platform for the documentation of these competencies and their progress through Industry placement, such that academic staff can chart the progress of students and employers can assess the competencies of graduates.

Chapter 14 summarises and links all the chapters under one theme and provides direction for the future coherent and standardized use of technology in education in a systematic manner instead of fragmented trials with various factors bringing in variations. It describes technology as integral component in the education of students in the allied health care curricula which includes dental technology, physiotherapy, pharmacy, nutrition and dietetics, nursing and medical laboratory science programs.

This Chapter summarises the array of digital technologies that have implemented for the education of allied health care students as documented in the Chapters in this book. The digital technologies have been used for curriculum design, to engage and facilitate the understanding of fundamental concepts in relevant to the disciplines, the development of active learning strategies as well as the design of critical thinking and clinical reasoning education. Online digital atlases and libraries are providing flexible resources for students to use as study tools or while on industry placement. Adaptive digital learning communication technologies are evolving as is the use of virtual reality for teaching. Communication technologies have become an essential component of the allied health care education as students are required to work with patients, other allied health care practitioners, clinical placement coordinators and academic staff. As students are developing skills for their profession, the digital technologies have provided a platform for the documentation of these competencies and their progress through Industry placement, such that academic staff can chart the progress of students and employers can assess the competencies of graduates.

Karun Raghuvanshi
Caterpillar of Australia Pty Ltd, Australia

Chapter 1
Introduction and Current Status of Technology in Teaching and Learning of Allied Healthcare Students:
Use of Technology in Teaching and Learning of Allied Healthcare Students

Roselyn Rose'Meyer
Griffith University, Australia

Indu Singh
Griffith University, Australia

ABSTRACT

Allied healthcare professionals are an integral part of multidisciplinary healthcare teams requiring highly skilled and competent members from every discipline. Clinical and allied health education in Australia is challenged by increasing student numbers, changing healthcare practices, and service pressures impacting the clinical training of students. There is a need to optimise the effectiveness and efficiency of the way students develop their professional skills. New technological approaches deliver student-centered education involving work-integrated learning. This chapter covers different strategies developed and implemented over time, merging various technologies in an innovative manner providing better standardized skills and competencies to more students within limited resources to prepare them for a global inter-professional multidisciplinary healthcare team providing efficient service to society. It will also provide future directions to adapt technology from the non-healthcare industry to healthcare training and share some strategies of bringing the workplace to the classroom.

DOI: 10.4018/978-1-5225-3850-9.ch001

INTRODUCTION

The Allied Health sciences covers health professionals who are not doctors, dentists or nurses. Occupations for the Allied Health specialists includes physiotherapy, occupational therapy, medical laboratory science, pharmacy, nutrition and dietetics or speech pathology. The role of allied health professionals can be to prevent, diagnose and treat a range of conditions and illnesses. They often work within multidisciplinary health teams to provide patient care. Undergraduate education for these professions involves teaching the theoretical knowledge that underpins their disciplines with the practical skills which can involve analysis or measurement of biospecimens, dispensing advice or medicines, or healing patients depending on their scope of practice.

We are seeing significant changes in the way we deliver learning, teaching and student support as an outcome of the speedy uptake of technologies such as artificial intelligence, cognitive computing, adaptive learning and data analytics. These technologies will provide a more custom-made learning experience for students irrespective of where they are located.

With increases in student numbers and rapid changes in workplace technology it is essential that students have the skills, knowledge and experience to succeed and adapt to change in their chosen careers.

As such, the delivery of educational resources using technology needs to be designed and developed so that students learn a number of skills including mastering abstract principles, remembering factual information, assimilating methods, techniques and approaches, reasoning and critical thinking, debating ideas, or developing behavior appropriate to specific situations.

BACKGROUND

This chapter will focus on original use of technology and information resources in the development of learning strategies for allied health students. Mentoring and training students for the world in which they will work is an essential role of the university. Firstly we will review the use of technology in the development of resources for online teaching, then the strategies that are being put in place for the education of allied health students.

MAIN FOCUS OF THE CHAPTER

Delivery of Information and Communication of Knowledge

Oral Communication of Information

Despite the evidence that students learn better when they are engaged in the learning process, tertiary education has historically centred on the delivery of content, where educators deploy conventional lectures to implement content-loaded, time constrained curricula. Over 30 years ago, the first introduction of technology for didactic teaching beyond the blackboard was the implementation of overhead projectors, which have been superseded by electronic projectors and presentational software such as PowerPoint®. Additionally, the introduction of lecture capture systems for recording and streaming classroom lectures followed the development of video compression technology and relatively low cost video servers almost two decades ago.

More recently, Webinars have been used to deliver lectures online, for example, in the education of public health practitioners (Jacob, Allen, Ahrendt, & Brownson, 2017). However, none of the aforementioned technologies has changed the oral basis of communication for teaching and the use of recordings to replace live lectures has not always been well received by students (Simcock, Chua, Hekman, Levin, & Brown, 2017). While many Universities persist with the delivery of content through lectures either in person or through recordings, it is obvious that despite students requesting face to face teaching, when attendance is not compulsory, and students become busy with assessment, employment and family requirements, they do not attend lectures as frequently. These problems have required the development of different strategies to deliver content and cultivate problem solving abilities, amongst other skill sets. The growth of technologies in education has allowed for advances in the presentation of learning resources through a blended learning environment with a combination of online resources and face to face teaching. This concept can be observed with the inverted or flipped mode class where content may be delivered with online mini-lectures and resources such as research papers, articles, videos and book chapters, coupled with face to face tutorials focusing on troubleshooting difficult concepts, problem solving and critical thinking. Use of the inverted classroom has been shown to increase student pharmacist knowledge and improve their clinical confidence in pharmacogenomics (Weitzel et al., 2016).

Published textbooks which have historically been the mainstay of technical resources purchased as part as the delivery of course materials, have been largely superseded by electronic books. Electronic books have been available in some form for several decades and have started to gain ascendency over the printed form.

The development of software for online learning design has created a digital space that enables educators to create interactive, media-rich content that is highly responsive. Smart Sparrow is an example of a learning design platform that allows educators to produce constructive, interactive and adaptive e-learning courseware. For example, Smart Sparrow has been used to create a Virtual Laboratories adaptive learning tool, aimed at developing pathology diagnosis skills in Science students (Polly, Marcus, Maguire, Belinson, & Velan, 2014).

Technology for the Distribution of Learning Resources

A Virtual Learning Environment (VLE), or learning platform, is an online system that allows educators to share their materials with their student's online and well known examples include Moodle and Blackboard. VLEs are also known as Course Management Systems (CMS) and Learning Management Systems (LMS). These systems support course assessment, student tracking, and collaboration and communication tools. As they are online they can be accessed both on and off-campus and can support student learning in a setting that is external to the lecture theatre at all times day and night, seven days a week. This enables institutions to teach not only on-campus and full-time students but also those who cannot regularly attend campus due to geographic or time restrictions.

International standards associated with VLEs assist in making content and assessments available across different platforms. Not only does this allow for student access within individual Universities, but can also facilitate cross institutional and international collaboration between students (Fossum, Fruhling, Moe, & Thompson, 2016).

Electronic Resources for Learning and Teaching

Due to the ability of the new generation of students to interact with and manage their electronic environment, there has been a substantial change in the way students study and learn. There is a wealth of information that is available on the internet and in such an environment, interpretation and the ability to assess the reliability of information is vital. While internet resources provide students with massive amounts of online information, guidance is still required for students to identify quality material and to isolate and assimilate the concepts into knowledge that is relevant to their disciplines and useful for their engagement as practicing professionals.

Alongside the expansion of materials available through the internet has been the proliferation of online course and materials available through Massive Open Online Courses (MOOCs) delivered by hosts including Coursera, Udacity, and FutureLearn. These mostly free online educational resources offer an assorted choice of courses from leading universities and cultural institutions from around the world. Courses are delivered in modular form and are available on mobile, tablet and desktop devices. MOOCs have been used to provide nutrition courses as a form of distance learning that is cost-effective and easily accessible as well as equitable way to deliver continuing education to nutrition and health professionals around the world including those in developing countries (Stark & Pope, 2014). Students are presented with options of unlimited participation in courses with the flexibility of delivery when students find it convenient to learn. Beyond being a source of free online course materials, the open content movement has evolved due to the need for access to education and learning, the mounting costs of education and student choice about when and how to learn.

Technology Platforms for the Delivery of Resources

Minicomputers

Prior to the release of smartphones, small handheld devices were originally a platform though which data could be provided. One device is the Raspberry Pi which is a credit-card-sized computer that inserts into a TV and a keyboard. This miniature computer had the capacity to replicate the functions of a desktop PC providing access to spreadsheets, word processing, browsing the internet, and playing games. A similar device for imparting information was the personal digital assistant (PDA), also known as a handheld PC and was a mobile device that functioned as a personal information manager. The PDA provided a quick reference to contacts and other lists that were useful in educational or clinical situations (Long et al., 2016). Handhelds have also been used in the classroom during formal instruction providing a mechanism by which students can participate in real-time surveys. They can be used for clinical education through aiding the calculation of clinical prediction rules or providing information related to adverse effects and drug interactions (Day-Black & Merrill, 2015). Handheld computers have also developed into an essential part of patient care and documentation through electronic order entry and patient tracking applications. Many of the platforms for the delivery of educational and clinical applications have become outmoded following the extensive uptake of smartphones and the abundance of applications that have been developed for these devices (Chen, Lieffers, Bauman, Hanning, & Allman-Farinelli, 2017).

Mobile Computing

We have now reached a point where digital information is accessible regardless of where we are located around the world or what device we are using. This has been achieved through the creation of browser-based software that is device-independent. There are multiple types of mobile devices that students can use to access the internet. Mobile computing, and the use of the network-capable devices, such as RPi, is being established and used by students on many high school campuses. As it is a relatively new technology being introduced in university teaching some challenges still remain, specifically with notions of privacy, control of access, cheating on assessment items and copying of information. However, the ever expanding array of applications and software, the use of technology for educational purposes is only limited by our inventiveness.

Technologies to Develop Problem Solving Skills and Working Collaboratively in Teams

Interprofessional Learning and Videoconferencing

As Allied Health Professionals are expected to work in teams to manage patients, they require the facilities to collaborate either face to face or using technology. Interprofessional learning provides an opportunity to work with students from other medical or allied health fields to discuss cases and solutions to medical problems to develop the communication skills vital for their employment. Video-conferencing using dedicated cable systems and dedicated conferencing rooms have been in use since the 1980s. Online forums for collaborations have since evolved with the development of web conferencing experiences for learning. An example is the browser-based web conferencing package Blackboard Collaborate that facilitates synchronous collaboration no matter where the student is located.

Technology to Promote Student Collaboration

Problem solving and collaboration for assessment items with a complete team of students who are designated to cover different tasks and aspects of a project can now be attained using digital internet sites that facilitate group work such as Quick lessons or Composica. Group interactions can also be promoted using social media, a sub-category of computer technology that provides a group of internet-based applications that can be used as a conduit to work towards educational tasks. Social media covers a wide range of technologies and platforms, including blogs, wikis, YouTube videos, Twitter, Skype and Facebook (Orr, Baram-Tsabari, & Landsman,

2016; Zitzelsberger, Campbell, Service, & Sanchez, 2015). These applications allow the exchange of user-generated content, and promote interactions among students as they can generate, distribute and discuss materials and concepts in virtual communities and networks.

Technologies for the Development of Practical or Clinical Techniques

Whether using laboratory equipment or working with patients, the training of allied health students has become a challenge due to the costs of practical classes and clinical placements with an increased student load. Students create their knowledge and learning based upon previous experiences, a process called constructivism (Cadorin, Bagnasco, Rocco, & Sasso, 2014), and the foundational assumptions of constructivism is that knowledge is constructed from experience and that learning results from a personal interpretation of knowledge. Furthermore learning is an active process in which meaning is developed on the basis of experience.

Online Laboratories and Simulations

The laboratory experience for many courses has more recently been moved into the online space. These laboratories allow computer-based and remote data acquisition, virtual simulations, and interactive tuition. Students can interact with these systems to generate and collect data that allows for analysis of results and better understanding of learning outcomes. Online laboratories replace what has conventionally been considered practical experience with an added advantage of a reduction in consumable waste and time required to generate usable data. Students using online learning laboratory software have achieved better learning outcomes than those receiving face-to-face instruction (Brinson, 2015). Much research has been conducted regarding the advantages and disadvantages of the internet and computer technology on laboratory teaching and learning (Preast, Danielson, Bender, & Bousson, 2007). The benefit of the online laboratories is that students can investigate scientific phenomena using the tools, data collection techniques, models, and theories of science in physical laboratories that support interactions with the material world or in virtual laboratories that take advantage of simulations of the real world laboratory environment (de Jong, Linn, & Zacharia, 2013).

Interactive simulations are programs that replicate an authentic system, event, or process and where learners interact with the simulation through guided enquiry, quizzes and exploration. Learning through simulation is an active learning strategy that encourages students to practice critical thinking skills and reflect on their actions. This strategy requires educators to shift from teacher-centered, lecture-focused classrooms to student-centered, active learning environments that are cost-effective and efficient and emphasize collaboration, critical thinking, and decision making skills. Simulations can replace laboratory activities that are considered dangerous, reduce the costs of lab equipment and supplies, lessen time spent on experiments, and allow teachers to interact with students without having to worry about the management and supervision of expensive or fragile experiment. Simulation experiences can be low-fidelity to high-fidelity based on the technology involved and degree they match reality (Cant & Cooper, 2010). Simulation has a positive impact on student learning and assists students to integrate classroom theory and clinical application (Lasater, Johnson, Ravert, & Rink, 2014; Yuan, Williams & Fang, 2012), however there are still limitations related to the incentive to participate in the sessions and provision of sufficient feedback by teaching staff (Nuzhat, Salem, Al Shehri, & Al Hamdan, 2014).

Virtual Reality or Mixed-Reality Learning Environment

Virtual reality (VR) is the use of computer graphics systems that amalgamate several display and interface devices to provide the effect of immersion in an interactive 3 dimensional (3D) computer-generated situation (Pan, Cheok, Yang, Zhu, & Shi). Virtual reality definition refers to the insertion of virtual computer graphics objects into a real 3D scene, or alternatively the inclusion of real world elements into a simulated environment. The 3D environment has been implemented to animate motion data for biomechanics students (Dixon, Loh, Michaud-Paquette, & Pearsall, 2017). The advantages of this technology is that it can give students access to laboratories that would not normally be accessible due to safety issues or equipment that is too expensive to be available in a teaching class.

Personal Learning Environments

Personal Learning Environments (PLE) are systems that help students to take control of and manage their own learning. They provide support for learners to stipulate their own learning objectives (with contribution from teachers), and manage their learning, both content and process. PebblePad is a PLE that enables students and staff to collect, curate, create, communicate and share achievements, personal capabilities and professional skills and can be used to create an eportfolio (Cordier et al., 2016). PLEs represent a shift away from the model in which students consume information through independent channels such as the library, a textbook, or learning management system, moving instead to a model where students draw connections from a growing matrix of resources according to their personal learning preference and needs.

CONCLUSION

Over the past 30 years there has been a steady rise in the use of technology for the practice of learning and teaching which has brought with it changes in the approach to educating allied health students. A range of platforms and software have made the delivery of learning resources more affordable and effective. The use of technology for educating medical and nursing undergraduate students is well documented whereas less in known regarding the utilisation of online or technical resources for the education of allied health students. The chapters in this book will detail new initiatives that have been developed for teaching this broad cohort of students and will provide insight into the potential use of technology for future training opportunities.

The chapters are broadly divided into the following areas of learning and teaching as follows:

Chapters 2 to 6 discuss curriculum design and the use of digital technologies for student learning and the development of critical thinking and clinical reasoning education.

Chapters 7 to 10 report on the use of digital technologies for the development of skills and competencies required for the allied health care student and how it can be applied for training in simulation and interprofessional learning.

Chapters 11 to 13 examine the use of digital technologies for Work Integrated learning and clinical placements and the documentation of these competencies for assessment and employment.

REFERENCES

Brinson, J. R. (2015). Learning outcome achievement in non-traditional (virtual and remote) versus traditional (hands-on) laboratories: A review of the empirical research. *Computers & Education*, *87*, 218–237. doi:10.1016/j.compedu.2015.07.003

Cadorin, L., Bagnasco, A., Rocco, G., & Sasso, L. (2014). An integrative review of the characteristics of meaningful learning in healthcare professionals to enlighten educational practices in health care. *Nursing Open*, *1*(1), 3–14. doi:10.1002/nop2.3 PMID:27708790

Cant, R. P., & Cooper, S. J. (2010). Simulation-based learning in nurse education: Systematic review. *Journal of Advanced Nursing*, *66*(1), 3–15. doi:10.1111/j.1365-2648.2009.05240.x PMID:20423432

Chen, J., Lieffers, J., Bauman, A., Hanning, R., & Allman-Farinelli, M. (2017). The use of smartphone health apps and other mobile health (mHealth) technologies in dietetic practice: A three country study. *Journal of Human Nutrition and Dietetics*, *30*(4), 439–452. doi:10.1111/jhn.12446 PMID:28116773

Cordier, R., McAuliffe, T., Wilson, N. J., Totino, R., Dender, A., Smith, C., & Stephens, M. (2016). The appropriateness and feasibility of an online e-Portfolio for assessment of undergraduate allied health students. *Australian Occupational Therapy Journal*, *63*(3), 154–163. doi:10.1111/1440-1630.12226 PMID:26449172

Day-Black, C., & Merrill, E. B. (2015). Using Mobile Devices in Nursing Education. *The ABNF Journal*, *26*(4), 78–84. PMID:26665501

de Jong, T., Linn, M. C., & Zacharia, Z. C. (2013). Physical and virtual laboratories in science and engineering education. *Science*, *340*(6130), 305–308. doi:10.1126/science.1230579 PMID:23599479

Dixon, P. C., Loh, J. J., Michaud-Paquette, Y., & Pearsall, D. J. (2017). biomechZoo: An open-source toolbox for the processing, analysis, and visualization of biomechanical movement data. *Computer Methods and Programs in Biomedicine*, *140*, 1–10. doi:10.1016/j.cmpb.2016.11.007 PMID:28254065

Fossum, M., Fruhling, A., Moe, C. E., & Thompson, C. B. (2016). Crossing Borders: An Online Interdisciplinary Course in Health Informatics for Students From Two Countries. *Computers, Informatics, Nursing*. doi:10.1097/cin.0000000000000323 PMID:28002116

Jacob, R. R., Allen, P. M., Ahrendt, L. J., & Brownson, R. C. (2017). Learning About and Using Research Evidence Among Public Health Practitioners. *Am J Prev Med*, *52*(3S3), S304-S308. doi: 10.1016/j.amepre.2016.10.010

Long, J. D., Gannaway, P., Ford, C., Doumit, R., Zeeni, N., Sukkarieh-Haraty, O., & Song, H. et al. (2016). Effectiveness of a Technology-Based Intervention to Teach Evidence-Based Practice: The EBR Tool. *Worldviews on Evidence-Based Nursing*, *13*(1), 59–65. doi:10.1111/wvn.12132 PMID:26773417

Nuzhat, A., Salem, R. O., Al Shehri, F. N., & Al Hamdan, N. (2014). Role and challenges of simulation in undergraduate curriculum. *Medical Teacher*, *36*(Suppl 1), S69–S73. doi:10.3109/0142159X.2014.886017 PMID:24617788

Orr, D., Baram-Tsabari, A., & Landsman, K. (2016). Social media as a platform for health-related public debates and discussions: The Polio vaccine on Facebook. *Israel Journal of Health Policy Research*, *5*(1), 34. doi:10.1186/s13584-016-0093-4 PMID:27843544

Pan, Z., Cheok, A. D., Yang, H., Zhu, J., & Shi, J. (2006). Virtual reality and mixed reality for virtual learning environments. *Computers & Graphics*, *30*(1), 8. doi:10.1016/j.cag.2005.10.004

Polly, P., Marcus, N., Maguire, D., Belinson, Z., & Velan, G. M. (2014). Evaluation of an adaptive virtual laboratory environment using Western Blotting for diagnosis of disease. *BMC Medical Education*, *14*(1), 222. doi:10.1186/1472-6920-14-222 PMID:25331335

Preast, V., Danielson, J., Bender, H., & Bousson, M. (2007). Effectiveness of a computer-based tutorial for teaching how to make a blood smear. *Veterinary Clinical Pathology*, *36*(3), 245–252. doi:10.1111/j.1939-165X.2007.tb00219.x PMID:17806072

Simcock, D. C., Chua, W. H., Hekman, M., Levin, M. T., & Brown, S. (2017). A survey of first-year biology student opinions regarding live lectures and recorded lectures as learning tools. *Advances in Physiology Education*, *41*(1), 69–76. doi:10.1152/advan.00117.2016 PMID:28143825

Stark, C. M., & Pope, J. (2014). Massive open online courses: How registered dietitians use MOOCs for nutrition education. *Journal of the Academy of Nutrition and Dietetics*, *114*(8), 1147–1155. doi:10.1016/j.jand.2014.04.001 PMID:24842306

Weitzel, K. W., McDonough, C. W., Elsey, A. R., Burkley, B., Cavallari, L. H., & Johnson, J. A. (2016). Effects of Using Personal Genotype Data on Student Learning and Attitudes in a Pharmacogenomics Course. *American Journal of Pharmaceutical Education*, *80*(7), 122. doi:10.5688/ajpe807122 PMID:27756930

Zitzelsberger, H., Campbell, K. A., Service, D., & Sanchez, O. (2015). Using wikis to stimulate collaborative learning in two online health sciences courses. *The Journal of Nursing Education*, *54*(6), 352–355. doi:10.3928/01484834-20150515-08 PMID:26057431

Chapter 2
The Scholarship of Learning and Teaching in the Dynamic Discipline of Pharmacology and Chemistry

Abdullah Karaksha
Griffith University, Australia

ABSTRACT

The scholarship of learning and teaching (SoLT) involves research into practices of teaching, learning, and curriculum. SoLT's main principle is that effective teachers in higher education should engage in scholarly teaching practices as a matter of course by staying in touch with the latest research developments in their discipline, integrating these developments into their curriculum, and routinely gathering and using student feedback to guide curriculum review and improvement. SoLT research focuses on understanding student learning in order to improve the teaching and learning experience for participants. SoLT principles are particularly important in pharmacology and chemistry education because they entail rich content that is rapidly changing. Over the years, the discipline of pharmacology has undergone rapid expansion and advancement: the number of United States Food and Drug Administration-approved drugs has increased exponentially, patients have become more educated, and our knowledge of the mechanisms underlying many adverse drug events and interactions has evolved.

DOI: 10.4018/978-1-5225-3850-9.ch002

INTRODUCTION

The scholarship of learning and teaching (SoLT) involves research into practices of teaching, learning and curriculum. SoLT's main principle is that effective teachers in higher education should engage in scholarly teaching practices as a matter of course, by staying in touch with the latest research developments in their discipline, integrating these developments into their curriculum, and routinely gathering and using student feedback to guide curriculum review and improvement. SoLT research focuses on understanding student learning in order to improve the teaching and learning experience for participants (Boyer, 1991; Buckridge, Krause, & Alexander, 2010; Grauerholz & Zipp, 2008). SoLT principles are particularly important in pharmacology and chemistry education, because they entail rich content that is rapidly changing (Gilbert & Treagust, 2009; Michel, Bischoff, & Jakobs, 2002). Over the years, the discipline of pharmacology has undergone rapid expansion and advancement - the number of United States Food and Drug Administration-approved drugs has increased exponentially, patients have become more educated and demanding, and our knowledge of the mechanisms underlying many adverse drug events and interactions have evolved (Zgheib, Simaan, & Sabra, 2011). Likewise, chemistry education has been intensively engaged in pure chemical education research – advancing fundamental and generic pedagogical knowledge. The advances have not been translated to the classroom, and chemistry education seems unsure of its direction (Bucat, 2004).

This expansion in our knowledge of the discipline has placed more pressure on academics to continuously incorporate new facts and principles and update their curricula (Bucat, 2004; Hughes, 2003). Moreover, students perceive pharmacology and chemistry as a more "difficult" learning area than other subjects in the undergraduate health curriculum (D. K. Badyal, S. Bala, & P. Kathuria, 2010; Sirhan, 2007; Wang, Hu, & Xi, 2012). Consequently, teaching pharmacology and chemistry curricula to students has been a challenge (D. Badyal, S. Bala, & P. Kathuria, 2010; Halliday, Devonshire, Greenfield, & Dommett, 2010) and up-to-date teaching methods, such as e-learning tools, have been proposed to keep the students engaged and up-to-date with the content (Beetham & Sharpe, 2013; McGil, 2011; Michel et al., 2002).

The objectives of this chapter were divided into two main streams:

- **Objective One:** To review and evaluate the implementation of commercially available e-learning tools in higher education.
- **Objective Two:** To identify the required educational theories and principles to design effective self-designed e-learning tools and the software needed to produce those tools.

E-LEARNING TOOLS: WHAT'S IN A NAME?

The term 'e-Learning tool' encompasses electronic devices that are focused on implementing technology-based solutions for improving student performance and learning experience. It can refer to instruction delivered on a computer by way of CD-ROM (offline content), the internet, or intranet for the use of technology in education and training, and can contain content such as videos, slides, photographs, and animations (Lewis, Davies, Jenkins, & Tait, 2005; Yelland, Tsembas, & Hall, 2008). There are a plethora of terms describing e-learning in the educational literature, placing it in the sub-category of 'educational technology' which describes the general processes and tools involved in addressing the educational needs of the student (Roblyer & Doering, 2010)—as well as 'multimedia learning'—which refers to the use of media tools, delivered online or offline (Shavinina & Loarer, 1999), aiming to generate or enhance learning. Multimedia tools integrate at least three of the following seven types of presentation: text, data, graphics, audio, photographic images, animation or moving pictures (Shavinina & Loarer, 1999). 'Online-learning' encompasses a range of technologies such as the world-wide-web, email, chat, newsgroups, text, audio and video conferencing delivered over computer networks (Yelland et al., 2008), while 'blended-learning' is used to describe the blend of conventional didactic lectures and online tools (Graham, 2006; Krause, 2009). Additionally, e-learning tools themselves can be described by the terms Computer-Assisted Instruction (CAI), Computer-Assisted Learning (CAL), Computer-Based Instruction (CBI) and Computer-Based Learning (CBL), which were initially used when personal computers were first available as a resource for the delivery of learning material (Carbonaro et al., 2008; Grigg & Stephens, 1998; Hughes, 2002; Lewis et al., 2005; Trigwell & Prosser, 1996). Moreover, some of these terms are still used to describe e-learning tools, to reflect the main function or mode of delivery; for example, e-learning tools delivered through the internet can be termed Web-Based Instruction (WBI) or Web-Based Learning (WBL) (Erickson, Chang, Johnson, & Gruppen, 2003; Lahaie, 2007), while e-learning tools used for delivery, marking and analysis of student assignments or examinations can be termed Computer-Assisted Assessment (CAA) (Adams, 2004; Lahaie, 2007). As there are many methods to deliver the teaching instruction using technology, e-learning tools are most commonly used as a more comprehensive term (Yelland et al., 2008). Thus, for the purpose of this book chapter, the term e-learning tool will be used to refer to this technology henceforth.

Significance of E-Learning Tools in Higher Education

The American Commission to Implement Change in Pharmaceutical Education (AACP) was initiated in 1989, with the task of developing a series of recommendations to guide pharmacy education as it evolved to meet the changing demands of the profession, the healthcare system, and society (AACP, 2011). The Commission concluded that there was an increased need for pharmacy schools to examine not only what they teach, but more importantly, how they teach and how students learn (AACP, 2011). It is therefore crucial for pharmacy educators to consult and reflect on known teaching theories in order to promote and develop new practices in the learning process. Moreover, the Higher Education Funding Council for England (HEFCE) poses the question: "How can higher education institutions become more flexible at a time of change while maximising the talent and commitment of the students?" (HEFCE, 2010). Both, the AACP recommendation and the HEFCE question, come in line with the findings of research into student engagement which suggest that student engagement with traditional didactic lectures, and attendance in traditional learning activities, has significantly declined (Barnett & Coate, 2005). Students are now entering higher education with a diverse range of backgrounds and skill sets which are very different from the 'traditional' university entrance criteria (Franklin & Van Harmelen, 2007). Moreover, increasing student numbers and ballooning financial costs of higher education have raised concerns about the quality of student learning and experience (Haggis, 2006; Kukulska-Hulme, 2012). At the same time, education has been undergoing a paradigm shift, moving away from *teaching-as-instruction* (what lecturers teach) towards *student-centred learning* approaches (what students do to learn) (Ramsden, 2003). Teaching is not seen as a method to transit information from teachers to students anymore. It is the time where teachers are playing the role of facilitators and students are taking more responsibility for their learning (Horgan, 2003). As a consequence, curricula have been redesigned around learning outcomes rather than content (Biggs, 2003). Moreover, the rapid expansion and innovation in technology, and the fact that students expect technology to be integrated into their learning experiences, (Berman, Fall, Maloney, & Levine, 2008; Yelland et al., 2008) have encouraged higher education institutions to incorporate technology-based teaching into their curriculum to increase student engagement (Cole, 2009; Rennie & Morrison, 2012).

The Commission placed great emphasis on the importance of developing and implementing educational plans and strategies to evolve students from *dependent* to *independent* learners (AACP, 2011). For dependent learners, teachers are the directors of learning and the student role is to respond to the direction brought by the teacher. In other words, teachers tell the student what, how and when the content is or has to be learnt (Martin, Prosser, Trigwell, Ramsden, & Benjamin, 2000; Moore, 1973).

Independent learners, on the other hand, are self-directing their learning activities; they can plan their study effectively without the need for teacher directions. For independent learners, the teachers' role is limited to providing information and advice when needed (Martin et al., 2000; Moore, 1973). The Commission also encourages academics to apply the concept of student-focused learning which places student as the focus of activities (Trigwell, Prosser, & Waterhouse, 1999). Students in this approach have to construct their own knowledge, and re-construct their previous knowledge to produce a new knowledge framework or conception with the teacher's role limited to encouraging and facilitating students to lead their self-directed learning (Trigwell et al., 1999). This approach to learning is usually associated with students developing a deeper approach to learning (attempting to make sense of content), rather than a surface approach (attempting to remember factual content) (Biggs & Tang, 2007b; Gibbs & Coffey, 2004). A deeper approach to learning is linked with students achieving superior learning outcomes, particularly in terms of understanding and developing new and more sophisticated conceptions of the subject (Gibbs & Coffey, 2004; Trigwell & Prosser, 1996). This is strongly supported by a large body of research (Biggs & Tang, 2007b; Gibbs & Coffey, 2004; Ramsden, 1992). For instance, one study showed that 90% of the participants who passed all their examinations in both experiment and normal studies, were classified as deep learners (Ramsden, 1992). Moreover, university students, from different disciplines, were more likely to outperform other students when they used a deep learning approach (Ramsden, 1992).

The abovementioned recommendations are particularly important in pharmacology education due to the rapid expansion of the pharmacology knowledge-base, an increased understanding of the mechanisms of drug action, discovery of novel drugs and therapeutic targets, and an increase in therapeutic classes and drugs available for the treatment of disease (Francis, Mauriello, Phillips, Englebardt, & Grayden, 2000). It is essential to keep adding this new knowledge into existing pharmacology curricula (Pahinis, Stokes, Walsh, & Cannavina, 2007), a task for which no additional time is usually allocated (Pahinis et al., 2007). Furthermore, academic staff are curtailed of some teaching time due to the emphasis on excellence in research that is imperative to achieve career progression (Hughes, 2003). Another challenge posed by rapidly increasing student numbers is the greater differences of academic ability and maturity at university entry and a more diverse range of student expectations, aspirations and outcomes (Hughes, 2003). Often, many students find that they are unable to participate in face-to-face teaching for geographic, financial, family or logistical reasons and consequently lose opportunities for study; while other preferentially choose to be self-learners and do not attend lectures (Barajas & Owen, 2000). The diversity of the international student cohort with the majority of these students being from a non-English speaking background poses further challenges (Hughes, 2003).

Digital native students (students ingrained in the advances in new technologies) who have novel learning styles that are non-linear and fluent in simulation-based virtual settings, consequently need more than the traditional teaching approaches to engage in the learning process (Prensky, 2009). It is likely that these factors, at least in part, hinder student learning, prevent true comprehension and understanding, and restrict integration of new knowledge into a student's existing knowledge-base or conceptual frame-work (Pahinis et al., 2007). As a result, teaching styles have changed and pharmacology educators have evolved and adopted a number of teaching strategies to address these challenges including: small group discussions, problem-based learning, peer teaching, recitation, simulations, and use of technology resources (AACP, 2011).

The focus of this chapter is about examining the effect of implementing e-learning tools as an innovative, interactive and flexible teaching method to be an important supplement of the existing curriculum in higher education. However, it is important to note that the use of e-learning tools in learning and teaching requires an intricate combination of content, pedagogy, and technological knowledge (Harris, Mishra, & Koehler, 2009; Roblyer & Doering, 2010). Educators, therefore, must be fluent in more than just the content to be taught and the technology to be used to deliver it but also in the learning and teaching pedagogy that underpins the strategy (Harris et al., 2009; Roblyer & Doering, 2010). These three critical elements need to converge and coalesce in order to design and deliver instruction effectively and optimally with technology (Harris et al., 2009; Roblyer & Doering, 2010). This approach is proposed for the development and use of e-learning tools by pharmacology educators to enhance the impact and learning experience for their students (Candler, Ihnat, & Huang, 2007; Hughes, 2002; Hughes, 2003). Additionally, e-learning tools have the potential to increase student knowledge and understanding of a particular subject, allow flexibility in learning, offer distance learning and enable them to direct their own learning (Lewis et al., 2005); thereby conforming to an optimal model for student-focused learning (Hughes, 2002; Hughes, 2003).

Evaluating the Benefits of E-Learning Tools on Student Learning

Many e-learning tools have been implemented and evaluated in dental, health science, nursing curricula and continuing professional education (Carbonaro et al., 2008; Francis et al., 2000; Lahaie, 2007). In addition, the use of e-learning tool resources is becoming widespread to support pharmacology teaching with some increase in resources in the last decade (Dewhurst & Norris, 2003; Hughes, 2003). However, those studies, investigations, projects and articles that have investigated aspects of this new teaching method, do not concur in their conclusions. For instance, some researchers proposed that e-learning tools support academics and educators to meet the growing needs and expectations for improving the quality of tertiary education (Candler et al., 2007; O'Shaughnessy, Haq, Maxwell, & Llewelyn, 2010; Walley, Bligh, Orme, & Breckenridge, 1994) and provide a number of advantages to students that help educators promote learning and improve education quality (Maxwell, 2012). Other authors have discounted such benefits and claim that the use of e-learning tools remains limited (Berman et al., 2008; MacLean, Scott, Marshall, & Asperen, 2011; Masters & Ellaway, 2008; Yelland et al., 2008). This discrepancy can be attributed to two major reasons: lack of underlying pedagogical principles, and a focus on differing e-learning tool aspects.

The first reason for the observed conflicting reports is that the majority of e-learning tools are designed with no specific focus on pedagogy. Pedagogical knowledge includes cognitive, social, and developmental theories of learning and how they apply to students in the classroom (Harris et al., 2009). These concepts are important to understand how students construct knowledge and learn. Consequently, e-learning tool designers should put as much emphasis on the educational theories that help students learn better as they do when designing the tools (Harris et al., 2009). Failing to do so may result in producing e-learning tools that are attractive to academics and students but in reality do not carry any true educational benefit on student learning (Yelland et al., 2008).

The second reason for the observed conflicting reports is the fact that these studies focus on widely different aspects of e-learning tools. Some studies have only assessed student preferences and their attitudes to the use of e-learning tools (Chen, Lambert, & Guidry, 2010; Euzent, Martin, Moskal, & Moskal, 2011; MacLean et al., 2011; Taplin, Low, & Brown, 2011), while others have examined student motivations for using online learning approaches, such as perceptions of flexibility or convenience (Horspool & Lange, 2010). While these studies have found that student attitudes towards e-learning tools are generally positive, student preferences for or against e-learning tools (and for that matter, the course in which the e-learning tools are applied) does not accurately reflect the impact of e-learning tools on student learning (Sun, Tsai, Finger, Chen, & Yeh, 2008). Other studies which chose to investigate the impact of the tools on learning by assessing student performance, however, took into account only the students' final grades in the course as their marker of performance and learning (Nieder, Borges, & Pearson, 2011; Sari, 2012; Williams, Birch, & Hancock, 2012). While exam grades determine whether a student passes or fails the course, students may pass a course and strategically perform well in the exams without deep understanding of the course content (Chan, Tsui, Chan, & Hong, 2002b).

A more comprehensive and objective approach to evaluate the impact of e-learning tools on student learning would be to assess students' levels of understanding of the learned content using an expansive analyses of performance at assessment tasks including the taxonomic classification of examination answers (more details are provided in case study three). To the best of our knowledge, no study to date has employed this approach to evaluate the impact of e-learning tools in higher education. Therefore, it would appear that no study focused on higher education has followed a holistic approach to evaluate the impact of technology on student learning, which might have contributed to the overly cautious implementation of e-learning tools in higher education settings (Berman et al., 2008). Hence, there is a pressing need for further scholarly research to address this critical gap in our knowledge and elucidate the true educational benefits of the e-learning tools on student learning experiences and level of understanding and harness the full potential of e-learning tools in tertiary education.

LEARNING THEORIES AND PEDAGOGICAL DESIGN TO CREATE IN-HOUSE E-LEARNING TOOLS

The decision to create our in-house e-learning tools was undertaken after attempts to source a commercially available or free access e-learning tools, which conformed to our educational needs, proved difficult. A significant limitation of commercially purchased e-learning tools is that the content will potentially be out of date after a relatively short period of time due to the rapid advancement in new knowledge in many scientific disciplines, particularly pharmacology (Barajas & Owen, 2000). The content of the e-learning tools should be aligned with the educational objectives and aims of the specific course that chooses to employ them, or they will fail to benefit student learning (Charsky & Ressler, 2011). In this regard, commercially available e-learning tools are typically generic and prescriptive to the discipline, profession, publisher or country of origin. Consequently, this section focused on defining the pedagogy[1] to create e-learning tools, designed and developed in-house that conform to our program's educational needs as well as our curricular requirements to align with the objectives of the courses to form a system which operates well for the benefit of students. They were also designed to be easily updatable without extra cost or the need for complex programming skills.

Therefore, a comprehensive review of the literature was conducted to define the appropriate educational principles that could be used as the cornerstone for the design of the e-learning tools. These principally related to cognitive load theory and Mayer's dual channel assumption (Mayer, 2001; Sweller, 1994). Cognitive load theory is based on information processing assumptions and refers to the total amount

Figure 1. Limitations of commercially available e-tools

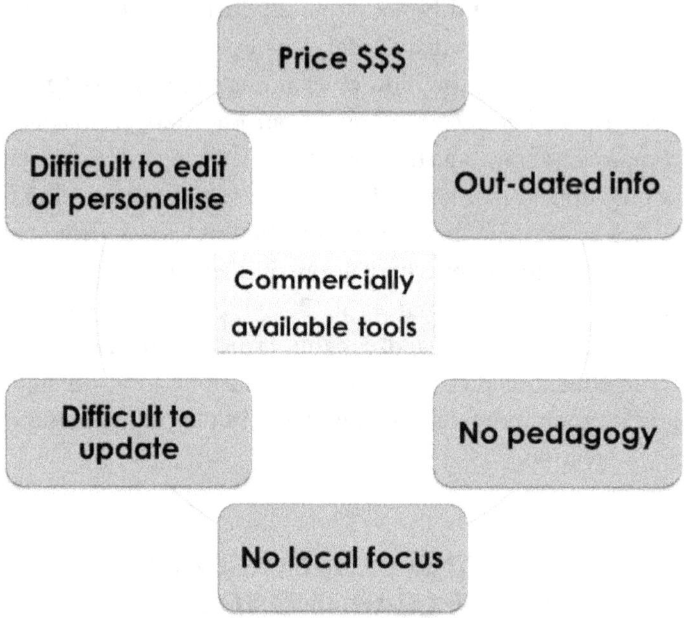

of mental activity imposed on working memory at an instant in time (Cooper, 1998; Grunwald & Charisse, 2006; Sweller, 1994). Cognitive load theory suggests that when large volumes of information are presented simultaneously, the learner can experience overload in their working memory, owing to limited capacity (Sweller, 1994). In effect, the learner becomes overwhelmed with what is presented, resulting in a loss of direction and focus (Sankey & Hill, 2005; Sweller, 1994). With respect to e-learning tools, the main factors influencing cognitive overload are designs incorporating text and animation (Stokes, 2002). Although these might focus the learner on the exciting aspects of the topic, the learner often bypasses thoughtful analysis of the underlying meaning (Stokes, 2002). According to cognitive load theory, too many distractions may impede learning (Doolittle, 2002). These were problems identified in many of the commercially available e-learning tools. In the same context, Mayer's dual coding (channel) theory suggests that the working memory consists of two distinct processing systems, auditory (verbal) and visual (nonverbal). The auditory system processes narrative information while the visual system processes images (animation) (Mayer, 2001). Fletcher (1990) found that students retain 20% of what they hear and 40% of what they see, but 75% of what they see, hear, and interact with (Fletcher, 1990). Additional teaching theories considered relevant, together with description and evidence, are provided in Table 1. This table was published in previous conference paper (Karaksha, Grant, Davey, & Anoopkumar-Dukie, 2011).

Table 1. Teaching theories and principles relevant to e-learning tool development

Teaching Theories and Principles	Description and Evidence
Multimedia Principle: Students learn better from words and pictures than from words alone (Mayer, 2001)	Mayer and Anderson (1992) concluded in their study that when animations were presented concurrently with narration, students demonstrated large improvements in problem-solving transfer over the no instruction group (Richard E Mayer & Anderson, 1992). Problem-solving transfer relates to 'factual /procedural knowledge' within Bloom's revised taxonomy (Anderson, Krathwohl, & Bloom, 2001). Mayer and Moreno (1998) also concluded that students who received both animation and narration outperformed those who received animation and on-screen text in retention testing (Mayer & Moreno, 1998).
Spatial Contiguity Principle: Students learn better when multiple source of information are integrated rather than separated (Mayer & Moreno, 2003)	The designed e-learning tool eliminates the need to collate information from different disciplines. Mayer and Moreno (1998) stated that students preformed significantly ($p<0.05$) worse in the retention test when they had to refer to different sources of information compared to the students who had to refer to only one information source (Mayer & Moreno, 1998).
Temporal Contiguity Principle: Students learn better when corresponding words and pictures are presented simultaneously rather than successively (Mayer & Moreno, 2003)	Moreno and Mayer (1999) demonstrated in their study that students who watched the animation concurrently with the narration, performed significantly better ($p<0.05$) in retention and problem solving tests from those who had them separately (Moreno & Mayer, 1999).
Coherence Principle: Students learn better when extraneous words, pictures, and sounds are excluded rather than included (Mayer, 2001)	Presentations that add 'bells and whistles' or extraneous information impede student learning and disrupt the process of organizing the material (Doolittle, 2002). Cooper (1998) showed that modifying the presented materials to obtain a lower level of extraneous cognitive load will aid learning if the resulting total cognitive load falls to a level that is within the bounds of mental resources (Cooper, 1998).
Modality Principle: **Students** learn better from animation and narration than from animation and onscreen text (Mayer, 2001)	Moreno and Mayer (1999) confirmed in their study that students who watched the animation and listened to the narration performed significantly better ($p<0.05$) in retention, matching and problem solving tests than those who watched the animation and read the on-screen text (Moreno & Mayer, 1999).
Individual Differences Principles: Design effects are stronger for low-knowledge learners than for high knowledge learns (Mayer, 2001)	Miclea et al (2008) suggested that novices (learners with low prior knowledge) may benefit more from e-learning tool than experts (learners with high prior knowledge) (Miclea, Miclea, & Ciuca, 2008).
Interactivity: Students learn better when they interact with learning materials rather than by receiving direct instruction (Mayer, 2001)	Moreno (2005) explained that students learn better when allowed to interact with e-learning tool (Pytlikzilling, Bodvarsson, & Bruning, 2005).

E-LEARNING TOOL DESIGN

Once the literature review identified the appropriate educational principles to underpin the e-learning tools, we undertook the design in two stages: storyboarding and animation. Stage one involved a brainstorming process to detail the concept of the tool, and make a storyboard to cover the main information needed for the desired concepts. It was critically important to verify that the objectives of the tools matched with the course learning objectives at this early stage. Stage two was to create the tool by making custom animations (sequenced in Microsoft PowerPoint 2010) using simple images and drawings. iSpring Pro 6.1.0 (iSpring Solutions, Inc United States) was then used to add narration, produce the embedded animation, and convert the animations into a Flash format (swf file) for ease of delivery through publication on the Blackboard™ course website. Tools were designed so that participants could easily control the speed of the final version of the tools, skip content, and move forward and backward as needed, to revisit specific concepts. The design of the e-learning tools incorporated the above mentioned educational theories. For example, cognitive load theory and Mayer's dual channel assumption) (Mayer, 2001) state that students learn better from a combination of words and pictures presented simultaneously when extraneous words, pictures, and sounds are excluded. Students also learn better when multiple sources of information are integrated, when animation and narration are combined, and when students can interact with learning materials.

There are three main advantages of custom-designed e-learning tools over the functionally limited commercially available tools. The first is that they were designed and developed incorporating the desired educational theories. The second is that the content and delivery are structured and moulded to the specific requirements of our specific pharmacology curriculum and learning and teaching needs. The third advantage of a custom tool is that educators can easily and economically update the content to encompass evolving course learning objectives, changing practices and new developments in drug discovery and applications.

To evaluate the effect of the proposed pedagogy, a series of three case studies were conducted.

Case Study One

An e-learning tool describing two gastrointestinal drug mechanisms of action was developed and delivered via a CD to participants. The study group comprised third year pharmacy students at Griffith University enrolled in pharmacology course in 2010. Seventy-five participants were randomly allocated into four groups, students who received the lecture and viewed the e-learning tool (n = 23), students who utilised the e-learning tool only (n = 22), students who received the lecture only (n = 13) and students who received no formal instruction (n = 17). Performance was assessed using multiple choice questions. Time taken to answer each question and the quiz as a whole was also compared between the four groups. Participant satisfaction with the tool was measured using a 5-point Likert scale (strongly agree, agree, neutral, disagree and strongly disagree).

Performance, as measured by mean test scores, was significantly greater ($p<0.05$) in the pharmacy student group that received the pharmacology content via the lecture and viewed the e-learning tool as compared with those who received the lecture only, or had neither. Results from the study revealed that student performance in the short-term knowledge retention quiz suggested that there was added educational value in supplementing the traditional pharmacology curricula with e-learning tools developed in-house. Moreover, the majority of students indicated satisfaction with the e-learning tool. Finally, student feedback and suggestions for improvement were taken on board to refine the design and delivery of the e-learning tools leading to the second study. For full details of this study, please refer to the following conference proceeding: (Karaksha et al., 2011).

Case Study Two

The second study was conducted by designing an e-learning tool, embedded as an animation in the lecture on the pharmacological mechanisms of action of gastrointestinal drugs for second year nursing students enrolled in a core pharmacology and pathophysiology course in 2011 at Griffith University. Forty-five nursing students voluntarily participated in the study and were divided into two groups: the intervention group, which attended a face-to-face lecture with embedded animation (n=25), and the control group, which accessed the didactic lecture online without the embedded animation (n=20). Student performance in short-term retention was assessed using two case-based quizzes. The first quiz comprised multiple choice and short answer questions on the pharmacology of gastrointestinal drugs (including the content reinforced by the embedded animation). The second quiz was on immunology and included multiple choice questions. A short survey was used to discriminate between the two groups, obtain students' demographic data and evaluate their preference towards online e-learning tools.

This study found no significant difference ($p>0.05$) in academic performance between the two nursing student cohorts who either attended the face-to-face lecture with the embedded animation or those who accessed the didactic lecture online without the embedded animation. The results also showed that students' performance correlated positively with their grade point average ($p<0.05$, $r = 0.63$) and that there was a strong association between attendance at lectures and performance in the quizzes ($p<0.05$). Another finding of this study was the significant relationship between non-attendance at lectures and preference for using online learning materials ($p<0.05$). For full details of the study, please refer to the following conference proceeding: (Karaksha, Grant, Davey, Anoopkumar-Dukie, & Nirthanan, 2013).

While the results of the two case studies on student performance revealed conflicting conclusions, there were several limitations that might have contributed to this inconsistency. The impact of e-learning tools on student learning in the studies was likely to have been blunted since these tools were used as an ad hoc rather than continuous supplementation to all lectures. Further, the concept of long-term knowledge retention following the use of the e-learning tool was also not assessed in the studies. The assessment items were either distributed on a CD (first study) or implemented online (second study) for the participants to access them from their computers. No control measures were taken for the assessment items and students could have compared or discussed responses to the questions, or have accessed their learning materials while taking the quizzes. Self-reporting bias is also a possibility. Therefore, to minimise these limitations, it was decided to design a comprehensive series of e-learning tools that could be used to supplement all the lectures in the pharmacology course and to evaluate student performance in the final summative examinations in the course as a means of assessing their level of understanding to determine the educational benefit of the e-learning tools.

Case Study Three

The e-learning tool design was refined and improved after each study, leading to the design of a series of 148 third generation e-learning tools describing the drug mechanisms of action for third year undergraduate pharmacology curriculum for pharmacy students at Griffith University, Australia. The e-learning tools were delivered as supplementary material to the Human Pharmacology I (3024PHM) and II (3028PHM) courses in 2012 and were uploaded to the courses' website (Blackboard™) for ease of access by students and for monitoring usage statistics. Two important outcomes with regard to the e-learning tools were evaluated at the end of the courses - student preference and engagement with the e-learning tools; and student performance in the final summative examinations

Student engagement and uptake of the e-learning tools during semester one and two of 2012 was assessed using a survey and usage statistics for the material which were delivered via the Blackboard™. Forty three students voluntarily participated in the survey, representing 54% of the total cohort. Of those, 23 students accessed the e-learning tools (group one) and the remaining did not use the e-learning tools (group two) during semester one.

Student performance in the final exams was assessed by conducting a qualitative and quantitative study. The study aimed to evaluate and compare the student level of understanding in the final examinations between the student cohort in 2012 (intervention group, n = 25), who studied the Human Pharmacology curriculum delivered via traditional face-to-face lectures which were supplemented with the e-learning tools, and the student cohort in 2011 (control group, n = 53) where the Human Pharmacology curriculum was delivered without the e-learning tools. To control for the differences in the level of difficulty of the content in exam questions between 2011 and 2012, the short and long answer questions were classified according to Bloom's revised taxonomy. Consequently, student answers were qualitatively evaluated using the Structure of the Observed Learning Outcomes (SOLO) taxonomy. SOLO provides a consistent framework through which to evaluate student responses and has been widely used in educational research as a means of determining the complexity and depth of student learning outcomes (Chan, Tsui, Chan, & Hong, 2002a). SOLO is a hierarchical model that is suitable for measuring learning outcomes of different kinds of subjects, among different levels of students and for all lengths of questions (Chan et al., 2002a).This taxonomy consists of five levels of increasing structural complexity: pre-structural, uni-structural, multi-structural, relational and extended abstract (Biggs & Tang, 2007a, 2010).

The key demographic variables (age, gender, and GPA) were also collected and compared between the two groups to control for the inherent ability of the participants.

Analysing student engagement with the e-learning tools revealed low usage during semester one in 2012. This was attributed to the majority of students (75%) either being unaware of, or forgetting about the embedded e-learning tools, while a few (20%) stated a lack of interest in accessing additional learning materials. E-learning tools usage significantly increased in semester two after using frequent email reminders and announcements (p=0.0001). Student qualitative comments indicated their positive preference towards the e-learning tools.

Overall, student attitudes towards the addition of e-learning tools into their learning and teaching experience was positive. Positive feedback from students included: "*I wouldn't pass without those e-learning tools. Great benefit, I passed the courses using them*". Moreover, student feedback also indicated that supplementing lectures with the e-learning tools gave them the flexibility to choose the learning method that best suited their needs. One student said in this regard; "*the e-tools were useful because they were graphic representations of drugs' mechanism of action - I'm a visual learner and remember and understand easier by looking at animations*". However, while the students had positive preference for technology, the majority (79%) were either neutral or not in favour of the substitution of didactic lectures entirely with online-learning tools. Therefore, the technology-based teaching methods are recommended to be used as supplement to, and not a substitution for face to face teaching. Another important finding in this study was that students do not purposefully engage with supplement teaching materials (like e-learning tools in this instance) unless they are consistently reminded and encouraged to do so. During semester one of this study, student engagement with and uptake of e-learning tools was poor. Analysing students' reasons for not accessing the e-learning tools during semester one showed that the majority either forgot or did not know about them, and only a few students indicated that they were not interested in accessing additional learning materials. This minority indicated that the lecture notes and textbook were enough support for their learning. "*[I] found lecture text to be enough*" and "*I did not want to use too many resources as I already understood everything*". To improve student uptake and engagement with the e-learning tools, a student-focused approach was followed in the second semester by sending frequent emails and announcements through the course website to emphasise the benefits of the e-learning tools and to remind the students about the importance of using these resources. This approach significantly increased the e-learning tools usage in semester two when compared with semester one, suggesting more student engagement with the tools.

While student engagement with the e-learning tools is an important measure of success of implementing e-learning tools, their true educational benefit can be only determined by evaluating students' level of understanding of the content as assessed by their performance in the final course examinations. In doing so, a comparison was undertaken between the performance of the student cohort in 2012 (intervention group), who studied the Human Pharmacology curriculum delivered via traditional face-to-face lectures which were supplemented with the e-learning tools, with student cohort performance from 2011 (control group) where the Human Pharmacology curriculum was delivered without the e-learning tools. As the comparison was conducted between two different academic cohorts, it was important to control for confounding factors such as the demographic variables and ensure that the assessment was comparable. There were no significant differences in the distribution of the key demographic variables between the groups suggesting that participants had similar characteristics across the two academic years. The structure, quality and level of difficulty of the summative exam was consistent across both years. As mentioned above, the level of understanding was checked using SOLO taxonomy.

Backward linear regression analysis was performed to model the level of student understanding while controlling for possible confounding variables during each semester (semester 1 and 2 in each academic year) separately. For semester one, four models were generated, with the most significant model containing the variables *intervention group* (control vs intervention) and *grade point average*, with the variables *domestic/international*, *age*, *gender* removed from the model. This model showed *grade point average* as the most significant predictor of level of understanding ($p<0.05$) and *intervention group* approaching significance as a predictor of level of understanding ($p=0.09$). Student background, age, and gender were not shown to be significant predictors ($p>0.05$). For semester two, again the model containing the variables *intervention group* and *grade point average* was the most significant of the four models generated. This model demonstrated *grade point average* as the most significant predictor of level of understanding ($p<0.05$); however, *intervention group* was also shown to be a highly significant predictor for semester two ($p<0.05$). These results were supported by correlation analysis of student level of understanding in the intervention group and e-learning tools usage. In both semesters, a strong positive correlation was observed; however in semester one the correlation was 77% compared to 88% in semester two (Karaksha, Grant, Anoopkumar-Dukie, Nirthanan, & Davey, 2013; Karaksha, Grant, Nirthanan, Davey, & Anoopkumar-Dukie, 2014).

CONCLUSION

The aims of this chapter were to evaluate commercially existing e-learning tools and then identify the required educational theories and principles to design effective self-designed e-learning tools and the software needed to produce those tools. The results of the first two case studies were used to refine the design of the e-learning tools to be more effective in their content, delivery and appeal, leading to the development of a comprehensive suite of e-learning tools which were utilised to supplement the Human Pharmacology curriculum in the undergraduate pharmacy program. Across the case studies, different student cohorts (Nursing, Pharmacy and Health Science students) showed positive preference and attitude towards the implementation of technology as a supplement to the traditional teaching methods. E-learning tools appeared to significantly improve student level of understanding as scored by the SOLO taxonomy when there was substantial engagement of students with the tools. The studies demonstrated that a holistic approach underpinned by educational pedagogy could be employed to objectively evaluate the impact of technology on student learning, effectively comparing different student cohorts using Bloom's revised taxonomy to classify exam questions into common learning dimensions, and using the SOLO taxonomy scoring to evaluate student level of understanding. This approach is superior to a simplistic comparison of summative exam grades as has been utilised in previous studies. The chapter has showed that a well-designed study was able to truly elucidate the educational benefits of the e-learning tools, and that well developed e-learning tools indeed added significant educational benefit to existing curricula by improving student level of understanding and perception.

REFERENCES

AACP. (2011). *American Association of Colleges of Pharmacy, Commission to Implement Change in Pharmaceutical Education "What is the Mission of Pharmaceutical Education?"*. Retrieved from www.aacp.org/resources/historicaldocuments/BackgroundPaper1.pdf

Adams, A. M. (2004). Pedagogical underpinnings of computer-based learning. *Journal of Advanced Nursing*, *46*(1), 5–12. doi:10.1111/j.1365-2648.2003.02960.x PMID:15030437

Anderson, L. W., Krathwohl, D. R., & Bloom, B. S. (2001). *A taxonomy for learning, teaching, and assessing: a revision of Bloom's taxonomy of educational objectives*. Longman.

Badyal, D., Bala, S., & Kathuria, P. (2010). Student evaluation of teaching and assessment methods in pharmacology. *Indian Journal of Pharmacology*, *42*(2), 87. doi:10.4103/0253-7613.64502 PMID:20711372

Badyal, D. K., Bala, S., & Kathuria, P. (2010). Student evaluation of teaching and assessment methods in pharmacology. *Indian Journal of Pharmacology*, *42*(2), 87. doi:10.4103/0253-7613.64502 PMID:20711372

Barajas, M., & Owen, M. (2000). Implementing Virtual Learning Environments: Looking for Holistic Approach. *Journal of Educational Technology & Society*, *3*(3), 39–53.

Barnett, R., & Coate, K. (2005). *Engaging the curriculum in higher education*. McGraw-Hill Education.

Beetham, H., & Sharpe, R. (2013). *Rethinking Pedagogy for a Digital Age: Designing for 21st Century Learning*. Routledge.

Berman, N., Fall, L., Maloney, C., & Levine, D. (2008). Computer-assisted instruction in clinical education: A roadmap to increasing CAI implementation. *Advances in Health Sciences Education: Theory and Practice*, *13*(3), 373–383. doi:10.1007/s10459-006-9041-3 PMID:17089076

Biggs, J. (2003). Setting the stage for effective teaching. In Teaching for quality learning at university: What the student does (2nd ed.; pp. 56-73). Buckingham, UK: SRHE and Open University Press.

Biggs, J., & Tang, C. (2007a). Designing Intended Learning Outcomes. In Teaching for Quality Learning at University (3rd ed.). Open University Press (McGraw-Hill Education).

Biggs, J., & Tang, C. (2007b). Teaching according to how students learn. In Teaching for quality learning at university (4th ed.; pp. 15-30). Berkshire, UK: Open University Press (McGraw-Hill Education).

Biggs, J., & Tang, C. (2010). *Applying constructive alignment to outcomes-based teaching and learning*. Paper presented at the Training material for "quality teaching for learning in higher education" workshop for master trainers, Ministry of Higher Education, Kuala Lumpur, Malaysia.

Boyer, E. L. (1991). Highlights of the Carnegie Report: The Scholarship of Teaching from "Scholarship Reconsidered: Priorities of the Professoriate". *College Teaching*, *39*(1), 11–13. doi:10.1080/87567555.1991.10532213

Bucat, R. (2004). Pedagogical content knowledge as a way forward: Applied research in chemistry education. *Chemistry Education Research and Practice*, *5*(3), 215–228. doi:10.1039/B4RP90025A

Buckridge, M., Krause, K.-L., & Alexander, H. (2010). *Scholarship of Learning and Teaching*. Retrieved from http://www.griffith.edu.au/__data/assets/pdf_file/0010/119467/SOLT-GPG.pdf

Candler, C., Ihnat, M., & Huang, G. (2007). Pharmacology education in undergraduate and graduate medical education in the United States. *Clinical Pharmacology and Therapeutics*, *82*(2), 134–137. doi:10.1038/sj.clpt.6100266 PMID:17632538

Carbonaro, M., King, S., Taylor, E., Satzinger, F., Snart, F., & Drummond, J. (2008). Integration of E-Learning Technologies in an Interprofessional Health Science Course. *Medical Teacher*, *30*(1), 25–33. doi:10.1080/01421590701753450 PMID:18278648

Chan, C. C., Tsui, M. S., Chan, M. Y. C., & Hong, J. H. (2002a). Applying the Structure of the Observed Learning Outcomes (SOLO) Taxonomy on Student's Learning Outcomes: An empirical study. *Assessment & Evaluation in Higher Education*, *27*(6), 511–527. doi:10.1080/0260293022000020282

Chan, C. C., Tsui, M. S., Chan, M. Y. C., & Hong, J. H. (2002b). Applying the Structure of the Observed Learning Outcomes (SOLO) Taxonomy on Student's Learning Outcomes: An empirical study. *Assessment & Evaluation in Higher Education*, *27*(6), 511–527. doi:10.1080/0260293022000020282

Charsky, D., & Ressler, W. (2011). "Games are made for fun": Lessons on the effects of concept maps in the classroom use of computer games. *Computers & Education*, *56*(3), 604–615. doi:10.1016/j.compedu.2010.10.001

Chen, P.-S. D., Lambert, A. D., & Guidry, K. R. (2010). Engaging online learners: The impact of Web-based learning technology on college student engagement. *Computers & Education*, *54*(4), 1222–1232. doi:10.1016/j.compedu.2009.11.008

Cole, M. (2009). Using Wiki technology to support student engagement: Lessons from the trenches. *Computers & Education*, *52*(1), 141–146. doi:10.1016/j.compedu.2008.07.003

Cooper, G. (1998). *Research into Cognitive Load Theory and Instructional Design at UNSW*. Retrieved from New South Wales, Australia: http://dwb4.unl.edu/Diss/Cooper/UNSW.htm

Dewhurst, D. G., & Norris, T. A. M. (2003). Helping teachers to embed e-learning materials into undergraduate pharmacology courses. *Bioscience Education*, *1*(1), 1–16. doi:10.3108/beej.2003.01010006

Doolittle, P. E. (2002). *Multimedia Learning: Empirical Results and Practical Applications*. Paper presented at the Irish Educational Technology Users' Conference, Carlow, Ireland.

Erickson, S. R., Chang, A., Johnson, C. E., & Gruppen, L. D. (2003). Lecture Versus Web Tutorial for Pharmacy Students' Learning of MDI Technique. *The Annals of Pharmacotherapy*, *37*(4), 500–505. doi:10.1345/aph.1C374 PMID:12659603

Euzent, P., Martin, T., Moskal, P., & Moskal, P. (2011). Assessing student performance and perceptions in lecture capture vs. face-to-face course delivery. *Journal of Information Technology Education*, *10*, 295–307.

Fletcher, J. D. (1990). *Effectiveness and Cost of Interactive Video Disk Instruction in Defense Training and Education*. Academic Press.

Francis, B., Mauriello, S. M., Phillips, C., Englebardt, S., & Grayden, S. K. (2000). Assessment of Online Continuing Dental Education in North Carolina. *The Journal of Continuing Education in the Health Professions*, *20*(2), 76–84.

Franklin, T., & Van Harmelen, M. (2007). *Web 2.0 for content for learning and teaching in higher education*. Retrieved from http://www.jisc.ac.uk/media/documents/programmes/digital_repositories/web2-content-learning-and-teaching.pdf

Gibbs, G., & Coffey, M. (2004). The Impact Of Training Of University Teachers on their Teaching Skills, their Approach to Teaching and the Approach to Learning of their Students. *Active Learning in Higher Education*, *5*(1), 87–100. doi:10.1177/1469787404040463

Gilbert, J. K., & Treagust, D. F. (2009). *Towards a coherent model for macro, submicro and symbolic representations in chemical education. In Multiple representations in chemical education* (pp. 333–350). Springer.

Graham, C. R. (2006). Blended learning systems. The handbook of blended learning, 3-21.

Grauerholz, L., & Zipp, J. F. (2008). How to do the Scholarship of Teaching and Learning. *Teaching Sociology*, *36*(1), 87–94. doi:10.1177/0092055X0803600111

Grigg, P., & Stephens, C. D. (1998). Computer-assisted learning in dentistry a view from the UK. *Journal of Dentistry*, *26*(5-6), 387–395. doi:10.1016/S0300-5712(98)00012-8 PMID:9699427

Grunwald, T., & Charisse, C.-M. (2006). Guidelines for Cognitively Efficient Multimedia Learning Tools: Educational Strategies, Cognitive Load, and Interface Design. *Academic Medicine*, *81*(3), 213–223. doi:10.1097/00001888-200603000-00003 PMID:16501261

Haggis, T. (2006). Pedagogies for diversity: Retaining critical challenge amidst fears of 'dumbing down'. *Studies in Higher Education*, *31*(5), 521–535. doi:10.1080/03075070600922709

Halliday, A. C., Devonshire, I. M., Greenfield, S. A., & Dommett, E. J. (2010). Teaching medical students basic neurotransmitter pharmacology using primary research resources. *Advances in Physiology Education*, *34*(4), 205–212. doi:10.1152/advan.00005.2010 PMID:21098388

Harris, J., Mishra, P., & Koehler, M. (2009). Teachers' technological pedagogical content knowledge and learning activity types: Curriculum-based technology integration reframed. *Journal of Research on Technology in Education*, *41*(4), 393–416. doi:10.1080/15391523.2009.10782536

HEFCE. (2010). *The higher education workforce framework*. Retrieved from Horgan, J. (2003). Lecturing for learning. In H. Fry, S. Ketteridge, & S. Marshall (Eds.), *A Handbook for Teaching and Learning in Higher Education* (2nd ed.; pp. 75–90). London: Kogan Page.

Horspool, A., & Lange, C. (2010). Applying the scholarship of teaching and learning: Student perceptions, behaviours and success online and face-to-face. *Assessment & Evaluation in Higher Education*, *37*(1), 73–88. doi:10.1080/02602938.2010.496532

Hughes, I. (2002). Computer-Based Learning - an Aid to Successful Teaching of Pharmacology? *Naunyn-Schmiedeberg's Archives of Pharmacology, 366*(1), 77–82. doi:10.1007/s00210-002-0552-z PMID:12107637

Hughes, I. (2003). Teaching Pharmacology in 2010 - New Knowledge, New Tools, New Attitudes. *Nihon yakurigaku zasshi. Folia pharmacologica Japonica, 122*(5), 411 - 418.

Karaksha, A., Grant, G., Anoopkumar-Dukie, S., Nirthanan, S. N., & Davey, A. K. (2013). Student engagement in pharmacology courses using online learning tools. *American Journal of Pharmaceutical Education, 77*(6), 125. doi:10.5688/ajpe776125 PMID:23966728

Karaksha, A., Grant, G., Davey, A., Anoopkumar-Dukie, S., & Nirthanan, S. (2013). Educational benefit of an embedded animation used as supplement to didactic lectures in nursing pharmacology courses. *Proceedings of the 7th International Technology, Education and Development Conference (INTED'13).*

Karaksha, A., Grant, G., Davey, A. K., & Anoopkumar-Dukie, S. (2011). Development and evaluation of computer-assisted learning (CAL) teaching tools compared to the conventional didactic lecture in pharmacology education. *Proceedings of EDULEARN11 Conference.*

Karaksha, A., Grant, G., Nirthanan, S. N., Davey, A. K., & Anoopkumar-Dukie, S. (2014). A Comparative Study to Evaluate the Educational Impact of E-Learning Tools on Griffith University Pharmacy Students' Level of Understanding Using Bloom's and SOLO Taxonomies. *Education Research International.*

Krause, K.-L. (2009). *GIHE Good Practice Guide on Blended Learning*. Retrieved from http://www.griffith.edu.au/gihe/pdf/gihe_tipsheet_web_bl.pdf

Kukulska-Hulme, A. (2012). How should the higher education workforce adapt to advancements in technology for teaching and learning? *The Internet and Higher Education, 15*(4), 247–254. doi:10.1016/j.iheduc.2011.12.002

Lahaie, U. (2007). Web-Based Instruction: Getting Faculty Onboard. *Journal of Professional Nursing, 26*(6), 335–342. doi:10.1016/j.profnurs.2007.01.024 PMID:18053959

Lewis, M. J., Davies, R., Jenkins, D., & Tait, M. I. (2005). A review of evaluative studies of computer-based learning in nursing education. *Nurse Education Today, 25*(8), 586–597. doi:10.1016/j.nedt.2005.09.006 PMID:16289489

MacLean, J., Scott, K., Marshall, T., & Asperen, P. (2011). Evaluation of an e-learning teaching resource: What is the medical student perspective? *Focus on Health Professional Education: A Multi-Disciplinary Journal, 13*(2), 53-63.

Martin, E., Prosser, M., Trigwell, K., Ramsden, P., & Benjamin, J. (2000). What university teachers teach and how they teach it. *Instructional Science, 28*(5), 387–412. doi:10.1023/A:1026559912774

Masters, K., & Ellaway, R. (2008). e-Learning in medical education Guide 32 Part 2: Technology, management and design. *Medical Teacher, 30*(5), 474–489. doi:10.1080/01421590802108349 PMID:18576186

Maxwell, S. R. J. (2012). An agenda for UK clinical pharmacology: How should teaching of undergraduates in clinical pharmacology and therapeutics be delivered and assessed? *British Journal of Clinical Pharmacology, 73*(6), 893–899. doi:10.1111/j.1365-2125.2012.04232.x PMID:22360965

Mayer, R. E. (2001). *Multimedia Learning*. Cambridge, UK: Cambridge University Press. doi:10.1017/CBO9781139164603

Mayer, R. E., & Anderson, R. B. (1992). The Instructive Animation: Helping Students Build Connections Between Words and Pictures in Multimedia Learning. *J Educ Psychol, 84*(4), 444–452. doi:10.1037/0022-0663.84.4.444

Mayer, R. E., & Moreno, R. (1998). A Split-Attention Effect in Multimedia Learning: Evidence for Dual Processing Systems in Working Memory. *J Educ Psychol, 90*(2), 312–320. doi:10.1037/0022-0663.90.2.312

Mayer, R. E., & Moreno, R. (2003). Nine Ways to Reduce Cognitive Load in Multimedia Learning. *Educational Psychologist, 38*(1), 43–52. doi:10.1207/S15326985EP3801_6

McGil, L. (2011). *Curriculum innovation: Pragmatic approaches to transforming learning and teaching through technologies*. Bristol, UK: JISC.

Michel, M. C., Bischoff, A., & Jakobs, K. H. (2002). Comparison of problem-and lecture-based pharmacology teaching. *Trends in Pharmacological Sciences, 23*(4), 168–170. doi:10.1016/S0165-6147(00)01940-4 PMID:11931991

Miclea, M., Miclea, S., & Ciuca, A. (2008). *Computer-Supported Psychotherapy Should Pay Attention To E-Learning*. Paper presented at the Cognitie, Creier, Comportament / Cognition, Brain, Behavior, Romanian Association for Cognitive Science.

Moore, M. G. (1973). *Speculations on a Definition of Independent Study.* Paper presented at the The Kellogg Invitational Conference (2nd), Vancouver, Canada.

Moreno, R., & Mayer, R. E. (1999). Cognitive Principles of Multimedia Learning: The Role of Modality and Contiguity. *J Educ Psychol, 91*(2), 358–368. doi:10.1037/0022-0663.91.2.358

Nieder, G. L., Borges, N. J., & Pearson, J. C. (2011). Medical student use of online lectures: Exam performance, learning styles, achievement motivation and gender. *The Journal of the International Association of Medical Science Educators: JIAMSE, 21*(3), 222–228. doi:10.1007/BF03341711

O'Shaughnessy, L., Haq, I., Maxwell, S., & Llewelyn, M. (2010). Teaching of clinical pharmacology and therapeutics in UK medical schools: Current status in 2009. *British Journal of Clinical Pharmacology, 70*(1), 143–148. doi:10.1111/j.1365-2125.2010.03665.x PMID:20642558

Pahinis, K., Stokes, C. W., Walsh, T. F., & Cannavina, G. (2007). Evaluating a Blended-Learning Course Taught to Different Groups of Learners in a Dental School. *Journal of Dental Education, 71*(2), 269–278. PMID:17314389

Prensky, M. (2009). H. sapiens digital: From digital immigrants and digital natives to digital wisdom. *Innovate: Journal of Online Education, 5*(3), 1–9.

Pytlikzilling, L. M., Bodvarsson, M., & Bruning, R. (2005). Technology-Based Education. Information Age Publishing.

Ramsden, P. (1992). *Learning to teach in higher education.* London: Routledge. doi:10.4324/9780203413937

Ramsden, P. (2003). Learning to teach in higher education: Approaches to learning (2nd ed.). London: Routledge Falmer.

Rennie, F., & Morrison, T. (2012). *E-learning and social networking handbook: Resources for higher education.* Routledge.

Roblyer, M. D., & Doering, A. H. (2010). *Integrating Educational Technology Into Teaching* (5th ed.). Allyn & Bacon.

Sankey, M., & Hill, R. S. (2005). *Multimodal design for hybrid learning materials in a second level economics course.* Paper presented at the the Eleventh Australasian Teaching Economics Conference: Innovation for Student Engagement in Economics, Sydney, Australia.

Sari, A. (2012). Impact of Determinants on Student Performance towards Information Communication Technology in Higher Education. *International Journal of Learning and Development*, *2*(2), 18–30. doi:10.5296/ijld.v2i2.1371

Shavinina, L., & Loarer, E. (1999). Psychological Evaluation of Educational Multimedia Applications. *European Psychologist*, *4*(1), 33–44. doi:10.1027//1016-9040.4.1.33

Sirhan, G. (2007). Learning difficulties in chemistry: An overview. *Journal of Turkish science education, 4*(2), 2.

Stokes, S. (2002). Visual Literacy in Teaching and Learning: A Literature Perspective. *Electronic Journal for the Integration of Technology in Education*, *1*(1), 10–19.

Sun, P.-C., Tsai, R. J., Finger, G., Chen, Y.-Y., & Yeh, D. (2008). What drives a successful e-Learning? An empirical investigation of the critical factors influencing learner satisfaction. *Computers & Education*, *50*(4), 1183–1202. doi:10.1016/j.compedu.2006.11.007

Sweller, J. (1994). Cognitive load theory, learning difficulty, and instructional design. *Learning and Instruction*, *4*(4), 295–312. doi:10.1016/0959-4752(94)90003-5

Taplin, R. H., Low, L. H., & Brown, A. M. (2011). Students' satisfaction and valuation of web-based lecture recording technologies. *Australasian Journal of Educational Technology*, *27*(2), 175–191. doi:10.14742/ajet.964

Trigwell, K., & Prosser, M. (1996). Congruence Between Intention and Strategy in University Science Teachers' Approaches to Teaching. *Higher Education*, *32*(1), 77–87. doi:10.1007/BF00139219

Trigwell, K., Prosser, M., & Waterhouse, F. (1999). Relations between teachers' approaches to teaching and students' approaches to learning. *Higher Education*, *37*(1), 57–70. doi:10.1023/A:1003548313194

Walley, T., Bligh, J., Orme, M., & Breckenridge, A. (1994). Clinical pharmacology and therapeutics in undergraduate medical education in the UK: The future. *British Journal of Clinical Pharmacology*, *37*(2), 137–143. doi:10.1111/j.1365-2125.1994.tb04253.x PMID:8186060

Wang, J., Hu, X., & Xi, J. (2012). Cooperative learning with role play in Chinese pharmacology education. *Indian Journal of Pharmacology*, *44*(2), 253–256. doi:10.4103/0253-7613.93862 PMID:22529486

Williams, A., Birch, E., & Hancock, P. (2012). The impact of online lecture recordings on student performance. *Australasian Journal of Educational Technology*, *28*(2), 199–213. doi:10.14742/ajet.869

Yelland, N., Tsembas, S., & Hall, L. (2008). E learning: Issues of pedagogy and practice for the information age. In P. Kell, W. Vialle, D. Konza, & G. Vogyl (Eds.), Introduction - learning and the learner: Exploring learning for new times (pp. 95-111). University of Wollongong.

Zgheib, N. K., Simaan, J. A., & Sabra, R. (2011). Using Team-based Learning to Teach Clinical Pharmacology in Medical School: Student Satisfaction and Improved Performance. *Journal of Clinical Pharmacology*, *51*(7), 1101–1111. doi:10.1177/0091270010375428 PMID:20671296

ENDNOTE

1 Pedagogy in this context refers to the teaching theories and principles that apply in designing e-learning tools.

Chapter 3
The Use of Digital Software Applications and Digital Atlases to Supplement Anatomy Teaching to Undergraduate Allied Health Students

Leanne C. Kenway
Griffith University, Australia

Mahmoud M. Bakr
Griffith University, Australia

ABSTRACT

Teaching anatomy has traditionally been restricted to didactic lectures and cadaveric dissection, where students are required to rote learn, without focus on analysis, conceptualisation, and clinical reasoning. A shift in pedagogical practices has occurred with rapidly developing online technologies now embedded within many university degree programs. Anatomy education has evolved to include new teaching modalities, such as computer-assisted learning including the use of 2D images or 3D models, web-based interactive games, virtual reality, augmented simulation, and haptics. Dissection courses have been found to be time-consuming and expensive, and in many universities, time committed to teaching is on the decline, there are increased costs associated with running body donation programs, and larger student numbers have led to fewer laboratory sessions available to students for learning. This chapter focuses on the use of digital atlases as a useful supplement to teaching anatomy in not only medical but all the allied health professions.

DOI: 10.4018/978-1-5225-3850-9.ch003

INTRODUCTION

Despite the fact that the study of anatomy is considered a cornerstone of medical practice for those with surgical specialties as well as for allied health professionals (Losco, Grant, Armson, Meyer, & Walker, 2017), there is a continuing debate as to the best way to teach it (Tam, Hart, Williams, Heylings, & Leinster, 2009).

Historically, teaching a basic science course such as anatomy has been restricted to didactic lectures and cadaveric dissection, relying largely on students rote learning without focus on analysis, conceptualisation and clinical reasoning (Kerby, Shukur, & Shalhoub, 2011; Sugand, Abrahams, & Khurana, 2010). Dissection courses have been found to be time-consuming and expensive, and in many universities, time committed to teaching is on the decline, there are increased costs associated with running body donation programmes and larger student numbers have led to fewer laboratory sessions available to students for learning (Drake, McBride, Lachman, & Pawlina, 2009; Turney, 2007). This has led to a shift in pedagogical practices, with the inclusion of new teaching modalities such as computer-assisted learning (Sugand et al., 2010; Turney, 2007), which may include interactive simulations with 2D images or 3D models, web-based games, virtual reality or online quizzes.

Increased numbers of digital natives - the millennials - raised with rapidly evolving technologies show a decreased tolerance for didactic lecture-style dissemination of course information (Prensky, 2001). Millenials, individuals born between 1982 and 2002 (Wilson & Gerber, 2008), have been exposed to information technology from a very young age, and comprise a large percentage of students currently enrolled in university degree programs. Consequently, many student cohorts are skilled in accessing and utilising new technologies to support their learning (Strauss & Howe, 1991), and splitting attention between styles of instruction, including multimedia, has been shown to help mentally integrate learning.

The majority of research investigating new innovative approaches to teaching anatomy have been undertaken in the area of medical education, and with mixed results (Abid et al., 2010; Codd & Choudhury, 2011; Donnelly, Patten, White, & Finn, 2009; Estevez, Lindgren, & Bergethon, 2010; Garg, Norman, Eva, Spero, & Sharan, 2002; Keedy et al., 2011; Marsh, Giffin, & Lowrie, 2008; Murakami et al., 2014; Nguyen, Nelson, & Wilson, 2012; Nicholson, Chalk, Funnell, & Daniel, 2006; Oh, Kim, & Choe, 2009; ten Brinke et al., 2014; Tworek, Jamniczky, Jacob, Hallgrímsson, & Wright, 2013). There are fewer studies investigating the use of digital technologies in teaching anatomy to each of the allied health professions (Bareither et al., 2013; Hoyek, Collet, Di Rienzo, De Almeida, & Guillot, 2014; Hu, Wilson, Ladak, Haase, & Fung, 2009; Karthikeyana & Ramalingamb, 2017; Levinson, Weaver, Garside, McGinn, & Norman, 2007; Lisk, McKee, Baskwill, & Agur, 2015; Mącznik, Ribeiro, & Baxter, 2015; Maggio, Hariton-Gross, & Gluch,

2012; Nguyen, Mulla, Nelson, & Wilson, 2014; Roach, Brandt, Moore, & Wilson, 2012; Shead, Roos, Olivier, & Ihunwo, 2016; Vuchkova, Maybury, & Farah, 2011). Students enrolled in schools of Dentistry, Physiotherapy, Speech Pathology, Occupational Therapy, Pharmacy, Nursing and Nutrition and Dietetics must take at least one course in basic Human Anatomy as part of their required curriculum, with some students requiring advanced human anatomy courses in later years before undertaking clinical placements.

In many cases, it is believed that traditional teaching methods are suited to practical disciplines and need to be retained, at least in part, rather than be replaced by entirely online courses. The study of anatomy, in particular, benefits from a blend of teaching approaches – traditional cadaveric prosections to be observed in the laboratory, where small table discussion and group interaction is promoted, supplemented by online activities to enhance and consolidate learning, provided that the activities are aligned with the designated learning outcomes. When studying anatomy, in addition to terminology, students learn visuospatial information, including the shape of anatomical structures, their respective positions in 3D space, and their location relative to other structures (Nguyen et al., 2014). Students must be able to visualize this 3D organization in their mind to fully understand the workings of and relationships that exist within the human body (Shaffer, 2004). While this has been the historical goal of the human dissection laboratory, there has been a rapid development of numerous digital anatomy teaching software packages that allow students to model and manipulate 2D and 3D anatomy presentations and images, linked with text-based content and quizzes (Tworek et al., 2013). The benefits of using technology to teach anatomy can extend beyond the walls of universities, as clinicians are now utilising multimedia packages to inform their patients of the anatomical structures involved in the injury, and the healing and rehabilitation processes. The aim is to increase patient knowledge and compliance with rehabilitation programs for a better long-term prognosis (G. Buchanan, Ma, & Rea, 2014).

Outcomes of studies investigating the impact of 3D models and digital applications on learning anatomy have been varied, along with the quality of studies published. Two recent reviews established that there was no solid evidence that 3D anatomy models (including digital and non-digital) were superior to traditional teaching methods of anatomy (Azer & Azer, 2016), and that there was insufficient evidence that computer-assisted learning techniques should replace traditional methods for teaching anatomy (Tam et al., 2009). However, a larger comprehensive review found evidence to support computer-assisted learning, in that it proved better overall than traditional teaching methods such as lectures and models, and in some cases prosections. It was concluded that computer-assisted learning is a valuable tool and the authors supported the use of complementary online learning tools as a supplement, rather than replacement for, laboratory dissection or prosection sessions to enhance teaching and learning of anatomy (Losco et al., 2017).

Social media applications have also been investigated as potential avenues to engage the millennial student, such as the use of YouTube as an online resource for video-sharing (Jaffar, 2012) and the creation of a faculty-administered Facebook page (Jaffar, 2014).

General Perspective

This chapter seeks to examine the use of online learning tools in anatomy education in the allied health sciences. Our objective, in particular, is to discuss the use of digital atlases, created with either 2D or 3D images, in teaching anatomy. Furthermore, should digital atlases replace or supplement more traditional methods of teaching anatomy, such as cadaveric dissection or examination of prosected specimens? Finally, we conclude with future considerations for the use of digital atlases.

BACKGROUND

Recent advances in digital technologies have enabled education systems to move from traditional classroom teaching models to a blended or 'e-learning' approach. Integration of these e-learning tools with contemporary face-to-face teaching can improve student outcomes, at the same time improving student access to education and training.

E-learning promotes active learning, self-directed and individually-paced learning. It is defined as "learning that is delivered, enabled or mediated using electronic technology for the explicit purpose of training organisations" (Sloman, 2009).

Evolution of Anatomy Learning and Teaching

Millenial students, 'digital natives', have grown up surrounded by and utilising developing technologies, and there is a recognisable shift in the style of course delivery suitable for demanding student engagement amongst this cohort. Traditional face-to-face lectures may, in some instances, be replaced with online recorded videos to disseminate basic anatomical information, and dissection/prosection laboratory time is becoming rarer due to cost, the time-consuming nature of running laboratories, increased student numbers and reduced course curriculum time (Shaffer, 2004). The traditional studying of human anatomy is undergoing a dynamic shift. Resources need to be developed utilising digital technologies that entice the millennial student, in order to enhance student engagement and achieve learning outcomes.

The learning and teaching of anatomy has evolved over centuries from viewing surface anatomy, to cadaveric dissection (as early as the 13th century), observing prosected cadaveric specimens, manipulation of plastic models, imaging modalities (ultrasound), radiology, CT scanning, MRI imaging, body painting for surface anatomy, e-learning using multimedia resources, haptic simulators, virtual reality (Sugand et al., 2010), and through social media (Foley, Maher, & Corrigan, 2014).

History of 3D Models

For centuries, 3D models made from wax, bronze and ivory were used for teaching anatomy. More recently, computer technology development has allowed the creation of virtual 3D medical models, which are visually rich and oftentimes interactive or animated.

In the 11th century, bronze models were used in China to teach acupuncture points (Xiannong, 2010). In the 16th century, Professor Andreas Vesalius wrote the illustrated anatomy texts *De Humani Corporis Fabrica libri septum*. The collection of seven books is based on his lectures, during which he deviated from common practice at the time by dissecting a corpse to illustrate what he was discussing (Cowen, MC. 1989). Human dissection became the primary source of anatomy education, however, access was limited due to scarce availability of bodies (for both religious and social reasons) and decomposition was a problem (due to a lack of effective preservation). Models were then created with fine anatomical details as an alternative teaching modality. From the 16th to the 18th century, models made of ivory were popular. In the 17th and 18th centuries, coloured waxes became popular as they were more 'realistic'. In the 19th century, papier-mache models were used in France. These were simpler in construction, therefore cheaper and more widely distributed. However, they did not last. The current choice of material for physical 3D models is plastic due do their cost-effective, ubiquitous and long-lasting nature.

With the onset of the digital age, 3D models began to be created virtually. 3D computer-generated imagery arose from its use in aerospace and the automobile industries, and blossomed in the entertainment industry. 3D medical models were created from data scanned from human specimens. This provided the advantage of being able to remotely view pathological specimens. Medical professionals now use computerised axial tomography (CaT) and magnetic resonance imaging (MRI) scans to derive the data to model diseased anatomy in live patients in 3D, which benefits in surgical training.

In terms of education, information gained from 3D models may be used in different ways – still pictures, animated sequences, video files, interactive 3D object or special files allow the learner to view the object from any angle. 3D models are viewed in a browser and can be rotated and observed from any angle. One advantage for using both 2-D and 3-D imagery in teaching and learning, is that the brain has a greater capacity for absorbing visual information (pictures) than textual information.

Commercial Digital Applications

Over the past decade, commercial digital applications have developed exponentially and become widely available for use on smart devices, android devices, or personal computers. Some of these digital programs or applications include, the Netter 3D atlas, Primal Pictures, Pocket Anatomy, Essential Anatomy, Complete Anatomy, Cyber-Anatomy, Snap Anatomy, Visible Body, Visible Human Project, A.D.A.M. Interactive Anatomy, Biodigital Human Platform, 3D Medical: Muscle System Pro III and Skeletal System Pro III and Anatronica. All are digital applications with detailed 3D graphics in layered human body systems. Users are able to rotate, zoom, pan and select anatomical structures. Bony landmarks of the skeletal system can be explored, nerves and arteries can be traced along their path back to their origins, and muscles can be removed one at a time, layer by layer. Incredibly detailed graphic images are colourful and vibrant, and each digital application is packed with thousands of anatomical structures displayed in 3D, enhancing student interest and learning.

The literature published to date overwhelmingly supports the notion that the learning and teaching of anatomy using online learning tools such as 2D, 3D or virtual reality is either superior to (Abid et al., 2010; Estevez et al., 2010; Glittenberg & Binder, 2006; Hampton & Sung, 2010; Hilbelink, 2007; Hoyek et al., 2014; Nicholson et al., 2006; Pani, Chariker, & Naaz, 2013; Pani et al., 2014; Stirling & Birt, 2014; Venkatiah, 2010) or at least equal to (Bukowski, 2002; Codd & Choudhury, 2011; Hopkins, Regehr, & Wilson, 2011; Keedy et al., 2011; Lisk et al., 2015; Lynn, Yenser, & Harman, 2015; Maggio et al., 2012; Metzler et al., 2012; Roach et al., 2012; Vuchkova et al., 2011), traditional methods of teaching such as lectures, chalk drawings, or cadaveric dissection/prosection in terms of student knowledge acquisition, retention or satisfaction. Several studies, however, have found disadvantages to learning anatomy using complex 3D or virtual reality tools compared with traditional static models (Khot, Quinlan, Norman, & Wainman, 2013), or more simple online interactive tasks (Levinson et al., 2007). It was suggested this may relate to the learners spatial ability, which may be hampered by more complex multimedia graphics. Although Hu and colleagues (Hu et al., 2009) reported poorer short-term learning outcomes for surgical students studying laryngeal anatomy of the larynx using a high fidelity complex 3D model compared with standard written instructions, long-term outcomes were equal between the two interventions, and students reported that they found the 3D model to be more enjoyable (Fritz et al., 2011). It is difficult to repeat methodology when little information regarding the detail of the digital instructions is described; what students were required to do with the information, how images were presented or if they had specific or generic instructions. No one method of teaching anatomy is 'the best' on its own, but digital technologies add value to the anatomy curriculum and overwhelmingly have a place as a supplement to teaching at the very least.

Whilst the release of Complete Anatomy has addressed the teething issues found in its predecessor, Essential Anatomy, it is currently only available on Windows 10 platform (not older), Mac and some newer versions of iPad, but not on iPhone. 3D4Medical, the creators of Complete Anatomy state that at the present time, it's not feasible to create an iPhone edition. Complete Anatomy is simply too comprehensive for the limited screen space on an iPhone – not surprising with over 9000 computer generated structures contained within the advanced layering system containing exploding skulls, moveable joints and contracting muscles. Essential Anatomy 5 is designed to provide the user with a general (essential) overview, while Complete Anatomy offers a more detailed (complete) thorough experience. Complete Anatomy includes several new tools and features along with a sharing platform that allows you to share dynamic content with groups and in the public arena.

Netter's 3D atlas contains the coloured illustrations of master medical artist Frank Netter, overlaid on clinically accurate models of human anatomy. Students can dissect, rotate, and peel models with over 7000 images to label. With so many detailed functions available, is the software user-friendly and easy to navigate? Is it possible that the mental effort required during the learning process is devoted to understanding the complex program and functionalities of the software, rather than the understanding of anatomy itself? This is especially important when considering learning outcomes for older students who did not grow up surrounded by technology and are not digital natives (the digital immigrants). Does the software usability influence learning outcomes? In a recent study comparing two interactive digital software programs, A.D.A.M. Interactive Anatomy (2D images) and Netter's 3D Interactive Anatomy, results indicated that the simple e-learning tool (A.D.A.M.) was as effective as more complex tools (Netter 3D) (Van Nuland & Rogers, 2016). The authors suggested that students with poor spatial ability were not disadvantaged academically. This study showed similar outcomes as other studies finding students using static images demonstrated similar learning outcomes with those using dynamic images (Levinson et al., 2007; Vogel-Walcutt, Gebrim, & Nicholson, 2010).

Western University in Ontario, Canada, designed and implemented a fully online course in Systemic Human Anatomy offered to third year undergraduate students as a foundation course in the Bachelor of Medical Sciences program (Attardi & Rogers, 2015). This was designed as an alternative to (and running concurrently with) the traditional offering of the same course delivered with face-to-face didactic lectures and in-person laboratories. The online anatomy course was delivered via Blackboard Collaborate, a collaborative software for both lecture content and the laboratory demonstrations. This involved a teaching assistant in real time video feed, an online chat among participants and live manipulation of a 3D virtual model, which the instructor broadcast from the desktop to the participant's computers. In addition, Attardi and Rogers (2015) undertook a review of 10 different commercial software programmes to determine suitability for demonstrating the three-dimensional virtual anatomical models. Netter's 3D Interactive anatomy was chosen, receiving the highest overall score based on five categories. These included the quality of the virtual models (resolution, visual clarity, accuracy and comprehensiveness of anatomical structures), volumetric data (models derived from data eg cadavers, Visible Human Project), manipulation of virtual models (ability to dissect or remove specific structures, to rotate models through a number of axes, view from different angles, speed of manipulation of model), program functionality (ease of use of menu and tools, ability to save and share dissections) and cost (licensing fee). Of the programmes evaluated, many did not afford the user several of these functionalities. Netter 3D Interactive Anatomy required a personal login to the instructor version or download of a desktop application based on payment of a licensing fee annually per student. Interestingly, none of the programmes that Attardi and Rogers reviewed was considered to have sufficient anatomical detail of the brainstem and cerebral structures, so that additional online resources needed to be created, resulting in the creation of a self-directed neuroanatomy website. Results showed that final grades were not different between students who enrolled in the traditional offering of Systemic Human Anatomy, or the online version. When student's prior academic records were correlated with final grade in the course, their previous academic success was more predictive of outcome, than the style of delivery of the course.

A recent review in Medical Teacher (Losco et al., 2017) provides evidence in support of use of the alternative online tools (particularly computer-assisted learning) in the teaching of anatomy as a supplement to, or in partial replacement of dissection. Interestingly, no significant differences were noted in learning outcomes between the 2D and 3D technologies reviewed overall, despite student satisfaction with 3D interventions being greater.

Limitations of Commercial Applications

These applications are developing rapidly, evolving constantly to meet the needs of the market. However, there are a number of limitations with many of the commercially available digital applications.

First, and foremost, the cost of initial investment in these programs is generally high. If the digital application is sourced externally and downloaded onto a personal device, often the very basic applications are free, but they do not contain detailed anatomy, nor is the functionality of the full program available. Higher quality applications with greater detail and more interactive options and structures come at a price. In addition, regular upgrades to the application can be obtained for an additional fee. If the digital software program is acquired by the university and embedded for use within the program for all students, the university purchases a licensing agreement for use of the digital software. This may relieve the student of any immediate cost, but is a considerable expense to the university, and often requires renewal annually. For example, Primal Pictures has a number of anatomical region-specific downloadable smart device applications available free of charge, which then accrue 'in-app' top up fees to be paid (around $65), and a full 3D Human Anatomy, Functional and Physiology Primal Pictures Package licenced to the university can cost in excess of $26,000USD annually. This allows unlimited user access, so that copyright is released, allowing staff and students full access to all images and animations.

Whilst the majority of university students may have a smart phone or device to run the applications, *not all do*. And in addition to this, those that do, do not necessarily have the funds to purchase the application, or update it as fast as the developers do. The authors believe that there is a need for a digital image repository that encourages active learning, is aligned with student learning objectives, outcomes and assessment, and should be made available to students *without additional cost* during their undergraduate years, allowing all students access during enrolment throughout their degree, regardless of socio-economic background.

Emerging Technologies for Teaching Anatomy at Griffith University

Griffith University has explored this approach in two courses to date, with integration of digital atlases, or an e-atlas, into the course curriculum. These 2D digital images provide a cost-effective resource available to all students from different socio-economic and educational backgrounds enrolled in the courses via the Blackboard software management/learning platform on any computer, and utilised as a resource for study.

Notably, successful student learning outcomes were achieved after institution of a digital atlas of cadavers of head and neck anatomy for first year students from the School of Dentistry and Oral Health at Griffith University, Australia (Bakr, Massey, & Massa, 2016a). A purpose-designed online digital library was implemented, with accompanying quiz bank, in addition to on-campus face-to-face traditional teaching. The success of this blended, or mixed mode, of delivery, was confirmed with significant improvement seen in laboratory grades (despite assessment using cadaveric resources, not the supplementary 2D online resources) and positive evaluation by students via a satisfaction survey. It was noted, however, that written assessments in final exams were not significantly improved.

This first year course for Dentistry students at Griffith University consisted of 3 hours of traditional didactic lectures and a single 2-hour practical laboratory session per week. Laboratories were augmented with the construction of 2D videos of head and neck anatomy, provided as online resources to support student learning. Importantly, this digital atlas of cadavers included photos of *all dry and wet specimens used in the practical sessions,* not coloured illustrations. Examples of two quiz images are shown in Figures 1 and 2. The atlas included self-directed online quizzes addressing all core knowledge and structures, previously only taught in laboratories, utilising select images from the atlas. Students were allowed multiple attempts at the quizzes, and once they correctly labelled 80% of structures, the 'trophy image' for that quiz was unlocked with all labelled components revealed. Examples of the corresponding trophy images are shown in Figures 3 and 4. Questions were styled similarly to those utilised in exams. Once all quizzes were successfully completed, students were provided with a comprehensive online digital library of images of head and neck anatomy to be used during self-directed revision prior to final exams.

Students also rated their perceived value of the digital cadaver atlas and evaluation of its use in the mix mode of delivery of on a 5 point Likert scale. Student rating of the course (SEC) increased significantly with introduction of the supplementary

Figure 1. Sample quiz images from the online digital head and neck anatomy library developed at the School of Dentistry and Oral Health - Griffith University, Australia. Anterior view of the maxilla

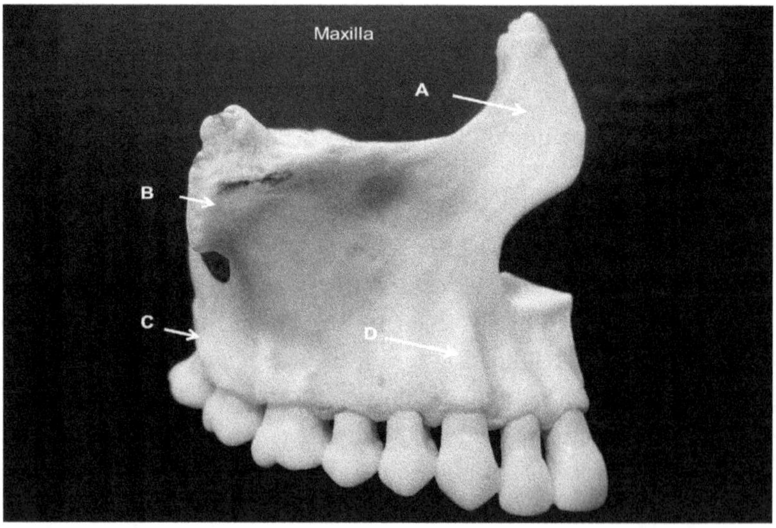

Figure 2. Lateral superficial view of the head

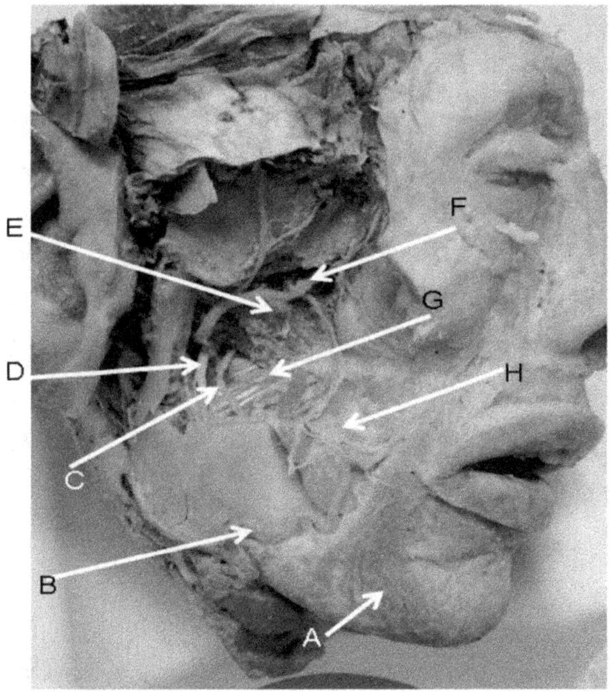

online resources. Approximately 10-17% of students remained 'neutral' as to whether the additional online resources were beneficial. 97% of students completed all online quizzes successfully and unlocked 'trophy images'. Although the average performance before and after utilising online resources was restricted to laboratory exam performance, and did not extend to the end of semester written exam, it did lead to increased numbers of students with high distinction grades and fewer students failing the course. In particular, students appreciated that all images were taken from similar or actual specimens used in their laboratory sessions, unlike the virtual images found in commercial applications. The element of familiarity with cadaveric images was found to assist in giving students a sense of confidence and security when revising for assessment.

The online digital atlas provided multiple advantages. After a small initial investment for development and production of the resource library, the digital archive of teaching resources was considered cost-effective. It was created with a longer expected life than the teaching life of human cadaveric material. In addition, the atlas allowed for revision of core anatomical knowledge and understanding, in a flexible

Figure 3. Sample fully labelled 'trophy' images unlocked once students successfully complete the relevant module with a mark of 80% or above. Images from the online digital head and neck anatomy library developed at the School of Dentistry and Oral Health - Griffith University, Australia. anterior view of the maxilla

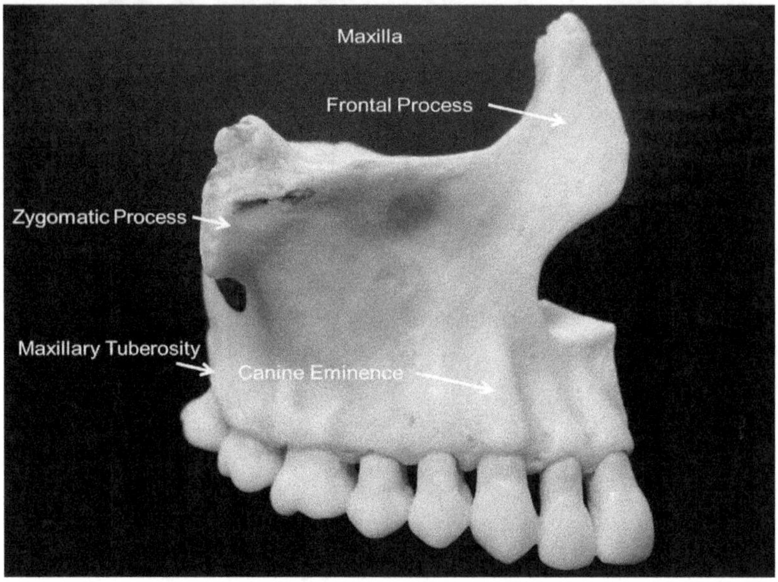

and private setting, with the potential to be used for ongoing professional education. Similar results were previously described by Sung and colleagues (Sung, Kwon, & Ryu, 2008) where the advantages of online digital resources included the provision of a cost-effective teaching resource after the initial development and production of the resource library, improved flexibility and availability of learning opportunities at any time including while students are off-campus (Sung et al., 2008).

Singh et al. (2016) designed an innovative tool to "take the classroom to the students" to enhance flexible learning, where the software is available on every computer on campus as well as on students' personal electronic devices. The e-Haem Atlas, an electronic haematology atlas, was developed for Griffith University Medical Laboratory Science students. The e-Haem atlas was developed using images of actual blood films of various disorders collected from Victoria, New South Wales and Queensland, allowing all students access to the same histology images, whether they had actually collected the sample or not and regardless of the location of the student's placement. Students had off-campus access to their online atlas for self-directed review at all times, allowing them to see samples from pathologies they may not have been exposed to on placement.

Figure 4. Lateral superficial view of the head

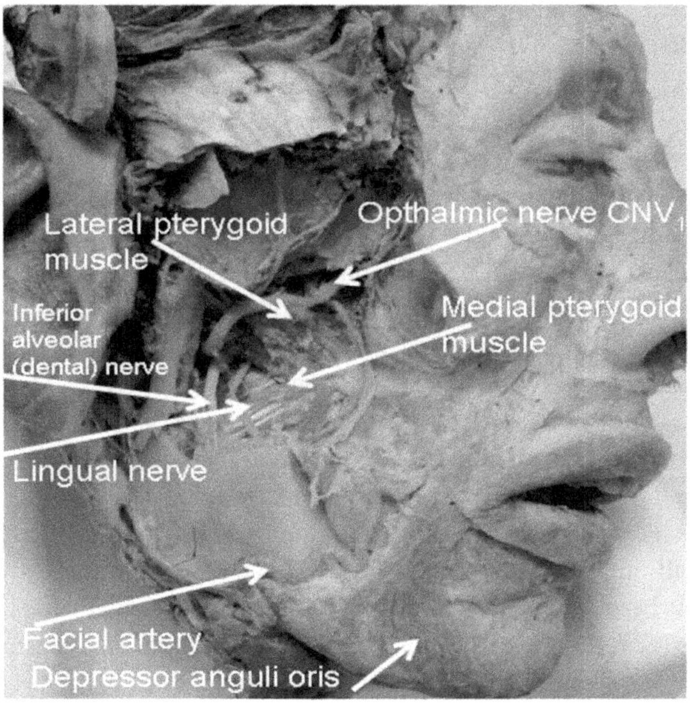

Social Media

Social media applications have also been investigated as potential avenues to engage the millennial student, such as the use of YouTube as an online resource for video-sharing (Jaffar, 2012) and the creation of a faculty-administered Facebook page (Jaffar, 2014). The University of Sharjah in the United Arab Emirates launched the Human Anatomy Education Channel on the video-sharing site, YouTube, containing videos emphasising applied aspects of anatomy (Jaffar, 2012). 98% of the medical students evaluated were found to use You Tube as an online information resource. Consequently, the Human Anatomy Education Page was then launched on Facebook and incorporated into the online resources available to the medical students. It was perceived as an effective contribution to learning and the Facebook "Insights" tool was able to record page interactions (Jaffar, 2014). When a group of first year and graduating allied health students from Thomas Jefferson University in Pennsylvania, United States of America, were surveyed investigating their media preferences, results indicated that they prefer online media as the primary source of information, with the majority of them utilising Facebook over Twitter or LinkedIn and other social networking sites (Giordano & Giordano, 2011). Since its inception in 2004,

Facebook has experienced a rapid growth in use, coinciding with increased access to free Wi-Fi and a boom in sales of mobile phones (Jaffar, 2014).

The advantages of integrating social media into teaching and learning are plentiful. It is convenient, as MOST students (medical) already have personal profiles (Hamat, Embi, & Abu Hassan, 2012). Collaborative learning may be fostered with peers (Magro, Sharp, Ryan, & Ryan, 2013), in an informal learning environment while motivating student engagement, which is supportive of innovative learning approaches (Idris & Wang, 2009). No negative impact was found on academic performance in a study by Pasek and colleagues (Pasek, More, & Hargittai, 2009), and information-related Facebook activities were actually correlated with higher grades (Junco, 2012). It was deemed an invaluable tool for arranging meetings and sharing information with peers, not only friends.

However, while most students in the study by Hamat and colleagues (Hamat et al., 2012) were found to already have a personal Facebook profile, not all did. If a Facebook page is not available to all enrolled learners, it loses its value. Traditional learning management systems engaged by the universities would guarantee automatic access for all students, regardless of social media involvement. Additionally, Facebook has been described by some as more of a distraction than a learning tool (Wise, Skues, & Williams, 2011), with a negative impact on academic performance (Kirschner & Karpinski, 2010). However, this was suggested to be based on student procrastination rather than poor academic ability. Concerns have also been raised regarding the danger of potential 'student/teacher' friendships on Facebook, as well as the risk of invasion of teacher privacy and cyber safety (Stanciu, Mihai, & Aleca, 2012).

Virtual Reality and Haptics

The latest trend in health education is the use of virtual and augmented reality as well as haptic simulation, which involves the use of the sense of touch and force feedback to simulate practical tasks and facilitate training of health practitioners on complex procedures in a risk-free virtual reality environment. Haptics and virtual reality can offer a lot of advantages over traditional teaching methods including cost-effectiveness, instant objective feedback provided by the virtual simulator software, building and development of new psychomotor skills while saving patients from the stresses involved with the possibility of trainees and novices making mistakes (Soumya & Ramachandra, 2011). Virtual reality 3D and haptic simulators have been used successfully in different fields of teaching health education including abdominal anatomy (Kinnison, Forrest, Frean, & Baillie, 2009), neuroanatomy (Estevez et al., 2010; Svirko & Mellanby, 2017), manual dexterity training (Wierinck, Puttamen, Swinnen, & van Steenberghe, 2005), restorative dental procedures (J. A. Buchanan,

2004) clinical examinations (T. Tanzawa et al., 2011) and medical emergencies (T. Tanzawa et al., 2012). Currently, the Simodont Dental Trainer is used for manual dexterity skill development, and teaching dental anatomy and pre-clinical restorative dentistry in the virtual simulation laboratory at Griffith University's School of Dentistry and Oral Health (Figure 5).

Virtual and augmented reality are proven to be very promising and engaging tools in anatomical science education, especially with the financial, ethical, and manpower restraints of the cadaver-based classes that are traditionally used across all health related disciplines (Moro, Stromberga, Raikos, & Stirling, 2017). However, virtual reality and haptics simulators could only be used as a supplementary tool augmenting the currently used traditional teaching methods and the available armamentarium for a more immersive and enriched learning experience. It should not be considered as a replacement of the human element which is very important in the educational process of health practitioners for a number of reasons, including the development of their decision-making and communication skills, which plays an integral component in the process of training future clinicians (Bakr, Massey, & Alexander, 2013, 2014, 2015).

Figure 5. The virtual simulation laboratory in the School of Dentistry and Oral Health, Griffith University, Australia. The Simodont Dental Trainer is being used for manual dexterity skill development, and teaching dental anatomy and pre-clinical restorative dentistry.

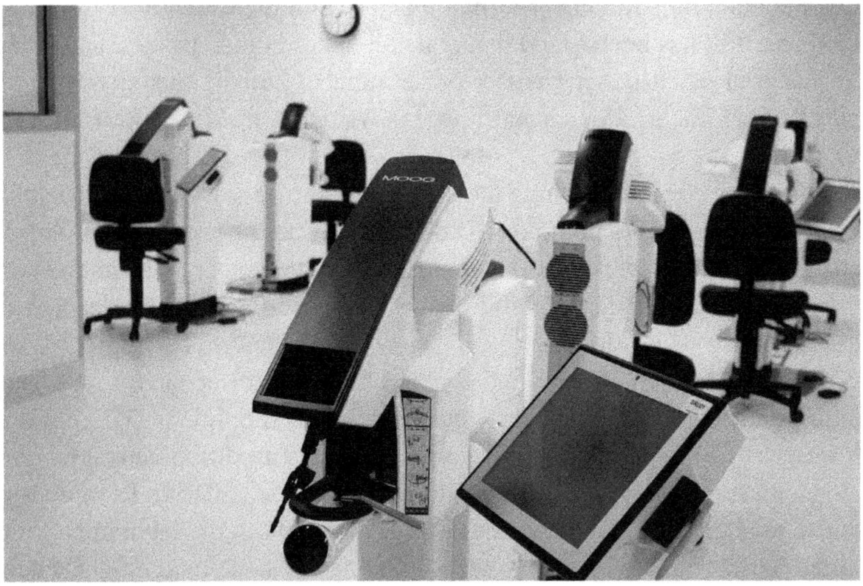

SUMMARY

In medical and allied health education, anatomy is a critical and integral keystone in undergraduate curricula, in the pre-clinical years. It forms the foundation of and scaffolds more specialised clinical knowledge in later years of undergraduate clinical degrees, such as Physiotherapy, Occupational Therapy, Speech Therapy, Nursing, Medical Imaging and postgraduate clinical degrees such as Dentistry (Bakr, Massey, & Massa, 2016b) and Medicine (Ahmed et al., 2010; Bagley, Gillott, & Gunasekera, 2011; Gupta, Morgan, Singh, & Ellis, 2008; Prince, Scherpbier, Van Mameren, Drukker, & Van Der Vleuten, 2005). A comprehensive understanding and knowledge of anatomy is essential to optimise safe clinical practice.

The majority of research-to-date investigating use of 3D applications and digital atlases when studying anatomy has focussed on the habits and outcomes of medical students, and not those enrolled in the allied health science disciplines. The research that *has* observed the teaching of anatomy to allied health students has in most instances combined a number of the allied health professions in the investigation, rather than evaluating each professional cohort individually. This has consequences in terms of student performance, as students in the different disciplines may utilise 2D or 3D digital atlases differently, depending on the necessary level of anatomical knowledge required, whether they will go on to study advanced anatomy courses in their degree program, as well as their cognitive ability to be able to utilise the software and visualise complex human anatomy, and then finally transfer that learning in relation to the human body.

The digital applications presented above include excellent graphics, but for the most part contain illustrations or virtual images, with the exception of the Visible Human Project. It has been found that real colours of human tissues, and studying human material has a better transfer of learning to human anatomy, than when studying animal material or virtual images (Waters, Van Meter, Perrotti, Drogo, & Cyr, 2005).

Additionally, simple e-learning tools presenting images in 2D have been found to be as effective as more complex 3D digital software programs (Van Nuland & Rogers, 2015), and students using static images have demonstrated similar learning outcomes with students using dynamic images. (Levinson et al., 2007; Vogel-Walcutt et al., 2010).

As a result, the School of Dentistry and Oral Health at Griffith University, Australia, launched a supplementary, purpose-designed online 2-D digital library using images of the wet and dry cadaveric specimens used in practical laboratory sessions for studying head and neck anatomy (Bakr et al., 2016a). Resources were developed to address core conceptual knowledge taught in the laboratory sessions supported by self-directed online quizzes utilising the same images. Once quizzes were successfully completed, students were provided with a comprehensive online digital library of images to be used as a reference at any time or place for self-directed study. The digital atlas overcomes barriers of limited cadaver availability, difficulty seeing specimens in large classes, extends the life expectancy of teaching specimens and provides standardised training for all students. The quizzes were designed to complement student identification skills gained in the anatomy laboratory, without need for demonstrator supervision during student self-study periods. Some students of the allied health sciences find entering an anatomy laboratory lined with cadaveric specimens rather confronting to both their visual and olfactory senses, and offering images of the same specimens in the form of a digital atlas may decrease discomfort and anxiety in these students.

Additional benefits of a purpose-designed digital atlas rather than the use of a commercial digital application, includes flexible, self-directed learning opportunities for all enrolled students via the university's software management system, Blackboard and ubiquitous delivery of resources. Student access is not dictated by their ownership of a smart device, nor their socio-economic background. The digital atlas helps build the student's cognitive skills via self-directed learning, a new focus on teaching pedagogy with increased pressure for students to work and spend more time involved in online learning.

Beyond the cost of its initial establishment, a digital library is cost-effective and sustainable, and able to be updated with additional resources as necessary. It allows students 24 hour access to an electronic anatomy atlas via Blackboard, and helps build student confidence when revising actual laboratory content. In this way, digital resources are aligned with learning outcomes and the specimens used in practical laboratory sessions and exams.

ISSUES, CONTROVERSIES, PROBLEMS

The major issues associated with utilising digital applications when teaching anatomy to allied health students relate to cost and accessibility. The cost of developing an accurate, effective, and interactive 3D model may not be justified, especially with constant development and upgrading. The initial setup when purchasing a commercial digital application is extremely costly to a university, requiring annual renewal and additional upgrades. If digital applications are not embedded internally within the program and are sourced externally by students, individuals purchase digital software for a fee, with additional fees to be paid upon upgrade. Whilst the majority of digital natives own smart devices such as phones, tablets or iPads, not all do. When a smart device is used as a learning tool, learning-space technology is delivered as software to the student computer rather than as hardware to the

University learning spaces. If all students had access to a smart device, as well as the funds to purchase and upgrade the applications on a regular basis, smart devices would provide a convenient, mobile learning platform. However, this is not the case. Consistency in student access to online resources is imperative for a successful learning and teaching environment, and unless all students have the same access to resources, its value cannot be properly evaluated, nor realised.

Information and communication technologies continue to develop at an exponential rate, with new digital software applications constantly appearing on the market. Deciding which application to choose is a difficult decision. Both 2D or static images, and 3D or animated applications have shown advantages and disadvantages in terms of student learning and transfer to student performance. Not only has the ever-increasing access to information technologies caused a digital divide, but also a cognitive divide between students based on digital literacy ie: digital natives vs digital immigrants.

Digital natives are used to receiving information at "twitch speed", and thrive on instant gratification and rewards. The current student population has grown up with the Internet, and they see virtual communication and accessing information online as routine (Green & Whitburn, 2016). The digital natives become engaged and active learners only when interactive technologies entice them. As more of the current student population are millennials, it is essential that the delivery of anatomy courses reflects a shift in pedagogy to address the changing needs of the students. They must be carefully designed if to be successfully self-directed, and not time-consuming and confusing (Smythe & Hughes, 2008).

Laboratory teaching hours of the basic sciences such as anatomy are decreasing, while student enrolment numbers are increasing. There is often minimal, if any, opportunity for students to re-visit the anatomical specimens for revision after the laboratory session. Prosected cadavers offer the anatomy student the chance to view normal human anomalies, as well as pathologies – an opportunity that is likely missed if only virtual images are studied. Many digital software programs are colourful and vibrant, but unrealistic, and virtual images do not reflect the dull colouration of cadaveric material in laboratory examinations.

Solutions and Recommendations for Future Research

Innovative tools take the classroom to the students to offer flexible learning where software is available on every computer on campus as well as personal devices. Therefore, there is a need for an accessible digital atlas, free of charge to existing students to serve as an archive and ongoing reference for students, beyond the laboratory.

It is important that the laboratory component of an anatomy course is retained if possible – the concepts of humanistic care, respect and empathy, and the appreciation of the gift of body donation are supported by small group discussion around the cadaver, and cannot be replaced by any digital application. It is recommended that online digital atlases are used as a supplement to the laboratory sessions, allowing for repeated observation and learning activities without the limitations of time and the shortage of cadavers.

At Griffith University, the digital head and neck cadaver library has been uniquely developed for students in the School of Dentistry and Oral Health. The dental digital atlas was developed in alignment with laboratory content, using images from cadaveric specimens and used for subsequent laboratory assessment. Familiarity of the digital cadaveric images resulted in successful student learning outcomes, with students performing better in the laboratory examinations after implementation of the digital atlas, as well as rating the atlas as having a positive impact on their learning (Bakr et al., 2016a).

For successful implementation of a digital anatomy repository, the approach must be planned. Clear and explicit expectations of the students need to be set - how to use the atlas, how to interact with the assigned activities, the relevancy, the purpose of the technology, any support options available, and a suggested timeline of expected interactions should be outlined.

Methodology that can be adapted for wider implementation would benefit several of the allied health professions. The digital cadaver library has proven successful within the dental program, but head and neck anatomy is also a foundation for speech therapy students studying anatomy.

Our intention now is to extend the scope of the digital head and neck anatomy atlas to include musculoskeletal anatomy of the upper and lower limbs for the foundation year anatomy course. This will provide the basis for scaffolding knowledge that will benefit physiotherapy, exercise science, and occupational therapy students who undertake advanced anatomy studies later in their programs. It is envisaged that students can utilise the e-atlas of anatomy across several courses as they transition through their degree programs at Griffith. We hope to progressively build a repository of digital anatomical images for the entire human body, to be used by all the allied health science students.

Development of game-based simulation modules will enhance student engagement online, particularly for those students who have an increasing expectation of the quality and type of technology used in learning resources. As graphics capabilities and desktop 3D learning environments continue to develop, programs will be far more intuitive, have much greater fidelity, and interactivity. The challenge is to keep abreast of these developments and utilise these capabilities combined with cadaveric images to improve student performance and satisfaction.

CONCLUSION

A standardised set of online learning tools are required to cater for students from various socio-economic backgrounds in the digital age. A multitude of commercial digital applications exist that aim to enhance learning and teaching of anatomy. Many of these are costly and not accessible by all students. Griffith University has successfully implemented the use of a digital atlas of head and neck anatomy embedded within the University's learning management system, Blackboard, to address this strategy, at the same time enhancing flexibility and autonomy in student learning.

The digital atlas is cost-effective and available to all students enrolled in the Dentistry program, reducing potential confusion arising from multiple external resources that may offer contradictory or misleading information. A purpose-designed, interactive learning environment has been created to support and supplement traditional learning resources, enhance student engagement, and provide digital images accessible by the entire student cohort. It provides flexibility for self-directed study, and accommodates a growing number of university students without additional stress on university infrastructure. Most importantly, digital images of the wet and dry specimens utilised in laboratory sessions throughout the course increases familiarity with course content and allows transfer of knowledge of human material to its application to the human body in a more realistic way. Virtual reality and haptic technologies could offer alternative solutions in the future in all fields of health education.

REFERENCES

Abid, B., Hentati, N., Chevallier, J.-M., Ghorbel, A., Delmas, V., & Douard, R. (2010). Traditional versus three-dimensional teaching of peritoneal embryogenesis: A comparative prospective study. *Surgical and Radiologic Anatomy*, *32*(7), 647–652. doi:10.1007/s00276-010-0653-1 PMID:20352215

Ahmed, K., Rowland, S., Patel, V., Khan, R. S., Ashrafian, H., Davies, D. C., & Paraskeva, P. A. et al. (2010). Is the structure of anatomy curriculum adequate for safe medical practice? *The Surgeon*, *8*(6), 318–324. doi:10.1016/j.surge.2010.06.005 PMID:20950770

Attardi, S. M., & Rogers, K. A. (2015). Design and implementation of an online systemic human anatomy course with laboratory. *Anatomical Sciences Education*, *8*(1), 53–62. doi:10.1002/ase.1465 PMID:24920278

Azer, S. A., & Azer, S. (2016). 3D Anatomy Models and Impact on Learning: A Review of the Quality of the Literature. *Health Profession Education*, *2*(2), 80–98. doi:10.1016/j.hpe.2016.05.002

Bagley, C. H., Gillott, E., & Gunasekera, A. (2011). Undergraduate Anatomy Teaching: Are we Failing a Generation of Future Surgeons? *The Bulletin of the Royal College of Surgeons of England*, *93*(1), 26–28. doi:10.1308/147363511X545456

Bakr, M. M., Massey, W. L., & Alexander, H. (2013). Evaluation of Simodont® Haptic 3D Virtual Reality Dental Training Simulator. *International Journal of Dental Clinics*, *5*(4).

Bakr, M. M., Massey, W. L., & Alexander, H. (2014). Students' Evaluation of a 3DVR Haptic Device (Simodont®). Does Early Exposure to Haptic Feedback During Preclinical Dental Education Enhance the Development of Psychomotor Skills? *International Journal of Dental Clinics*, *6*(2), 1–7.

Bakr, M. M., Massey, W. L., & Alexander, H. (2015). Can Virtual Simulators Replace Traditional Preclinical Teaching Methods: A Students' Perspective? *International Journal of Dentistry and Oral Health*, *2*(1). doi:10.16966/2378-7090.149

Bakr, M. M., Massey, W. L., & Massa, H. M. (2016a). Digital Cadavers: Online 2D Learning Resources Enhance Student Learning in Practical Head and Neck Anatomy within Dental Programs. *Education Research International*, *10*. doi:10.1155/2016/8506251

Bakr, M. M., Massey, W. L., & Massa, H. M. (2016b). Flipping a Dental Anatomy Course: A Retrospective Study Over Four Years. *Education Research International*, *9*. doi:10.1155/2016/7097398

Bareither, M. L., Arbel, V., Growe, M., Muszczynski, E., Rudd, A., & Marone, J. R. (2013). Clay modeling versus written modules as effective interventions in understanding human anatomy. *Anatomical Sciences Education*, *6*(3), 170–176. doi:10.1002/ase.1321 PMID:23027681

Buchanan, G., Ma, M., & Rea, P. M. (2014). A multimedia package for patient understanding and rehabilitation of non-contact anterior cruciate ligament injuries. *International Journal of Medical Imaging*, *2*(3), 44–53. doi:10.11648/j.ijmi.20140203.11

Buchanan, J. A. (2004). Experience with Virtual Reality-Based Technology in Teaching Restorative Dental Procedures. *Journal of Dental Education*, *68*(12). PMID:15576814

Bukowski, E. L. (2002). Assessment outcomes: Computerised instruction in a human gross anatomy course. *Journal of Allied Health*, *31*(3), 153–158. PMID:12227266

Codd, A. M., & Choudhury, B. (2011). Virtual reality anatomy: Is it comparable with traditional methods in the teaching of human forearm musculoskeletal anatomy? *Anatomical Sciences Education*, *4*(3), 119–125. doi:10.1002/ase.214 PMID:21480538

Donnelly, L., Patten, D., White, P., & Finn, G. (2009). Virtual human dissector as a learning tool for studying cross-sectional anatomy. *Medical Teacher*, *31*(6), 553–555. doi:10.1080/01421590802512953 PMID:19288305

Drake, R. L., McBride, J. M., Lachman, N., & Pawlina, W. (2009). Medical education in the anatomical sciences: The winds of change continue to blow. *Anatomical Sciences Education*, *2*(6), 253–259. doi:10.1002/ase.117 PMID:19890982

Estevez, M. E., Lindgren, K. A., & Bergethon, P. R. (2010). A Novel Three-Dimensional Tool for Teaching Human Neuroanatomy. *Anatomical Sciences Education*, *3*(6), 309–317. doi:10.1002/ase.186 PMID:20939033

Foley, N. M., Maher, B. M., & Corrigan, M. A. (2014). Social Media and Tomorrow's Medical Students—How Do They Fit? *Journal of Surgical Education*, *71*(3), 385–390. doi:10.1016/j.jsurg.2013.10.008 PMID:24797855

Fritz, D., Hu, A., Wilson, T., Ladak, H., Haase, P., & Fung, K. (2011). Long-term retention of a 3-dimensional educational computer model of the larynx: A follow-up study. *Archives of Otolaryngology--Head & Neck Surgery*, *137*(6), 598–603. doi:10.1001/archoto.2011.76 PMID:21690512

Garg, A. X., Norman, G. R., Eva, K. W., Spero, L., & Sharan, S. (2002). Is There Any Real Virtue of Virtual Reality?: The Minor Role of Multiple Orientations in Learning Anatomy from Computers. *Academic Medicine*, *77*(10Supplement), S97–S99. doi:10.1097/00001888-200210001-00030 PMID:12377717

Giordano, C., & Giordano, C. (2011). Health Professions Students' Use of Social Media. *Journal of Allied Health*, *40*(2), 78–81. PMID:21695367

Glittenberg, C., & Binder, S. (2006). Using 3D computer simulations to enhance ophthalmic training. *Ophthalmic & Physiological Optics*, *26*(1), 40–49. doi:10.1111/j.1475-1313.2005.00358.x PMID:16390481

Green, R. A., & Whitburn, L. Y. (2016). Impact of introduction of blended learning in gross anatomy on student outcomes. *Anatomical Sciences Education*, *9*(5), 422–430. doi:10.1002/ase.1602 PMID:26929149

Gupta, Y., Morgan, M., Singh, A., & Ellis, H. (2008). Junior doctors' knowledge of applied clinical anatomy. *Clinical Anatomy (New York, N.Y.)*, *21*(4), 334–338. doi:10.1002/ca.20628 PMID:18428998

Hamat, A., Embi, M. A., & Abu Hassan, H. (2012). The Use of Social Networking Sites among Malaysian University Students. *International Education Studies*, *5*(3), 56–66. doi:10.5539/ies.v5n3p56

Hampton, B. S., & Sung, V. W. (2010). Improving medical student knowledge of female pelvic floor dysfunction and anatomy: A randomized trial. *American Journal of Obstetrics and Gynecology*, *202*(6), 601.e601–601.e608. doi:10.1016/j.ajog.2009.08.038 PMID:20430356

Hilbelink, A. J. (2007). *The effectiveness and user perception of 3-dimensional digital human anatomy in an online undergraduate anatomy laboratory.* University of South Florida, Scholar Commons.

Hopkins, R., Regehr, G., & Wilson, T. D. (2011). Exploring the Changing Learning Environment of the Gross Anatomy Lab. *Academic Medicine*, *86*(7), 883–888. doi:10.1097/ACM.0b013e31821de30f PMID:21617516

Hoyek, N., Collet, C., Di Rienzo, F., De Almeida, M., & Guillot, A. (2014). Effectiveness of three-dimensional digital animation in teaching human anatomy in an authentic classroom context. *Anatomical Sciences Education*, *7*(6), 430–437. doi:10.1002/ase.1446 PMID:24678034

Hu, A., Wilson, T., Ladak, H., Haase, P., & Fung, K. (2009). Three-dimensional educational computer model of the larynx: Voicing a new direction. *Archives of Otolaryngology--Head & Neck Surgery*, *135*(7), 677–681. doi:10.1001/archoto.2009.68 PMID:19620589

Idris, Y., & Wang, Q. (2009). Affordances of Facebook for Learning. *International Journal of Continuing Engineering Education and Lifelong Learning*, *19*(2/3), 247–255. doi:10.1504/IJCEELL.2009.025031

Jaffar, A. A. (2012). YouTube: An emerging tool in anatomy education. *Anatomical Sciences Education*, *5*(3), 158–164. doi:10.1002/ase.1268 PMID:22383096

Jaffar, A. A. (2014). Exploring the use of a facebook page in anatomy education. *Anatomical Sciences Education*, *7*(3), 199–208. doi:10.1002/ase.1404 PMID:24022984

Junco, R. (2012). Too much face and not enough books: The relationship between multiple indices of Facebook use and academic performance. *Computers in Human Behavior*, *28*(1), 187–198. doi:10.1016/j.chb.2011.08.026

Karthikeyana, P., & Ramalingamb, K. P. (2017). E-learning initiatives in delivering the undergraduate physiotherapy education program in Papua New Guinea. *Asia Pacific Journal of Contemporary Education and Communication Technology (APJCECT), 3*(1).

Keedy, A. W., Durack, J. C., Sandhu, P., Chen, E. M., O'Sullivan, P. S., & Breiman, R. S. (2011). Comparison of traditional methods with 3D computer models in the instruction of hepatobiliary anatomy. *Anatomical Sciences Education*, *4*(2), 84–91. doi:10.1002/ase.212 PMID:21412990

Kerby, J., Shukur, Z. N., & Shalhoub, J. (2011). The relationships between learning outcomes and methods of teaching anatomy as perceived by medical students. *Clinical Anatomy (New York, N.Y.)*, *24*(4), 489–497. doi:10.1002/ca.21059 PMID:20949485

Khot, Z., Quinlan, K., Norman, G. R., & Wainman, B. (2013). The relative effectiveness of computer-based and traditional resources for education in anatomy. *Anatomical Sciences Education*, *6*(4), 211–215. doi:10.1002/ase.1355 PMID:23509000

Kinnison, T., Forrest, N. D., Frean, S. P., & Baillie, S. (2009). Teaching Bovine Abdominal Anatomy: Use of a Haptic Simulator. *Anatomical Sciences Education*, *2*(6), 280–285. doi:10.1002/ase.109 PMID:19780149

Kirschner, P. A., & Karpinski, A. C. (2010). Facebook® and academic performance. *Computers in Human Behavior*, *26*(6), 1237–1245. doi:10.1016/j.chb.2010.03.024

Levinson, A. J., Weaver, B., Garside, S., McGinn, H., & Norman, G. R. (2007). Virtual reality and brain anatomy: A randomised trial of e-learning instructional designs. *Medical Education*, *41*(5), 495–501. doi:10.1111/j.1365-2929.2006.02694.x PMID:17470079

Lisk, K., McKee, P., Baskwill, A., & Agur, A. M. R. (2015). Student perceptions and effectiveness of an innovative learning tool: Anatomy Glove Learning System. *Anatomical Sciences Education*, *8*(2), 140–148. doi:10.1002/ase.1459 PMID:24757171

Losco, C. D., Grant, W. D., Armson, A., Meyer, A. J., & Walker, B. F. (2017). Effective methods of teaching and learning in anatomy as a basic science: A BEME systematic review: BEME guide no. 44. *Medical Teacher*, *39*(3), 234–243. doi:10.1080/0142159X.2016.1271944 PMID:28129720

Lynn, V. A., Yenser, A., & Harman, R. (2015). Body apps: iPads for undergrad Anatomy and Physiology students. *College & Research Libraries News*, *76*(3), 149–152. doi:10.5860/crln.76.3.9281

Mącznik, A. K., Ribeiro, D. C., & Baxter, G. D. (2015). Online technology use in physiotherapy teaching and learning: A systematic review of effectiveness and users' perceptions. *BMC Medical Education*, *15*(1), 160. doi:10.1186/s12909-015-0429-8 PMID:26415677

Maggio, M. P., Hariton-Gross, K., & Gluch, J. (2012). The Use of Independent, Interactive Media for Education in Dental Morphology. *Journal of Dental Education*, *76*(11), 1497–1511. PMID:23144486

Magro, M., Sharp, J., Ryan, K., & Ryan, S. (2013). Investigating Ways to Use Facebook at the University Level: A Delphi Study. *Proceedings of the Informing Science and Information Technology Education Conference 2013*. https://www.learntechlib.org/p/114656

Marsh, K. R., Giffin, B. F., & Lowrie, D. J. Jr. (2008). Medical student retention of embryonic development: Impact of the dimensions added by multimedia tutorials. *Anatomical Sciences Education*, *1*(6), 252–257. doi:10.1002/ase.56 PMID:19109854

Metzler, R., Stein, D., Tetzlaff, R., Bruckner, T., Meinzer, H.-P., Büchler, M. W., & Fischer, L. et al. (2012). Teaching on Three-Dimensional Presentation Does Not Improve the Understanding of According CT Images: A Randomized Controlled Study. *Teaching and Learning in Medicine*, *24*(2), 140–148. doi:10.1080/10401334.2012.664963 PMID:22490095

Moro, C., Stromberga, Z., Raikos, A., & Stirling, A. (2017). The Effectiveness of Virtual and Augmented Reality in Health Sciences and Medical Anatomy. *Anatomical Sciences Education*. doi:10.1002/ase.1696 PMID:28419750

Murakami, T., Tajika, Y., Ueno, H., Awata, S., Hirasawa, S., Sugimoto, M., & Yorifuji, H. et al. (2014). An integrated teaching method of gross anatomy and computed tomography radiology. *Anatomical Sciences Education*, *7*(6), 438–449. doi:10.1002/ase.1430 PMID:24443310

Nguyen, N., Mulla, A., Nelson, A. J., & Wilson, T. D. (2014). Visuospatial anatomy comprehension: The role of spatial visualization ability and problem-solving strategies. *Anatomical Sciences Education*, *7*(4), 280–288. doi:10.1002/ase.1415 PMID:24124041

Nguyen, N., Nelson, A. J., & Wilson, T. D. (2012). Computer visualizations: Factors that influence spatial anatomy comprehension. *Anatomical Sciences Education*, *5*(2), 98–108. doi:10.1002/ase.1258 PMID:22232125

Nicholson, D. T., Chalk, C., Funnell, W. R. J., & Daniel, S. J. (2006). Can virtual reality improve anatomy education? A randomised controlled study of a computer-generated three-dimensional anatomical ear model. *Medical Education*, *40*(11), 1081–1087. doi:10.1111/j.1365-2929.2006.02611.x PMID:17054617

Oh, C.-S., Kim, J.-Y., & Choe, Y. H. (2009). Learning of cross-sectional anatomy using clay models. *Anatomical Sciences Education*, *2*(4), 156–159. doi:10.1002/ase.92 PMID:19588481

Pani, J. R., Chariker, J. H., & Naaz, F. (2013). Computer-Based Learning: Interleaving Whole and Sectional Representation of Neuroanatomy. *Anatomical Sciences Education*, *6*(1), 11–18. doi:10.1002/ase.1297 PMID:22761001

Pani, J. R., Chariker, J. H., Naaz, F., Mattingly, W., Roberts, J., & Sephton, S. E. (2014). Learning with interactive computer graphics in the undergraduate neuroscience classroom. *Advances in Health Sciences Education: Theory and Practice*, *19*(4), 507–528. doi:10.1007/s10459-013-9483-3 PMID:24449123

Pasek, J., More, E., & Hargittai, E. (2009). Facebook and Academic Performance: Reconciling a Media Sensation with Data. *First Monday Peer-Reviewed Journal on the Internet, 14*(5).

Prensky, M. (2001). Digital Natives, Digital Immigrants Part 1. *On the Horizon*, *9*(5), 1–6. doi:10.1108/10748120110424816

Prince, K. J. A. H., Scherpbier, A. J. A. A., Van Mameren, H., Drukker, J., & Van Der Vleuten, C. P. M. (2005). Do students have sufficient knowledge of clinical anatomy? *Medical Education*, *39*(3), 326–332. doi:10.1111/j.1365-2929.2005.02096.x PMID:15733169

Roach, V. A., Brandt, M. G., Moore, C. C., & Wilson, T. D. (2012). Is three-dimensional videography the cutting edge of surgical skill acquisition? *Anatomical Sciences Education*, *5*(3), 138–145. doi:10.1002/ase.1262 PMID:22278856

Shaffer, K. (2004). Teaching anatomy in the digital world. *The New England Journal of Medicine*, *351*(13), 1279–1281. doi:10.1056/NEJMp048100 PMID:15385652

Shead, D., Roos, R., Olivier, B., & Ihunwo, A. O. (2016). Gross anatomy curricula and pedagogical approaches for undergraduate physiotherapy students: A scoping review protocol. *JBI Database of Systematic Reviews and Implementation Reports*, *14*(10), 98–104. doi:10.11124/JBISRIR-2016-003164 PMID:27846120

Sloman, M. (2009). Learning and technology - What have we learnt? *Impact: Journal of Applied Research in Workplace E-learning*, *1*(1), 12–26.

Smythe, G., & Hughes, D. (2008). Self-directed learning in gross human anatomy: Assessment outcomes and student perceptions. *Anatomical Sciences Education*, *1*(4), 145–153. doi:10.1002/ase.33 PMID:19177401

Soumya, B. G., & Ramachandra, S. S. (2011). Haptics Application in Dentistry: Is the Time Poised Yet? *Dental Hypotheses*, *19*. doi:10.5436/j.dehy.2011.2.00019

Stanciu, A., Mihai, F., & Aleca, O. (2012). Social Networking as an Alternative Environment for Education. *Accounting and Information Management Systems*, *11*(1), 56–75.

Stirling, A., & Birt, J. (2014). An enriched multimedia eBook application to facilitate learning of anatomy. *Anatomical Sciences Education*, *7*(1), 19–27. doi:10.1002/ase.1373 PMID:23650104

Strauss, W., & Howe, N. (1991). *Generations: The History of America's Future, 1584 to 2069*. HarperCollins.

Sugand, K., Abrahams, P., & Khurana, A. (2010). The anatomy of anatomy: A review for its modernization. *Anatomical Sciences Education*, *3*(2), 83–93. doi:10.1002/ase.139 PMID:20205265

Sung, Y. H., Kwon, I. G., & Ryu, E. (2008). Blended learning on medication administration for new nurses: Integration of e-learning and face-to-face instruction in the classroom. *Nurse Education Today*, *28*(8), 943–952. doi:10.1016/j.nedt.2008.05.007 PMID:18599162

Svirko, E., & Mellanby, J. (2017). Teaching Neuroanatomy Using Computer-Aided Learning: What Makes for Successful Outcomes? *Anatomical Sciences Education*. doi:10.1002/ase.1694 PMID:28431201

Tam, M. D. B. S., Hart, A. R., Williams, S., Heylings, D., & Leinster, S. (2009). Is learning anatomy facilitated by computer-aided learning? A review of the literature. *Medical Teacher*, *31*(9), e393–e396. doi:10.1080/01421590802650092 PMID:19811174

Tanzawa, T., Futaki, K., Kurabayashi, H., Goto, K., Yoshihama, Y., Hasegawa, T., & Maki, K. et al. (2012). Medical Emergency Education Using a Robot Patient in a Dental Setting. *European Journal of Dental Education*. doi:10.1111/j.1600-0579.2012.00770.x PMID:23279398

Tanzawa, T., Futaki, K., Tani, C., Hasegawa, T., Yamamoto, M., Miyazaki, T., & Maki, K. (2011). Introduction of a Robot Patient into Dental Education. *European Journal of Dental Education*, *16*(1), e195–e199. doi:10.1111/j.1600-0579.2011.00697.x PMID:22251346

ten Brinke, B., Klitsie, P. J., Timman, R., Busschbach, J. J. V., Lange, J. F., & Kleinrensink, G.-J. (2014). Anatomy Education and Classroom Versus Laparoscopic Dissection-Based Training: A Randomized Study at One Medical School. *Academic Medicine*, *89*(5), 806–810. doi:10.1097/ACM.0000000000000223 PMID:24667502

Turney, B. W. (2007). Anatomy in a Modern Medical Curriculum. *Annals of the Royal College of Surgeons of England*, *89*(2), 104–107. doi:10.1308/003588407X168244 PMID:17346399

Tworek, J. K., Jamniczky, H. A., Jacob, C., Hallgrímsson, B., & Wright, B. (2013). The LINDSAY Virtual Human Project: An immersive approach to anatomy and physiology. *Anatomical Sciences Education*, *6*(1), 19–28. doi:10.1002/ase.1301 PMID:22791664

Van Nuland, S. E., & Rogers, K. A. (2015). The anatomy of e-learning tools: Does software usability influence learning outcomes? *Anatomical Sciences Education*, *9*(4), 378–390. doi:10.1002/ase.1589 PMID:26671838

Van Nuland, S. E., & Rogers, K. A. (2016). The anatomy of E-Learning tools: Does software usability influence learning outcomes? *Anatomical Sciences Education*, *9*(4), 378–390. doi:10.1002/ase.1589 PMID:26671838

Venkatiah, J. (2010). Computer-assisted modules to enhance the learning of anatomy by dissection. *Medical Education*, *44*(5), 523–524. doi:10.1111/j.1365-2923.2010.03657.x PMID:20519005

Vogel-Walcutt, J. J., Gebrim, J. B., & Nicholson, D. (2010). Animated versus static images of team processes to affect knowledge acquisition and learning efficiency. *Journal of Online Teaching and Learning*, *6*(1), 163–173.

Vuchkova, J., Maybury, T. S., & Farah, C. S. (2011). Testing the Educational Potential of 3D Visualization Software in Oral Radiographic Interpretation. *Journal of Dental Education*, *75*(11), 1417–1425. PMID:22058390

Waters, J. R., Van Meter, P., Perrotti, W., Drogo, S., & Cyr, R. J. (2005). Cat dissection vs. sculpting human structures in clay: An analysis of two approaches to undergraduate human anatomy laboratory education. *Advances in Physiology Education*, *29*(1), 27–34. doi:10.1152/advan.00033.2004 PMID:15718380

Wierinck, E., Puttamen, V., Swinnen, S., & van Steenberghe, D. (2005). Effect of Augmented Visual Feedback from a Virtual Reality Simulation System on Manual Dexterity Training. *European Journal of Dental Education*, *9*(1), 10–16. doi:10.1111/j.1600-0579.2004.00351.x PMID:15642018

Wilson, M., & Gerber, L. E. (2008). How Generational Theory can Improve Teaching: Strategies for Working with the "Millennials". *Currents in Teaching and Learning*, *1*(1).

Wise, L., Skues, J., & Williams, B. (2011). *Facebook in Higher Education Promotes Social but not Academic Engagement.* Paper presented at the Annual Australasian Society of Computers in Learning in Tertiary Education (ASCILITE) 2011, Hobart, Australia.

Xiannong, C. (2010). *Chinese acupuncture and moxibustion* (3rd ed.). Beijing: Foreign Languages Press.

Chapter 4
Evolving Dietetics Education to Respond to Emerging Technologies in Nutritional Genomics

Natalie Jane Colson
Griffith University, Australia

Melissa Adamski
Monash University, Australia

ABSTRACT

Nutritional genomics is a fast-growing area of precision medicine. It is expected that dietitians will be key players in this area. This chapter discusses the current state of industry, from research to the availability of commercial products, their regulation, and consumer perceptions. Current issues and controversies surrounding the readiness, availability, and delivery of this technology to consumers are examined, and finally, an education framework describing core competencies is presented. The framework aims to provide dietitians with the necessary tools to evaluate and make decisions on the potential for translation of this technology to clinical practice for disease prevention and management.

DOI: 10.4018/978-1-5225-3850-9.ch004

INTRODUCTION

This chapter will examine emerging technologies in the field of nutritional genomics, the study of interaction between diet, the genome and health, and discuss the importance of evolving dietetics education in the context of dietitians being key players in the delivery of this technology to consumers. Although it has been argued that the evidence base for translating the outcomes of nutritional genomics research into personalized nutritional advice is immature, nutritional genomics tests are now available to the public and are being used in health care. Dietitians are well placed as leaders in the nutrition field to further the understanding of translation of the science into practice, and to provide guidance for the development and delivery of this technology in an evidence based way due to their expertise in nutrition and biomedical science. It is clear that in order for this to occur, dietetics education needs to evolve to enable dietitians to be competent and confident in all aspects of genetic driven nutrition care including accessing digital databases, ethical and legal considerations, interpreting complex genetic information contextualized within the nutrition care process, determining the clinical utility of various nutritional genetics tests for different clients, and effectively educating clients about the information that the data reveals.

BACKGROUND

Nutritional Genomics

Nutritional genomics is a term used to describe the bi-directional interaction between dietary components, the genome and health outcomes. It includes nutrigenomics which describes the effect of dietary components on the genome (via transcription, protein expression, epigenetic alterations, genomic stability) and nutrigenetics, which describes how individual genetic variation impacts the metabolic response to diet, potentially influencing health status and disease risk (Ferguson et al., 2016). It should be noted that the term nutrigenomics is sometimes used as an interchangeable inclusive term to describe nutritional genomics (Muller & Kersten, 2003).

The nutrigenomic effects of dietary components such as bioactive compounds, macronutrients and micronutrients have been confirmed in many human, animal and cell studies as have the effects of altering dietary energy content. For example, bioactive compounds such as flavonoids have been shown to alter the expression of genes in metabolic and other signalling pathways related to glucose homeostasis (Babu, Liu, & Gilbert, 2013). In animals, a high fat diet induces the adaptive response of hyperlipidemia and atherogenesis through the PPAR group of nuclear receptors, which act as nutrient sensors and influence gene expression in metabolically active organs (Lin et al., 2005), while in obese humans or those with metabolic syndrome, dietary restriction has been shown to alter the expression of key genes in adipose tissue (Dahlman et al., 2005; Kallio et al., 2007). All are examples of acute changes in gene expression in response to short-term dietary alterations. Clinical usefulness, which is yet to be demonstrated, will depend on the potential for long-term downstream effects that affect health.

A classic example of nutrigenetics is the rare disease called phenylketonuria (PKU), where mutations in the *PAH* gene, which codes for phenylalanine hydroxylase, cause reduced metabolism of phenylalanine and abnormal build up to potentially toxic levels (Blau, 2016). Without treatment by dietary restriction, irreversible brain damage can occur. In contrast to single gene diseases like PKU, multifactorial diseases such as diabetes, hypertension and inflammatory bowel disease usually involve multiple low risk common gene variants, frequently single nucleotide polymorphisms (termed SNPs), which typically interact with environmental factors such as diet and lifestyle to alter overall risk of disease development and progression. As a consequence, the actual impact of single gene variation in complex disorders is often less clear.

An example is type 2 diabetes (T2D) where the gene *TCF7L2*, encoding transcription factor 7-like 2, a key player in the signalling pathway regulating insulin secretion in the pancreas, has been implicated as the strongest locus to date for T2D risk. The associated risk alleles occur in up to 30% of the general population, and have been reported to double the risk of T2D in some populations (Tong et al., 2009) but not all (Qi, Wang, Strizich, & Wang, 2015). Studies examining genotype diet interaction have shown a possible interaction with diet (fibre, glycaemic load, Mediterranean style) (Cornelis, Qi, Kraft, & Hu, 2009; Roswall et al., 2014), however a study examining genetic risk along with modifiable lifestyle factors demonstrated that body mass index (BMI) and waist measurement were the strongest influencers on T2D risk regardless of genetic susceptibility (Langenberg et al., 2014). More recently it has been shown that *TCF7L2* genetic risk for T2D has a stronger predictive value when examined in a specific non-obese genetic risk score panel, illustrating gene x gene x obese state interactions (Corella et al., 2016). Although lifestyle interventions are currently more relevant for T2D than genotype directed interventions, better understanding of genotype, phenotype and environmental interactions could lead to personalized genetic risk driven nutrition advice.

Hypertension is another multifactorial disease with dietary and lifestyle determinants along with a well-recognised genetic susceptibility. Epidemiological studies have shown that a functional variant in the gene for the folate-metabolizing enzyme methylenetetrahydrofolate reductase (MTHFR) increases the risk of hypertension by 24–87% in a number of populations and that this risk may be mediated by riboflavin (McNulty, Strain, Hughes, & Ward, 2017). Randomised controlled trials have shown a lowering of blood pressure of 6-13 mmHg in those with the risk genotype supplemented with riboflavin (Horigan et al., 2010; Wilson et al., 2013; Wilson et al., 2012). Optimising riboflavin status could therefore be a potential targeted intervention for hypertensive individuals with the *MTHFR* risk genotype.

Over 160 gene variants have been implicated in inflammatory bowel disease along with environmental factors, including the microbiome. There is evidence for interactions between certain gene variants and micronutrients such as selenium, along with the possibility that variants affecting inflammation and vitamin D and zinc absorption may also play a role (Kostic, Xavier, & Gevers, 2014). The complete picture and how it translates to clinical applications so far remains unclear. Future research may reveal genotype x phenotype x dietary interactions that could lead to a personalized approach to management.

The above examples demonstrate the complex nature of nutrient gene interactions, and the need for a full understanding of how the changes related to gene variation and dietary factors influence metabolic pathways and health. As both nutrigenomics and nutrigenetics usually involve complex signalling pathways, it has been argued that a complete understanding of the potential modifiable impact on health may require an integrated approach involving other 'omics' such as transcriptomics, metabolomics, proteomics and microbiomics to follow the pathway from gene/nutrient through transcription and translation, metabolic end product and possible interaction with the microbiome through to eventual health outcome (Fenech et al., 2011).

Nutritional genomics is a fast growing field with great interest in the potential for developing a personalised approach to prescribing the most optimal diet for individuals based on their personal genetic profile. It has been argued that while there is still much to uncover, some specific gene–diet interactions may already have sufficient evidence for clinical application (Gorman, Mathers, Grimaldi, Ahlgren, & Nordstrom, 2013), although this has been disputed (Covolo, Rubinelli, Ceretti, & Gelatti, 2015; Pavlidis, Nebel, Katsila, & Patrinos, 2016)

ISSUES, CONTROVERSIES, PROBLEMS

Nutritional Genomics Services

Commercial companies have responded to this emerging technology and over the past decade nutritional genomics tests have become available to the public (Gorman et al., 2013). A Google search conducted in March 2017 using the term 'nutritional genomics testing' brought up over 517,000 results advertising or discussing nutritional genomics testing services. It should be noted that many services use the term nutrigenomics to describe nutrigenetic testing. Business models included direct to consumer (DTC) testing services, with results provided directly to the consumer by biotechnology companies or laboratories, or results generated and interpreted by biotechnology companies or laboratories and communicated by a practitioner such as a naturopath, nutritionist or dietitian, or biotechnology companies or laboratories providing genetic information directly to the health practitioner for their interpretation. Many DTC services claim to provide dietary recommendations based on personal genetic profile to maintain or improve long-term health outcomes. Claims include information on metabolic rate, best type of physical activity, how to optimise sports performance and reduce injury risk, body composition and weight loss. Some also recommend personalised supplements (Sterling, 2008).

Consumer Acceptance

An important consideration for the success of genotype driven nutrition advice is consumer acceptance. A number of studies have examined consumer reactions towards genetic testing and nutritional genomics to determine consumer interest and willingness to undergo genetic testing and follow personalised dietary and lifestyle advice. A pan-European survey of almost 6000 individuals indicated that 27% would be willing to undertake nutrigenetic testing for personalised nutrition advice. Notably those who were aware that they were at risk of chronic disease were more likely to utilise the technology (Stewart-Knox et al., 2009). This was confirmed in a 2013 review, which reported willingness to undergo genetic testing for disease prevention at 48-85% across a number of studies (Fallaize, Macready, Butler, Ellis, & Lovegrove, 2013). Another study ran a controlled trial of genetic based nutrition advice to determine perceptions of personalised nutrition and who should produce and deliver the information. Participants considered a university research laboratory or health care professional to be the best sources for obtaining accurate personal genetic information, and considered dietitians to be the best source of nutrigenetic advice, followed by medical doctors (Nielsen, Shih, & El-Sohemy, 2014).

Concerns About Regulation

While there is undoubtedly consumer interest in personalised lifestyle and nutrition advice, concerns have been raised about potential deficiencies in regulation of health-related genetic testing (Li et al., 2014). There are obvious difficulties with creating international standards that regulate the online DTC market, while local practitioner delivered advice may have similar issues as genetic test results may come from an offshore site. In 2006 the United States Government Accountability Office (GAO) examined four random DTC nutrigenetic tests by creating fictitious consumer profiles and reported that all misled consumers by making predictions that were medically unproven and further, that the information provided to consumers was misleading and ambiguous. It was reported that in two instances, expensive and unnecessary supplements were recommended (Kutz, 2006). In 2013, the US Food and Drug Administration (FDA) raised concerns over the marketing by one company of health-related genetic tests due to the risk that false results could cause consumers to undergo unnecessary health procedures. The company was ordered to cease marketing these products (U.S. Food and Drug Administration, 2013). This company has since obtained FDA approval to market specific DTC genetic carrier screening tests (U.S. Food & Drug Administration, 2015) and certain disease risk markers (Maxmen, 2017), highlighting the importance of working with government and regulatory agencies, particularly in the DTC market.

Concerns About Evidence Base

Concerns have been raised about whether genes or gene panels in commercial nutrigenetic tests are associated with the particular nutrition related health issue and whether there are evidence-based clinical guidelines about use of the tests. A 2015 meta-analysis examined 38 genes in commercially available nutrigenetic tests to examine potential associations with nutrition related pathologies in data from over 500,000 individuals. The authors concluded that no significant association could be found with any of the genes and pathologies and argued that commercially available nutrigenetic tests were not based on sound evidence. (Pavlidis et al., 2015). Concerns were also raised about who was the most suited health professional to interpret and deliver results from such tests (Pavlidis et al., 2015).

Some nutrigenetic tests determine nutrition related disease risk based on a panel of SNPs and there may be uncertainty and lack of clarity about how the genetic risk is calculated from the panel, how the panel is determined and what evidence exists for the determination of risk genotypes (Covolo et al., 2015; Pavlidis et al., 2016). One study examining concordance rates between DTC tests found large differences between disease risks calculated by different companies, likely due to different SNPs used and different reference populations (Imai, Kricka, & Fortina, 2011). In their 2016 review on nutritional genomics, Pavlidis and colleagues describe the need for transparent, multi-levelled, independent evaluation of the body of evidence for recommending nutrigenetic tests (Pavlidis et al., 2016).

Ethical, Social Concerns

The addition of incorporating genetic information into dietetics practice introduces new challenges which require new skills. The use of genetics in medicine is not new, however traditionally, specially trained medical specialists and healthcare professionals discussed, recommended and advised on genetic testing. With the growing body of research and access to genetic information, healthcare professionals not traditionally trained to discuss and interpret genetic information are increasingly becoming involved (Kohlmeier et al., 2016). While many healthcare professionals, such as dietitians, are trained in the areas of molecular biology, this may not include training in the application, interpretation and practical considerations (i.e. social, ethical and legal issues) of using genetics within clinical practice. Dietitians using nutritional genomics in practice may be unaware of social, ethical and legal concerns which may impact on evidenced based practice and patient safety (Camp & Trujillo, 2014).

There is also the consideration of whether genetic knowledge will result in changes in dietary and lifestyle behaviour. The Food4Me project examines consumer knowledge of personalised nutrition for potential application of individualised nutrition advice (Food4me). Two recent Food4me studies examined the effect of electronically provided genetic knowledge on behaviour. One examined genetic susceptibility for cardiovascular health and folate intake while the other examined genetic knowledge about obesity risk and physical activity. Both results showed that knowledge of genetic susceptibility had no impact on either folate intake (O'Donovan et al., 2016) in one study or physical activity in the other (Marsaux et al., 2016). Similar results were seen in two recent meta-analyses examining the effect of communicating genetic risk on health behaviour (Hollands et al., 2016; Li, Ye, Whelan, & Truby, 2016). One important limitation of these studies to detect motivation to change are that advice is usually not provided face to face and is provided free of charge. It is possible that motivation to change may be stronger in individuals who pay for and receive face-to-face genotype driven nutrition advice by a health professional such as a dietitian.

Position by the Academy of Nutrition and Dietetics

In 2014, the Academy of Nutrition and Dietetics released their position statement on nutritional genomics, stating that

The practical application of nutritional genomics for complex chronic disease is an emerging science and the use of nutrigenetic testing to provide dietary advice is not ready for routine dietetics practice. Registered dietitian nutritionists need basic competency in genetics as a foundation for understanding nutritional genomics; proficiency requires advanced knowledge and skills.

Direct-to-consumer genetic testing is not closely regulated in the United States and may not be accompanied by access to health care practitioners. Applying nutritional genomics in clinical practice through the use of genetic testing requires that registered dietitian nutritionists understand, interpret, and communicate complex test results in which the actual risk of developing a disease may not be known. The practical application of nutritional genomics in dietetics practice will require an evidence-based approach to validate that personalized recommendations result in health benefits to individuals and do not cause harm (Camp & Trujillo, 2014).

More recently, in their visioning report, which defines future practice areas and identifies education needs for future dietetics practitioners, the Academy of Nutrition and Dietetics recognized the continuing advances in nutritional genomics and identified genetic driven personalized health care as one of the key change drivers for future practice. Dietitians were seen as playing a significant role in personalized genetic predisposition nutrition interventions and counselling. The academy reported that specialized skills and advanced knowledge, such as the technical skills to interpret nutritional genomics tests for nutrition advice, were integral for dietitians to work in this area (Kicklighter et al., 2017).

Dietitian Involvement, Knowledge, Confidence

Despite concerns over the use of genotypic information in personalized nutrition due to overstated health claims, mistaken interpretations, ethical concerns including products that may exploit the consumer, and the difficulty of proving cause and effect, (Gorman et al., 2013) this is a rapidly advancing field and dietitians are predicted to be key players in the development and delivery of this technology (Kicklighter et al., 2017). Dietitians are recognised for their expertise in nutrition and biomedical science and are therefore well placed to lead the way in genetic driven nutrition care in an evidence based manner. Some dietitians are already involved in offering this technology to consumers via commercial products or by requests for interpretation of DTC results (personal communication). Dietitians need to position themselves appropriately as leaders in the delivery of evidence based nutrition advice in order to critically evaluate services and communicate findings to advise industry, government, regulatory bodies, consumers and the public. Dietitian confidence and competence are key components of this role.

A review of dietitian knowledge, confidence and education in nutritional genomics was published in 2014 (Wright, 2014). The authors examined 18 studies across the USA, UK, Canada, Australia and the Netherlands and demonstrated low levels of knowledge and confidence in the understanding and application of nutritional genomics. There was also limited evidence of suitable teaching and curriculum development strategies to improve dietitian knowledge of nutritional genomics and to translate it to clinical practice. Another study, which interviewed dietetics leaders in Australia and the UK (Li et al., 2014), similarly identified a knowledge and confidence gap, and the need for an interdisciplinary approach involving government and industry experts to facilitate incorporation of the science into practice. Dietetics students in Canada also reported minimal knowledge of nutritional genomics but a desire to learn, and positive attitudes towards incorporation into dietetics education (Horne, Madill, & O'Connor, 2016).

It is clear that in order for this to occur, dietetics education needs to evolve to enable dietitians to be competent and confident in interpreting complex genetic and personal information (e.g. anthropometric, biochemistry, food preferences), to be able to determine the clinical utility of various nutritional genetics tests for different clients, to effectively educate clients about the information that the data reveals, and to advise industry and other stakeholders.

SOLUTIONS AND RECOMMENDATIONS

Dietitians Need Several Skills

Interpreting Complex Genetic and Personal Information

To critically analyse genetic research and information, and interpret results of genetic tests including those performed by commercial providers (e.g. DTC), dietitians should be competent in understanding and synthesizing complex genetic information along with phenotypic and other client information. In order to do this, dietitians need robust training in the science and application of genetics, along with the science of nutritional genomics. Dietitians need to know how to access, interpret and analyse genetic and other peer-reviewed scientific publications, and how to access gene databases and interpret the information therein. Dietitians need to know how to search the literature on relevant genes and associated conditions and how to synthesise and translate all relevant information into healthcare practice. As leaders in the application of nutrition science to healthcare practice, dietitians should also contribute to the literature base, assisting geneticists with an understanding of how genetic influence may affect personal nutrition requirements.

The importance of competence in all aspects of nutritional genomics can be seen in the following example. There is a claimed nutrigenetic effect of coffee consumption on heart disease where individuals with the Cytochrome P450 1A2 (*CYP1A2)* rs762551 C/A C allele, suggested to determine slow caffeine metabolism, are purported to have an increased risk of heart attack with high caffeine consumption

(Cornelis, El-Sohemy, Kabagambe, & Campos, 2006). The Cytochrome P450 1A2 (CYP1A2) enzyme is responsible for most caffeine metabolism (Kalow & Tang, 1993). The *CYP1A2* rs762551 (C/A) SNP aka. [-163 C/A] is a Tag SNP that represents several haplotypes (Lim et al., 2010). The rs762551 A allele has been associated with faster caffeine metabolism compared to the C allele in some studies (Djordjevic, Ghotbi, Jankovic, & Aklillu, 2010; Ghotbi et al., 2007), but it is not consistent across all populations (Aklillu et al., 2003; Gervasini et al., 2013) possibly due to different haplotypes represented by -163C/A. Therefore care needs to be taken when interpreting genetic research in specific populations for use as a genetic test to guide nutrition recommendations for the general population, or alternatively, those in specific subgroups not included in the original research. This example illustrates the need for dietitians to be able to examine and interpret the literature in order to recognise such limitations with use of genetics tests.

Determining Clinical Utility

The clinical utility of a test or technology relates to its health care value (Burke, 2004). Dietitians need the skills and tools to determine the clinical utility of nutritional genomics tests, which is ultimately whether the test is likely to improve health outcomes. The clinical utility of nutritional genomic testing will be influenced by a number of additional factors and these are illustrated in Figure 1. These may include information on the gene and the variant, analytic validity, clinical validity, clinical impact, evidence for a nutrigenetic effect and ethical, legal and social issues. These are discussed further below.

Evaluating Evidence for a Nutrigenetic Effect

As discussed earlier, dietitians require the skills and training to read and critically analyse scientific papers and explore research studies that will provide evidence for a proposed nutritional genomic (nutrigenetic) effect. For example, case/control or cohort studies may provide evidence for aetiology or harm/benefit, while trials may provide evidence for treatment/intervention, such as whether a dietary modification for individuals with a particular genetic risk improves health outcomes. Dietitians should be conscious of the hierarchy of evidence for evidence based decision making, for example the importance of systematic reviews and independent replication of studies. The hierarchy of evidence for assessing qualitative health research (Daly et al., 2007) and The Australian National Health and Medical Research Council (NHMRC) levels of evidence and grades for recommendations for development of guidelines (National Health and Medical Research Council (NHMRC) Australia, 2015) are useful tools for assessing the quality of evidence for clinical practice.

Figure 1. Aspects important in determining the clinical utility of genetic driven nutrition care

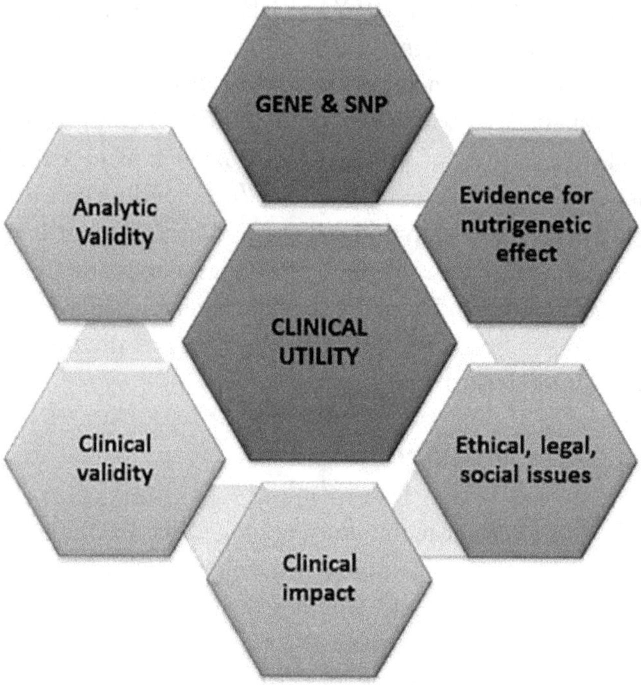

Analytic Validity, Clinical Validity, Clinical Impact

Analytic validity regarding genetic testing relates to the ability of a test to accurately determine a specific genotype. There are many factors dietitians need to take into consideration with genetic tests to understand more about the accuracy of the tests. These include how the sample is obtained, transported, labelled and recorded, how the sample is prepared and analyzed, and how the results are interpreted and reported. Currently two scenarios are common regarding providers of genetic tests. One involves the company outsourcing the testing of the DNA to an external laboratory, while the other involves the company conducting the analysis of the DNA themselves using their own internal laboratory (Trent, 2014). Dietitians need to consider both scenarios to understand how and where a patient's DNA sample may be transported, prepared, analyzed, interpreted and reported. If a company outsources the DNA analysis, the sample may be sent overseas where regulations for genetic testing may differ. To accurately advise patients about how their DNA sample will be handled, and obtain information about the analytical validity of a genetic test, dietitians should research the company providing the test and laboratory analyzing the sample. This should include considering the country the company and laboratory are located in, and comparing the regulatory standards of that country. This can assist dietitians to understand and advise on analytical validity.

Clinical validity relates to a test's ability to detect those with and without disease/condition or risk (Burke, 2004). The example described earlier where particular variants in the gene *TCF7L2* have been implicated as the strongest locus to date for T2D risk, is a good case in point of a genetic test that would have low clinical validity at present. Although this gene variant has been reported to double the risk of T2D in some populations (Tong et al., 2009), it has no effect in others (Qi et al., 2015). To date, body mass index (BMI) and waist measurement have been shown to be stronger predictors for T2D risk (Langenberg et al., 2014) and therefore, until more information is known about genetic risk for diabetes, the focus of intervention should be on waist measurements and BMI. Clinical impact describes whether a treatment or intervention has any effects, positive or negative. In this particular example focusing on healthy BMI and waist measurements to reduce diabetes risk would likely have more clinical impact than a genetic test for suggested *TCF7L2* diabetes risk variants. The clinical impact of nutritional genomic tests is also likely to be closely linked to whether genetic knowledge will result in changes in dietary and lifestyle behaviour.

Ethical Legal Social Issues

Ethical, legal and social issues (ELSI) are important for dietitians to consider when discussing or advising on nutritional genomic tests. Three areas for dietitians to consider are the ELSI associated with the communication of nutrigenetic information within nutrition and dietetics practice, integration of genetic information into the dietetic and nutrition consultation and nutrigenetic tests and the genetic testing process.

Communication of Nutritional Genomic Information

There are many factors to consider when communicating nutritional genomic information. Dietitians are trained to communicate nutrition science and recommendations to patients, however communicating and interpreting genetic information is not traditionally part of training. Dietitians should be aware of ELSI associated with communicating genetic information; the shared nature of genetic information (National Health and Medical Research Council (NHMRC), 2010; National Health and Medical Research Council (NHMRC) Australia, 2013; NSW Government Health Centre for Genetics Education, 2016) and communicating adequate information for patients to provide informed consent to testing (Genetic Alliance; The New England Public Health Genetics Education Collaborative.

Washington (DC), 2010; NSW Government Health Centre for Genetics Education, 2016), and the potential psychosocial/psychological impact of receiving genetic information (Genetic Alliance; The New England Public Health Genetics Education Collaborative. Washington (DC), 2010; Reilly & Debusk, 2008). Individuals respond to information differently, including the information provided in nutrigenetic test results (National Health and Medical Research Council (NHMRC), 2010; Reilly & Debusk, 2008). Furthermore, there are also discrimination considerations as genetic information may play a role in predicting future health events (Genetic Alliance; The New England Public Health Genetics Education Collaborative. Washington (DC), 2010; National Health and Medical Research Council (NHMRC) Australia, 2013; NSW Government Health Centre for Genetics Education, 2016; Reilly & Debusk, 2008).

Integration of Genetic Information Into Dietetic and Nutrition Consultations

Dietitians are aware of the need to keep patient medical records confidential, including tests results which may include genetic information. However, there may be additional factors to consider with the handling of genetic information. Dietitians should consider the shared nature of genetics and what that may mean for confidentiality and issues relating to disclosure of high risk results for family members (Genetic Alliance; The New England Public Health Genetics Education Collaborative. Washington (DC), 2010; Reilly & Debusk, 2008). There are also questions around unexpected genetic results or incidental findings and whether these should be communicated to the client (Camp & Trujillo, 2014; Reilly & Debusk, 2008). These are just some of the issues dietitians need to consider before communicating nutritional genomic information. A multidisciplinary approach collaborating with genetic counsellors, clinical geneticists, geneticists and primary care physicians is an important consideration in nutrition practice involving genetic testing (Camp & Trujillo, 2014).

Nutrigenetic Tests and the Genetic Testing Process

Traditionally genetic tests have been available through medical professionals, however this landscape is changing. While medical professionals specialising in genetics are still a pathway for people to access genetic tests, people can now access genetic tests through healthcare professionals not traditionally trained in the area of genetics, or online through the internet, bypassing a healthcare practitioner altogether. With the increasing availability of genetic tests, dietitians should consider a number of ethical, legal and social issues associated with tests and their providers. Issues such as privacy policies relating to DNA storage, sample access, results access, and third party access (Ahlgren et al., 2013; NSW Government Health Centre for Genetics Education, 2016; Reilly & Debusk, 2008), regulation and quality assurance standards (National Health and Medical Research Council (NHMRC) Australia, 2013), and as discussed earlier, analytic and clinical validity, clinical impact (Camp & Trujillo, 2014; Genetic Alliance; The New England Public Health Genetics Education Collaborative. Washington (DC), 2010; National Health and Medical Research Council (NHMRC) Australia, 2013) and the transparency of evidence, including translation of research findings to certain subgroups (Nordstrom et al., 2013).

Proposed Framework to Include in Dietetic Education

To address the need for comprehensive knowledge upskilling in dietetics education in the area of nutritional genomics, the authors propose a set of five core competencies that all dietitians should possess to practice with expertise and develop leadership in the area of nutritional genomics. These are summarised in Figure 2 and further described below. Development of these competencies could be included within current dietetic curricula or as a suite of stand-alone courses for those wishing to develop advanced competency in the area. The authors suggest delivery strategies should include case studies and simulated client learning experiences.

Figure 2. Core competencies for dietetic education to facilitate competent practice in the area of nutritional genomic. ELSI = Ethical Legal Social Issues

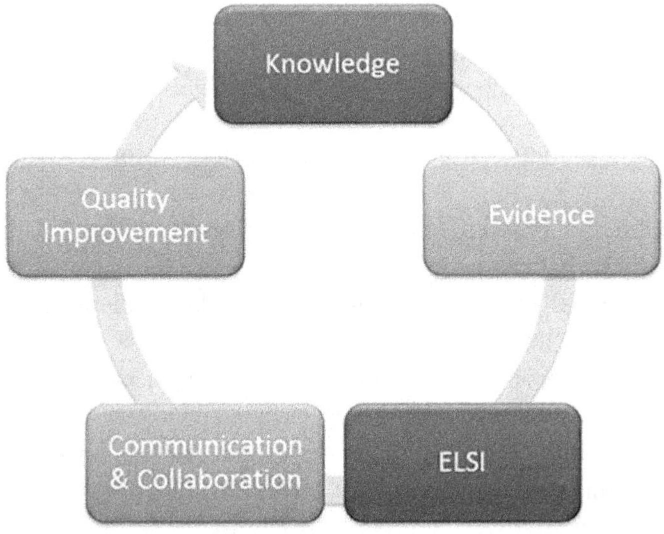

Knowledge

Dietitians should have an understanding of:

- **The Chromosomal and Molecular Basis of Inheritance:** Cell division, the cell cycle and control, meiosis and sexual reproduction, genetic variation due to sexual reproduction; the structure and function of nucleic acids, Mendel's laws and complex inheritance patterns e.g. epistasis, pleiotropy, multiple alleles, co-dominance, incomplete dominance, polygenic inheritance with examples, linked genes and haplotypes.
- The Genetic Basis of Disease including single gene disorders and complex disease, the role of genetic and environmental factors in complex disease, different types of DNA and chromosomal mutations and their effects, genome variation, population genetics and sources of genetic variation.
- Gene expression and regulation protein synthesis, the impact of diet and other modifiable factors on gene expression.
- Gene technology and how genetic variation is determined, interpretation of genetic test results.
- **Nutrigenetics and Nutrigenomics:** Definition, examples of genetic conditions where nutritional management is important - including classic single gene conditions such as inborn errors of metabolism as well as polygenic multifactorial conditions, interpretation of nutrigenetic test results, where to find information on gene function, role in disease, gene variation, impact of gene variation.

Evidence

Dietitians should be able to:

- Undertake a literature search to examine evidence for the clinical utility of genetic tests.
- Understand the different methodology of study designs and populations sampled and what can be inferred from results.
- Examine, critically review and summarize available scientific studies relating to a nutrigenetic test.
- Apply accepted tools for assessing the quality of research studies and levels of evidence.
- Integrate evidence, genetic, phenotypic and clinical information to make informed clinical decisions.

- Use professional judgement to support (or refute) the use of nutrigenetics tests for individuals.
- Understand the limitations and benefits of nutrigenetic testing for individual clients.
- Apply clinical decision making in the absence of strong evidence, with consideration for harm/benefit aspects.

Ethical, Legal, Social Issues

Dietitians should be able to

- Understand and communicate the nature of specific tests, pro and cons, risks, benefits and limitations of nutrigenetic tests, including applicability of specific results to individuals.
- Communicate alternatives to nutritional genomic tests.
- Use clinical judgement to determine if a nutrigenetic test is warranted.
- Communicate how the test sample will be obtained, the test rationale, how and where the results will be analysed, whether the sample will be stored/ discarded, and who can access results.
- Communicate genetic information in plain language.
- Understand the concept of informed consent and obligations regarding disclosure of information provided by the test to third parties such as insurance companies and family members.
- Understand the potential psychological impact of nutrigenetic test results.
- Consider the potential impact of nutritional genomic test results on behaviour change.
- Understand the concept of conflict of interest regarding nutritional genomic testing and obligations regarding financial gain from this type of testing or results being used for research.
- Understand the importance of researching the business and professional practices of nutrigenetic services.

Communication and Collaboration

Dietitians Should

- Understand the importance of a multi-disciplinary approach regarding the practice of nutritional genomics.

- Understand the obligation to refer clients to the appropriate professional and/ or service providers e.g. genetic counsellors when needs are beyond their scope of practice regarding nutrigenetic tests and their results.
- Understand the importance of collaboration with other health professionals in the management of clients regarding nutritional genomics tests.
- Understand the significance of engaging with policymakers and industry to influence decisions involving nutritional genomics.
- Be able to engage in active discussions with others to establish practices to best meet and serve the needs of the client and the population.

Quality Improvement

Dietitians should

- Understand the importance of staying up to date with the literature and practice of nutritional genomics and demonstrate an understanding of the application of evidence to practice.
- Understand the importance of complying with national, state and local legislation, policies and standards regarding nutritional genomic and genetic testing.
- Know how and where to access national and international regulations regarding nutritional genomic and genetic testing that is performed offshore.

CASE STUDY

The following Case Study provides an example of how a dietitian could apply the five core competencies proposed in this chapter to a client consultation concerning nutritional genetics.

A new client is concerned about results of an *MTHFR* gene test from a direct-to-consumer (DTC) provider. The client had the genetic test because they have been 'unwell' for a number of years, and their current healthcare professionals have not been able to provide a diagnosis. The client had read online that the *MTHFR* gene may be the cause of many different diseases and believed that knowing the results may provide some answers. The client purchased an online genetic test without any medical advice, and the result showed the client as TT homozygous at the *MTHFR* C677T locus. The DTC provider has suggested that based on these results, the client has a defect in the ability to use folic acid and therefore has an increased risk of a number of diseases. The client has been advised to avoid folic acid and purchase and consume 1mg of methylfolate daily. The client is now extremely concerned about the results and believes they have a 'genetic mutation' which may be causing them to feel unwell, however they are confused and don't understand what to do with the results. The client wishes to obtain advice from a dietitian on how to proceed with the nutrition recommendations.

For background information on the role of the *MTHFR* gene and enzyme, and the impact of variants, the dietitian could access the freely available OMIM (Online Mendelian Inheritance in Man) database, which describes Mendelian disorders and focuses on genotype and phenotype relationships and the impact of variants https://www.ncbi.nlm.nih.gov/omim/ Each OMIM entry has links to other genetic databases (Hamosh, Scott, Amberger, Bocchini, & McKusick, 2005).

The dietitian can further examine the variant using its rs number (Reference SNP) obtained from the OMIM search. The dietitian may access Ensembl genome browser http://www.ensembl.org/Homo_sapiens/Variation searching the rs number (in this instance rs1801133) (Aken et al., 2016). The phenotypes and relevant literature would be described and linked in this search.

The dietitian can examine the latest literature about the impact of *MTHFR* gene variation on the ability to use folic acid. A literature search may be undertaken using the National Centre for Biotechnology Information Pubmed Database https://www.ncbi.nlm.nih.gov/pubmed/ ("National Center for Biotechnology Information (NCBI)[Internet]. Bethesda (MD)," 1988). The dietitian may initially look for Level 1 evidence such as a systematic review and/or meta-analysis. The proposed search terms could be: MTHFR, systematic review, meta-analysis, folate, folic acid.

At this stage, the dietitian should have determined that the *MTHFR* C677T variant is associated with reduced enzyme activity and increased thermolability, and that it has a relatively high frequency throughout the world. Folate (including the synthetic form of folic acid) at a recommended daily intake (RDI) acts to stabilize the thermolabile enzyme with the 677C-T variation (Colson, Naug, Nikbakht, Zhang, & McCormack, 2017; Frosst et al., 1995; Hamosh et al., 2005).

Finally, the dietitian should examine relevant practice guidelines and position statements of various relevant bodies such as the Royal College of Pathologists of Australia at https://www.rcpa.edu.au (The Royal College of Pathologists of Australasia. Genetic Advisory Committee), the NSW Government Centre for Genetics Education at http://www.genetics.edu.au/health-professionals/ (NSW Health Centre for Genetics Education), or the American College of Medical Genetics (Hickey, Curry, & Toriello, 2013).

The dietitian is now armed with the knowledge and evidence to use professional judgement to provide advice to the client on the recommendations given by the DTC provider, and communicate the meaning and any possible implications of the gene variant to the client. With the client's consent, the dietitian could work with the client's general practitioner to examine folate related biochemistry to ensure that the client has adequate folate status and is not impacted by the genetic variant. The dietitian may also like to consider referral to a genetic counsellor, if appropriate, to further explain the genetic information and its implications.

FUTURE DIRECTIONS

In the emerging science of nutritional genomics it will be important to continue to monitor and evaluate the standards for nutritional genomics services and delivery, including robust and reproducible science, all aspects of the testing process and delivery, and the integration into clinical health care practice. A future challenge will be the interpretation and integration of additional information into a health professional's clinical assessment, for example other genetic markers and their interactions, biomarkers from other omics-based tests, along with other personal information such as microbiome composition. It is likely that bioinformatics will be an integral component of this process and dietitians can play a key role as part of a multidisciplinary team in translating this information into clinical practice.

In order to practice in this emerging area, it is crucial for students and new practitioners to develop a strong knowledge base and demonstrate competency. It is also important for practitioners and influencers in the area to formalise their knowledge base and skills and maintain current by keeping up with new progress in the area. Thus the development of undergraduate dietetics training curricula along with professional development modules with accreditation by professional bodies are a way forward to ensure competency in translation of the science and delivery to the health care industry.

It should be acknowledged that one of the critical barriers to this science is whether it influences positive behaviour change in individuals. Consequently, to determine the impact of this technology on the wider society, it will be essential to monitor response to personalised nutrition and whether it creates a positive effect on dietary and lifestyle change, nutrition status and disease prevention.

CONCLUSION

Nutritional genomics is an area of precision medicine that has the potential to create a more personalised approach to dietary management and health risk. Dietitians are well placed to be leaders in the discipline as clinical practitioners, academicians, consultants and researchers due to their expertise in the application of nutrition science to healthcare practice. However in order to develop professional competency in the area of nutritional genomics, dietetics education needs to evolve to include a number of key skills and competencies relevant to this practice. The authors propose five core competencies that are integral to successful practice in the discipline and propose that these be included in undergraduate dietetics curricula or as separate professional development/graduate programs.

REFERENCES

Ahlgren, J., Nordgren, A., Perrudin, M., Ronteltap, A., Savigny, J., van Trijp, H., & Gorman, U. et al. (2013). Consumers on the Internet: Ethical and legal aspects of commercialization of personalized nutrition. *Genes & Nutrition*, *8*(4), 349–355. doi:10.1007/s12263-013-0331-0 PMID:23471853

Aken, B. L., Ayling, S., Barrell, D., Clarke, L., Curwen, V., Fairley, S., & Searle, S. M. et al. (2016). The Ensembl gene annotation system. *Database (Oxford)*, *2016*, baw093. doi:10.1093/database/baw093 PMID:27337980

Aklillu, E., Carrillo, J. A., Makonnen, E., Hellman, K., Pitarque, M., Bertilsson, L., & Ingelman-Sundberg, M. (2003). Genetic polymorphism of CYP1A2 in Ethiopians affecting induction and expression: Characterization of novel haplotypes with single-nucleotide polymorphisms in intron 1. *Molecular Pharmacology*, *64*(3), 659–669. doi:10.1124/mol.64.3.659 PMID:12920202

Babu, P. V., Liu, D., & Gilbert, E. R. (2013). Recent advances in understanding the anti-diabetic actions of dietary flavonoids. *The Journal of Nutritional Biochemistry*, *24*(11), 1777–1789. doi:10.1016/j.jnutbio.2013.06.003 PMID:24029069

Blau, N. (2016). Genetics of Phenylketonuria: Then and Now. *Human Mutation*, *37*(6), 508–515. doi:10.1002/humu.22980 PMID:26919687

Burke, W. (2004). Clinical validity and clinical utility of genetic tests. Curr Protoc Hum Genet, 9. doi:10.1002/0471142905.hg0915s42

Camp, K. M., & Trujillo, E. (2014). Position of the Academy of Nutrition and Dietetics: Nutritional genomics. *Journal of the Academy of Nutrition and Dietetics*, *114*(2), 299–312. doi:10.1016/j.jand.2013.12.001 PMID:24439821

Colson, N. J., Naug, H. L., Nikbakht, E., Zhang, P., & McCormack, J. (2017). The impact of MTHFR 677 C/T genotypes on folate status markers: A meta-analysis of folic acid intervention studies. *European Journal of Nutrition*, *56*(1), 247–260. doi:10.1007/s00394-015-1076-x PMID:26497154

Corella, D., Coltell, O., Sorli, J. V., Estruch, R., Quiles, L., Martinez-Gonzalez, M. A., & Ordovas, J. M. et al. (2016). Polymorphism of the Transcription Factor 7-Like 2 Gene (TCF7L2) Interacts with Obesity on Type-2 Diabetes in the PREDIMED Study Emphasizing the Heterogeneity of Genetic Variants in Type-2 Diabetes Risk Prediction: Time for Obesity-Specific Genetic Risk Scores. *Nutrients*, *8*(12), 793. doi:10.3390/nu8120793 PMID:27929407

Cornelis, M. C., El-Sohemy, A., Kabagambe, E. K., & Campos, H. (2006). Coffee, CYP1A2 genotype, and risk of myocardial infarction. *Journal of the American Medical Association*, *295*(10), 1135–1141. doi:10.1001/jama.295.10.1135 PMID:16522833

Cornelis, M. C., Qi, L., Kraft, P., & Hu, F. B. (2009). TCF7L2, dietary carbohydrate, and risk of type 2 diabetes in US women. *The American Journal of Clinical Nutrition*, *89*(4), 1256–1262. doi:10.3945/ajcn.2008.27058 PMID:19211816

Covolo, L., Rubinelli, S., Ceretti, E., & Gelatti, U. (2015). Internet-Based Direct-to-Consumer Genetic Testing: A Systematic Review. *Journal of Medical Internet Research*, *17*(12), e279. doi:10.2196/jmir.4378 PMID:26677835

Dahlman, I., Linder, K., Arvidsson Nordstrom, E., Andersson, I., Liden, J., Verdich, C., & Arner, P. et al. (2005). Changes in adipose tissue gene expression with energy-restricted diets in obese women. *The American Journal of Clinical Nutrition*, *81*(6), 1275–1285. PMID:15941876

Daly, J., Willis, K., Small, R., Green, J., Welch, N., Kealy, M., & Hughes, E. (2007). A hierarchy of evidence for assessing qualitative health research. *Journal of Clinical Epidemiology*, *60*(1), 43–49. doi:10.1016/j.jclinepi.2006.03.014 PMID:17161753

Djordjevic, N., Ghotbi, R., Jankovic, S., & Aklillu, E. (2010). Induction of CYP1A2 by heavy coffee consumption is associated with the CYP1A2 -163C>A polymorphism. *European Journal of Clinical Pharmacology*, *66*(7), 697–703. doi:10.1007/s00228-010-0823-4 PMID:20390257

Fallaize, R., Macready, A. L., Butler, L. T., Ellis, J. A., & Lovegrove, J. A. (2013). An insight into the public acceptance of nutrigenomic-based personalised nutrition. *Nutrition Research Reviews*, *26*(1), 39–48. doi:10.1017/S0954422413000024 PMID:23561449

Fenech, M., El-Sohemy, A., Cahill, L., Ferguson, L. R., French, T. A., Tai, E. S., & Head, R. et al. (2011). Nutrigenetics and nutrigenomics: Viewpoints on the current status and applications in nutrition research and practice. *Journal of Nutrigenetics and Nutrigenomics*, *4*(2), 69–89. doi:10.1159/000327772 PMID:21625170

Ferguson, L. R., De Caterina, R., Gorman, U., Allayee, H., Kohlmeier, M., Prasad, C., & Martinez, J. A. et al. (2016). Guide and Position of the International Society of Nutrigenetics/Nutrigenomics on Personalised Nutrition: Part 1 - Fields of Precision Nutrition. *Journal of Nutrigenetics and Nutrigenomics*, *9*(1), 12–27. doi:10.1159/000445350 PMID:27169401

Food4me. (n.d.). *An integrated analysis of opportunities and challenges for personalised nutrition*. Retrieved from www.food4me.org

Frosst, P., Blom, H. J., Milos, R., Goyette, P., Sheppard, C. A., Matthews, R. G., & Rozen, R. et al. (1995). A candidate genetic risk factor for vascular disease: A common mutation in methylenetetrahydrofolate reductase. *Nature Genetics*, *10*(1), 111–113. doi:10.1038/ng0595-111 PMID:7647779

Genetic Alliance, & the New England Public Health Genetics Education Collaborative. (2010). *Understanding Genetics: A New England Guide for Patients and Health Professionals*. Retrieved from https://www.ncbi.nlm.nih.gov/books/NBK132187/

Gervasini, G., Ghotbi, R., Aklillu, E., San Jose, C., Cabanillas, A., Kishikawa, J., & Carrillo, J. A. et al. (2013). Haplotypes in the 5′-untranslated region of the CYP1A2 gene are inversely associated with lung cancer risk but do not correlate with caffeine metabolism. *Environmental and Molecular Mutagenesis*, *54*(2), 124–132. doi:10.1002/em.21747 PMID:23138776

Ghotbi, R., Christensen, M., Roh, H. K., Ingelman-Sundberg, M., Aklillu, E., & Bertilsson, L. (2007). Comparisons of CYP1A2 genetic polymorphisms, enzyme activity and the genotype-phenotype relationship in Swedes and Koreans. *European Journal of Clinical Pharmacology*, *63*(6), 537–546. doi:10.1007/s00228-007-0288-2 PMID:17370067

Gorman, U., Mathers, J. C., Grimaldi, K. A., Ahlgren, J., & Nordstrom, K. (2013). Do we know enough? A scientific and ethical analysis of the basis for genetic-based personalized nutrition. *Genes & Nutrition*, *8*(4), 373–381. doi:10.1007/s12263-013-0338-6 PMID:23471854

Hamosh, A., Scott, A. F., Amberger, J. S., Bocchini, C. A., & McKusick, V. A. (2005). Online Mendelian Inheritance in Man (OMIM), a knowledgebase of human genes and genetic disorders. *Nucleic Acids Research*, *33*(Database issue), D514–D517. doi:10.1093/nar/gki033 PMID:15608251

Hickey, S. E., Curry, C. J., & Toriello, H. V. (2013). ACMG Practice Guideline: Lack of evidence for MTHFR polymorphism testing. *Genetics in Medicine*, *15*(2), 153–156. doi:10.1038/gim.2012.165 PMID:23288205

Hollands, G. J., French, D. P., Griffin, S. J., Prevost, A. T., Sutton, S., King, S., & Marteau, T. M. (2016). The impact of communicating genetic risks of disease on risk-reducing health behaviour: Systematic review with meta-analysis. *BMJ (Clinical Research Ed.)*, *352*, i1102. doi:10.1136/bmj.i1102 PMID:26979548

Horigan, G., McNulty, H., Ward, M., Strain, J. J., Purvis, J., & Scott, J. M. (2010). Riboflavin lowers blood pressure in cardiovascular disease patients homozygous for the 677C-->T polymorphism in MTHFR. *Journal of Hypertension*, *28*(3), 478–486. doi:10.1097/HJH.0b013e328334c126 PMID:19952781

Horne, J., Madill, J., & O'Connor, C. (2016). Exploring Knowledge and Attitudes of Personal Nutrigenomics Testing among Dietetic Students and its Value as a Component of Dietetic Education and Practice. *The Canadian Journal of Clinical Nutrition*, *4*(1), 50–62. doi:10.14206/canad.j.clin.nutr.2016.01.07

Imai, K., Kricka, L. J., & Fortina, P. (2011). Concordance study of 3 direct-to-consumer genetic-testing services. *Clinical Chemistry*, *57*(3), 518–521. doi:10.1373/clinchem.2010.158220 PMID:21159896

Kallio, P., Kolehmainen, M., Laaksonen, D. E., Kekalainen, J., Salopuro, T., Sivenius, K., & Poutanen, K. S. et al. (2007). Dietary carbohydrate modification induces alterations in gene expression in abdominal subcutaneous adipose tissue in persons with the metabolic syndrome: The FUNGENUT Study. *The American Journal of Clinical Nutrition*, *85*(5), 1417–1427. PMID:17490981

Kalow, W., & Tang, B. K. (1993). The use of caffeine for enzyme assays: A critical appraisal. *Clinical Pharmacology and Therapeutics*, *53*(5), 503–514. doi:10.1038/clpt.1993.63 PMID:8491061

Kicklighter, J. R., Dorner, B., Hunter, A. M., Kyle, M., Pflugh Prescott, M., Roberts, S., & Byrne, C. et al. (2017). Visioning Report 2017: A Preferred Path Forward for the Nutrition and Dietetics Profession. *Journal of the Academy of Nutrition and Dietetics*, *117*(1), 110–127. doi:10.1016/j.jand.2016.09.027 PMID:28010848

Kohlmeier, M., De Caterina, R., Ferguson, L. R., Gorman, U., Allayee, H., Prasad, C., & Martinez, J. A. et al. (2016). Guide and Position of the International Society of Nutrigenetics/Nutrigenomics on Personalized Nutrition: Part 2 - Ethics, Challenges and Endeavors of Precision Nutrition. *Journal of Nutrigenetics and Nutrigenomics*, *9*(1), 28–46. doi:10.1159/000446347 PMID:27286972

Kostic, A. D., Xavier, R. J., & Gevers, D. (2014). The microbiome in inflammatory bowel disease: Current status and the future ahead. *Gastroenterology*, *146*(6), 1489–1499. doi:10.1053/j.gastro.2014.02.009 PMID:24560869

Kutz, G. (2006). *Nutrigenetic Testing Tests Purchased from Four Web Sites Mislead Consumers. Statement of Gregory Kutz, Managing Director Forensic Audits and Special Investigations.* Retrieved from http://www.gao.gov/assets/120/114612.pdf

Langenberg, C., Sharp, S. J., Franks, P. W., Scott, R. A., Deloukas, P., Forouhi, N. G., & Wareham, N. J. et al. (2014). Gene-lifestyle interaction and type 2 diabetes: The EPIC interact case-cohort study. *PLoS Medicine*, *11*(5), e1001647. doi:10.1371/journal.pmed.1001647 PMID:24845081

Li, S. X., Collins, J., Lawson, S., Thomas, J., Truby, H., Whelan, K., & Palermo, C. (2014). A preliminary qualitative exploration of dietitians' engagement with genetics and nutritional genomics: Perspectives from international leaders. *Journal of Allied Health*, *43*(4), 221–228. PMID:25433186

Li, S. X., Ye, Z., Whelan, K., & Truby, H. (2016). The effect of communicating the genetic risk of cardiometabolic disorders on motivation and actual engagement in preventative lifestyle modification and clinical outcome: A systematic review and meta-analysis of randomised controlled trials. *British Journal of Nutrition*, *116*(5), 924–934. doi:10.1017/S0007114516002488 PMID:27405704

Lim, J. S., Singh, O., Ramasamy, R. D., Ramasamy, S., Subramanian, K., Lee, E. J., & Chowbay, B. (2010). Pharmacogenetics of CYP1A2, novel polymorphisms and haplotypes in three distinct Asian populations. *Drug Metabolism and Pharmacokinetics*, *25*(6), 616–623. doi:10.2133/dmpk.DMPK-10-SC-051 PMID:20930417

Lin, J., Yang, R., Tarr, P. T., Wu, P. H., Handschin, C., Li, S., & Spiegelman, B. M. et al. (2005). Hyperlipidemic effects of dietary saturated fats mediated through PGC-1beta coactivation of SREBP. *Cell*, *120*(2), 261–273. doi:10.1016/j.cell.2004.11.043 PMID:15680331

Marsaux, C. F., Celis-Morales, C., Livingstone, K. M., Fallaize, R., Kolossa, S., Hallmann, J., & Saris, W. H. et al. (2016). Changes in Physical Activity Following a Genetic-Based Internet-Delivered Personalized Intervention: Randomized Controlled Trial (Food4Me). *Journal of Medical Internet Research, 18*(2), e30. doi:10.2196/jmir.5198 PMID:26851191

Maxmen, A. (2017). 23andMe given green-light to sell DNA tests for 10 diseases. *Nature news.* Retrieved from http://www.nature.com/news/23andme-given-green-light-to-sell-dna-tests-for-10-diseases-1.21802

McNulty, H., Strain, J. J., Hughes, C. F., & Ward, M. (2017). Riboflavin, MTHFR genotype and blood pressure: A personalized approach to prevention and treatment of hypertension. *Molecular Aspects of Medicine*, *53*, 2–9. doi:10.1016/j.mam.2016.10.002 PMID:27720779

Muller, M., & Kersten, S. (2003). Nutrigenomics: Goals and strategies. *Nature Reviews. Genetics*, *4*(4), 315–322. doi:10.1038/nrg1047 PMID:12671662

National Center for Biotechnology Information (NCBI). (1988). Retrieved from National Library of Medicine (US): https://www.ncbi.nlm.nih.gov/

National Health and Medical Research Council (NHMRC). (2010). *Medical Genetic Testing Information for Health Professionals*. Retrieved from https://www.nhmrc.gov.au/_files_nhmrc/publications/attachments/e99.pdf

National Health and Medical Research Council (NHMRC). (2013). *Discussing Direct-to-Consumer Genetic DNA Testing with Patients: A Short Guide for Health Professionals*. Retrieved from https://www.nhmrc.gov.au/_files_nhmrc/publications/attachments/g7_discussing_direct_to_consumer_genetic_testing_patients.pdf

National Health and Medical Research Council (NHMRC). (2015). *NHMRC additional levels of evidence and grades for recommendations for developers of guidelines*. Retrieved from https://www.nhmrc.gov.au/_files_nhmrc/file/guidelines/developers/nhmrc_levels_grades_evidence_120423.pdf

Nielsen, D. E., Shih, S., & El-Sohemy, A. (2014). Perceptions of genetic testing for personalized nutrition: A randomized trial of DNA-based dietary advice. *Journal of Nutrigenetics and Nutrigenomics*, *7*(2), 94–104. doi:10.1159/000365508 PMID:25170902

Nordstrom, K., Juth, N., Kjellstrom, S., Meijboom, F. L., & Gorman, U. (2013). Values at stake: Autonomy, responsibility, and trustworthiness in relation to genetic testing and personalized nutrition advice. *Genes & Nutrition*, *8*(4), 365–372. doi:10.1007/s12263-013-0337-7 PMID:23504640

NSW Government Health Centre for Genetics Education. (2016). *Ethical Issues in Human Genetics and Genomics*. Retrieved from http://www.genetics.edu.au/Publications-and-Resources/Genetics-Fact-Sheets/FactSheetELSI

NSW Health Centre for Genetics Education. (n.d.). *About MTHFR - Information for GPs*. Retrieved from http://www.genetics.edu.au/health-professionals/mthfr-dna-test

O'Donovan, C. B., Walsh, M. C., Forster, H., Woolhead, C., Celis-Morales, C., Fallaize, R., & Gibney, E. R. et al. (2016). The impact of MTHFR 677C --> T risk knowledge on changes in folate intake: Findings from the Food4Me study. *Genes & Nutrition*, *11*(1), 25. doi:10.1186/s12263-016-0539-x PMID:27708721

Pavlidis, C., Lanara, Z., Balasopoulou, A., Nebel, J. C., Katsila, T., & Patrinos, G. P. (2015). Meta-Analysis of Genes in Commercially Available Nutrigenomic Tests Denotes Lack of Association with Dietary Intake and Nutrient-Related Pathologies. *OMICS: A Journal of Integrative Biology*, *19*(9), 512–520. doi:10.1089/omi.2015.0109 PMID:26348710

Pavlidis, C., Nebel, J. C., Katsila, T., & Patrinos, G. P. (2016). Nutrigenomics 2.0: The Need for Ongoing and Independent Evaluation and Synthesis of Commercial Nutrigenomics Tests' Scientific Knowledge Base for Responsible Innovation. *OMICS: A Journal of Integrative Biology*, *20*(2), 65–68. doi:10.1089/omi.2015.0170 PMID:26689492

Qi, Q., Wang, X., Strizich, G., & Wang, T. (2015). Genetic Determinants of Type 2 Diabetes in Asians. *International Journal of Diabetology & Vascular Disease Research*, (Suppl 1). doi:10.19070/2328-353X-SI01001 PMID:27583258

Reilly, P. R., & Debusk, R. M. (2008). Ethical and legal issues in nutritional genomics. *Journal of the American Dietetic Association*, *108*(1), 36–40. doi:10.1016/j.jada.2007.10.016 PMID:18155987

Roswall, N., Angquist, L., Ahluwalia, T. S., Romaguera, D., Larsen, S. C., Ostergaard, J. N., & Tjonneland, A. et al. (2014). Association between Mediterranean and Nordic diet scores and changes in weight and waist circumference: Influence of FTO and TCF7L2 loci. *The American Journal of Clinical Nutrition*, *100*(4), 1188–1197. doi:10.3945/ajcn.114.089706 PMID:25099543

Royal College of Pathologists of Australasia, & the Genetic Advisory Committee. (n.d.). *Position Statement MTHFR Genetic Tests*. Retrieved from https://www.rcpa.edu.au/Library/College-Policies/Position-Statements/MTHFR-Genetic-Tests

Sterling, R. (2008). The on-line promotion and sale of nutrigenomic services. *Genetics in Medicine*, *10*(11), 784–796. doi:10.1097/GIM.0b013e31818c0441 PMID:18941418

Stewart-Knox, B. J., Bunting, B. P., Gilpin, S., Parr, H. J., Pinhao, S., Strain, J. J., & Gibney, M. et al. (2009). Attitudes toward genetic testing and personalised nutrition in a representative sample of European consumers. *British Journal of Nutrition*, *101*(7), 982–989. doi:10.1017/S0007114508055657 PMID:18775102

Tong, Y., Lin, Y., Zhang, Y., Yang, J., Zhang, Y., Liu, H., & Zhang, B. (2009). Association between TCF7L2 gene polymorphisms and susceptibility to type 2 diabetes mellitus: A large Human Genome Epidemiology (HuGE) review and meta-analysis. *BMC Medical Genetics*, *10*(1), 15. doi:10.1186/1471-2350-10-15 PMID:19228405

Trent, R. (2014). Direct-to-consumer DNA testing and the general practitioner. *Australian Family Physician*, *43*(7), 436–439. PMID:25006602

U.S. Food and Drug Administration. (2013). *Inspections, Compliance, Enforcement, and Criminal Investigations*. Retrieved from https://www.fda.gov/iceci/enforcementactions/warningletters/2013/ucm376296.htm

U.S. Food and Drug Administration. (2015). *FDA permits marketing of first direct-to-consumer genetic carrier test for Bloom syndrome*. Retrieved from https://www.fda.gov/NewsEvents/Newsroom/PressAnnouncements/ucm435003.htm

Wilson, C. P., McNulty, H., Ward, M., Strain, J. J., Trouton, T. G., Hoeft, B. A., & Scott, J. M. et al. (2013). Blood pressure in treated hypertensive individuals with the MTHFR 677TT genotype is responsive to intervention with riboflavin: Findings of a targeted randomized trial. *Hypertension*, *61*(6), 1302–1308. doi:10.1161/HYPERTENSIONAHA.111.01047 PMID:23608654

Wilson, C. P., Ward, M., McNulty, H., Strain, J. J., Trouton, T. G., Horigan, G., & Scott, J. M. et al. (2012). Riboflavin offers a targeted strategy for managing hypertension in patients with the MTHFR 677TT genotype: A 4-y follow-up. *The American Journal of Clinical Nutrition*, *95*(3), 766–772. doi:10.3945/ajcn.111.026245 PMID:22277556

Wright, O. R. (2014). Systematic review of knowledge, confidence and education in nutritional genomics for students and professionals in nutrition and dietetics. *Journal of Human Nutrition and Dietetics*, *27*(3), 298–307. doi:10.1111/jhn.12132 PMID:23781868

Chapter 5
The Use of an Online Adaptive Learning Platform as an Adjunct to Live Simulated Clinical Encounters

Neil Tuttle
Griffith University, Australia

ABSTRACT

Adaptive learning platforms that individualize each learner's experience according to their input have only recently become widely accessible. This chapter illustrates some of the potential of adaptive learning platforms and describes a case study where this emerging technology has been used with physiotherapy students in a simulated clinical setting. Aspects of patient care scenarios presented with an adaptive learning platform were interleaved with live simulated patient interactions. Evaluation of the projects and the benefits and challenges of using adaptive learning platforms in biomedical education are discussed.

INTRODUCTION

The intention underlying adaptive learning is to provide an environment which fits learning experiences to the needs of the students by responding or adapting to that individual student's needs and input. Adaptive learning is often considered to involve interactions with computers, but the idea that education is individualized and that an educational input is dependent on the output from the individual learner existed long before the advent of computers. In Socratic teaching, for example each

DOI: 10.4018/978-1-5225-3850-9.ch005

question is informed by the response of the learner. Similarly, in the Oxford tutorial method the directions of the small group discussions are dependent on responses of the learners. Another historical version of individualized education was described in John Stuart Mills' 1873 Autobiography (http://www.gutenberg.org/ebooks/10378) accessed March 6, 2017) where Mills, on daily walks with his father would summarize his previous days reading. These summaries led to discussions, what would now be called teaching moments, and suggestions of further reading. As time went on, Mills taught his younger sister what he was learning with the interesting twist that the sister would recount her learning to the father and the father feedback to both his son and daughter on the learning. All of these methods seem to be effective, are highly individualized and learner-centred, but are difficult to apply with large numbers of students.

In any group of students, there will be individuals with different needs and understandings; and who learn at different rates or from different frameworks. A challenge when teaching large numbers of students is how to present the material to maximize the learning of all students without leaving some students behind and/or risking boredom in others. It is not possible for all students to have the amount of time from an individual mentor that John Stuart Mills had, so attempts were made to develop automated ways of assisting student learning. The earliest learning machines are the precursors to today's computer based adaptive learning. Learning machines were defined as "an automatic or self-controlling device that (a) presents a unit of information .., (b) provides some means for the learner to respond to the information, and (c) provides feedback about the correctness of the learner's responses." (Benjamin, 1988) By this definition the earliest learning machines were produced in the 1920's by Pressey (Benjamin, 1988). His machines required students to respond to a multiple choice question; once a correct response had been selected they could move on to the next question. The number of attempts and the number of correct responses could be recorded and a reward of sweets could be provided to the student after a predetermined number of correct responses. Nonetheless, B. F. Skinner is often credited with the earliest learning machine in the 1950's. These devices required the student to enter the text of an answer and assisted students with a series of small hints until the student produced the correct answer. Importantly these hints occurred regardless of which incorrect answer was written and were not specific to the answer provided by the student. There was considerable controversy about the early teaching machines and their use all but died out by the mid 1960's, just as computers were about to come into common use.

The development, diversity, and theoretical underpinning of computer based education over the last forty years is far beyond the scope of this chapter, but it is worth briefly considering some of the influences. With the increasing sophistication and accessibility of computers from the late 1970's, there were two streams that contributed to an increased interest in computer based learning, computer games and dedicated educational software programs. Early computer games were developed as arcade games prior to becoming more accessible on home computers or game consoles played through television sets. Although not initially designed for learning, even the earliest computer games fulfil Benjamin's definition – they presented information, the user could respond, and the user received feedback from their response (consider Pacman scores or losing a life). The input from the user had a wide variety of options and resulted in complex output. Computer games added the element of the future pathway altering depending on the user's input. For example, a lower degree of skill resulted in losing a 'life' and having to re-do the simpler tasks until reaching the higher degree of skill and progressing to another level. The early video games have matured into what are now called serious games with objectives beyond entertainment. The development of educational software ran parallel to early computer games (Molnar, 1997). Early educational materials provided self-paced programs and feedback on responses, but generally had a single linear pathway. Gradually educational software also began to include a branching type of structure that was common in computer games where different pathways occurred in response to the users input. Interestingly a similar branching occurred in the 'choose your own adventure' stories in traditional book formats that were popular around the same time. Throughout this time, software development remained the province of the skilled computer programmer.

It is only in the past decade that the software and programming necessary to develop computer based educational materials that are truly adaptive has become accessible to academics or teachers without extensive programming skills. There are now a number of software platforms that can provide feedback to the learner, allow branching pathways to provide extra information when needed, and enable learners to progress through material at different rates. The addition in some of these platforms of the ability to very specifically track student performance both on an individual and group level provides educators with information to refine both the content on the platform and other aspects of their teaching.

In the remainder of this chapter we describe one application of computer based adaptive learning using the Smartsparrow platform [https://www.smartsparrow.com/]. The application presented challenges, but produced particular benefits. One of the greatest challenges was that in order for the student experience to be fluid, the concepts and processes being communicated needed to have a far greater degree of clarity and precision than would be necessary with traditional teaching methods. Although the author and his team are experienced in both the practice and teaching of the topics, development of the applications required us to dissect the material in entirely new ways.

BACKGROUND

Using an Adaptive Learning Platrorm as Part of a Hybrid Simulated Learning Enviroment to Prepare Physiotherapy Students for Clinical Placements

Clinical education is a form of work integrated learning that is an essential component in all physiotherapy educational programs (WCPT, 2011). During traditional clinical education, students see real patients in real clinical settings under progressively reducing levels of supervision (Franzone et al., 2015). In addition to traditional placements, some work integrated learning in Physiotherapy education occurs in simulated learning environments (SLEs). Patient-centred SLEs which include live actors portraying patients are increasingly being used to supplement clinical placements or to replace a percentage of traditional clinical placement hours and have been shown to 1) be able to replace up to 25% of clinical placement time with simulation without detrimental effects (Watson et al., 2012). See Chapter [11] for or a more detailed discussion of the role of clinical placements in Physiotherapy education and of the place simulation plays.

The patient-centred type of simulation used in this way to supplement clinical education is expensive and highly focused so tends to be used to simulate a limited number of discrete events or situations. The discrete events of actual patient care such as taking a history or performing a physical assessment do not however exist in isolation. Rather patient care includes gathering and processing preliminary information, a series of discrete events that make up an occasion of service, a number of occasions of service, and tasks such as communicating with other health professionals between occasions of service. A challenge in using live patient centred simulation, is to ensure that a sufficient range of situations are addressed and the discrete events are placed as part of a continuum of patient care.

One way of amplifying the effectiveness of live simulated learning activities is provide supplementary background and/or follow-up information to enhance the time spent in the live simulation. This supplementary material can be presented in a variety of ways ranging from hard-copy documents to multimedia presentations. Regardless of how well the material is presented, student engagement will be limited as long as they are passive recipients of information. Alternatively the supplementary material can become part of a hybrid simulation where students actively problem-solve and interact with aspects of the scenario that lead up to and follow the aspects being simulated by live interaction. Adaptive learning platforms (ALPs) can provide one way of actively engaging students by enabling them to interact with and receive guidance and feedback as they work independently through aspects of scenarios.

We integrated an adaptive learning platform with live simulations in a module to assist Physiotherapy students to transition from classroom learning to clinical placements. Students learn the building blocks of clinical practice in their on-campus learning, but putting these pieces together into integrated therapeutic encounters can be challenging for students and typically occurs on clinical placement. Particularly with the increasing demand for a limited pool of clinical placements it is useful for students to be better prepared when they commence their placements. We therefore implemented Transition to Placement (T2P) modules immediately before clinical placements to assist students to be more work-ready prior to their clinical placements. During the T2P modules, students work through simulated patient scenarios linking the various elements and eventually 'put it all together' into an integrated therapeutic encounter. The T2P modules were not part of summative assessment and as an overriding principle, it was assumed that the learners were intelligent, well-trained, cared about doing their best, and wanted to improve (Rudolph, Simon, Raemer, & Eppich, 2008).

The concept development, the overall structure of the simulated learning module, and an evaluation of its effectiveness is described in more depth in Chapter [11]. The integration of an adaptive learning platform with the live SLEs enabled a much larger number of scenarios to be worked through and ensured that the live SLEs could be more efficient and focused.

The aims of this chapter is to describe the development and implementation of an adaptive learning platform for the development of lessons to assist clinical reasoning.

Using an Adaptive Learning Platform to Develop Clinical Reasoning

Clinical reasoning is a term used to describe the process physiotherapists and all health professionals use to inform decisions within their therapeutic interactions. These decisions are not simply deciding on a patient's diagnosis and treatment regime (Doody & McAteer, 2002) but include constructing a meaning and determining appropriate conceptual and action responses on a moment to moment basis. An excellent description of the thinking involved in the reasoning processes has been presented by Del Mar and colleagues (Del Mar, Doust, & Glasziou, 2006).

Within Physiotherapy, the therapeutic interaction is typically divided into three parts; all of which involve clinical reasoning - taking a history, physical assessment and providing treatment. Unlike other areas of health care where responses to treatment may take days or weeks, the response to many physiotherapy treatments occur immediately. This immediacy of response enables the cyclical reasoning process to be compressed. For example, even within a given occasion of service, the patient's subjective and objective responses to each element of the overall intervention are re-evaluated to inform the modification and progression of the treatment plan (Tuttle, 2009). Such re-assessments typically occur multiple times within a treatment session as well as between occasions of service.

A template was developed within an adaptive learning platform that was intended to be able to be used for any scenario involving a patient with a musculoskeletal condition. Although all aspects from one scenario will be used as an example in this chapter, during the T2P modules as described in Chapter [10], some aspects of each scenario were presented in the adaptive learning platform while other aspects were undertaken as live SLEs. The interleafing of online modules with live patient centred simulation enabled the live interactions to be more focused, but also enabled more time to be spent considering the transitions between the different areas. For example, discussions could include how did the findings from the history inform a physical assessment that would be performed live or how did a live physical assessment inform the selection of treatment section that would subsequently be performed online.

The History

Prior to taking a history the student or clinician should know what information needs to be obtained and in the following discussion this will be presumed to be the case. The skills needed to take a history can be divided into two components, communication skills to obtain the information and clinical reasoning to interpret and respond to the information. Communication skills would be addressed in live simulations. The aspect that needed to be addressed using the ALP was the reasoning process during the history. Perhaps the most obvious approach to using an online module to model taking a history would be for students to type in (or speak using voice recognition) a question, receive an answer, ask the next question, and so on. The number of possible questions a student might ask however was too vast for us to even consider being able to program answers to them all. One way of narrowing the options would have been to provide a list of questions from which students could choose. Realistically, patient's responses would vary depending on what questions had been asked before and in what order. Again, this approach would have led to a level of complexity that was beyond our resources.

Rather than model the questions asked, we focused on the progressive interpretation of the information being received. The student was presented with a small amount of information such as a brief referral letter which was followed by a ranking screen (Figure 1) where they needed to rank the likelihood of possible diagnoses, contributing factors, treatment options, sinister pathologies (red flags)

and contributing psychosocial factors (yellow flags). We consider that each piece of information that a clinician receives should have the potential to change their thinking in some way (Del Mar et al., 2006) so after providing a small amount of additional information such as the area of the patient's symptoms, the student is returned to the ranking screen. This process of progressive disclosure followed by the opportunity for the student to revise their interpretation continued until all of the information that would normally be obtained during the history had been disclosed. Students were then provided with feedback on how each disclosure of information altered the likelihood of the various options that they could use to compare with their responses.

Planning and Conducting the Physical Assessment

Most clinicians move directly from taking a history to their physical assessment, but for students the decisions of what to include in the physical assessment needs to be explicit. The next stage of the scenarios represented in the ALP was therefore planning the physical assessment. There are a finite number of joints, muscles and connective tissues and a finite number of tests that can be used for each. The number of options is relatively large reaching several hundred, but it was possible to include all of the common options in an ordered branching structure that the students could choose from. In the ALP students can select functional tests or written outcome measures from a list that is specific for that scenario. There are then screens for different systems that might be assessed including articular, muscular, neurological, and neurodynamic systems. Each system screen includes multiple choice options for the student to select regions they would choose to assess. Each selected region will open another multiple choice screen for the student to select the specific tests they would choose to perform for that region in that system. Tests that would constitute a routine test for each system-region are pre-selected, but the students can increase or decrease the tests they would choose to perform with that patient. An example of these screens is shown in Figure 1.

Once the student has selected items for each region and each system, they are presented with a list of their selections ordered as would typically occur in clinical practice – functional tests followed by tests that would be performed in standing, sitting, lying supine, lying prone, and tests performed in other positions. If for that scenario, the student will be performing those tests in a live simulation, they can print out the list, use as a reference to discuss their decisions with their facilitator prior undertaking a live physical assessment. Otherwise, the student will be presented with the results of those assessments for that patient in the order the tests would be conducted clinically as described above.

Planning and Conducting the Treatment

Once a student has completed their physical assessment either with the ALP or a SLE, they are ready to progress to the treatment stage. The difficulty with modelling Physiotherapy treatment in an ALP is similar to that with modelling taking a history. Unlike medicine where there are a relatively small number of treatment options and dosages for a given condition, in Physiotherapy there are typically several treatment options with each option having multiple variations in application and dosage. Unfortunately, it is not generally possible at the outset to determine with any certainty which option will produce superior outcomes. The method for overcoming this uncertainty is taught in all schools of Physiotherapy in Australia (Hahne, Keating, & Wilson, 2004) and probably most schools internationally is supported by findings that the response to a given treatment is the best predictor of future response to that treatment (Hahne et al., 2004; Tuttle, 2005). The method is to assess the response to each intervention very specifically, then modify or progress the treatment based on that response; with this process of assessment, treatment and reassessment occurring multiple times within a given treatment session.. The clinical reasoning process of refining treatment based on a patient's response is arguably a clearer process than the reasoning involved in initial treatment selection, but it remains one of the most challenging aspects of musculoskeletal physiotherapy to teach.

In the treatment section of the ALP students make selections from a range of options, but are ultimately directed down a single common pathway. First students select from a range of possible tests they will use to evaluate the effectiveness of their intervention. Some of these such as maintaining a position for a period of time or the level of their resting pain are known to not be good predictors of treatment effectiveness. If students select these poor predictors, they receive immediate feedback of the reasons why this may not be the best choice. When students select one of at least two options which could be reasonable choices, they receive feedback that reflects the level of uncertainty. The feedback is typically in the form of *Good choice. Either A or C are reasonable option. The advantages of A are..., while the disadvantages are .... For B the advantages and disadvantages are .... In this case we will select B*. The students then select their first choice of treatment and again receive feedback indicating which choices are not preferred, the level of uncertainty, advantages and disadvantages, and a selected option.

Students are then provided with the patient's response and asked to decide if they will change their reassessment and how they would modify their treatment in light of the patient's response. Again they receive feedback on their choices including a level of uncertainty, but directing them to one option. This process is repeated several times within that simulated treatment session. Through a similar process students

are guided through when to finish that treatment session, what home program and education they will provide, and when the patient will be reviewed.

Students then usually plan a follow-up treatment that they discuss with their SLE facilitator and they may see that patient for a live follow-up treatment in the live SLE the next day.

Evaluation

Evaluation of the entire T2P module which contained this ALP component is discussed in Chapter [11]. During the first iteration of the T2P module, the ALP was used for half of the ten patient scenarios while traditional paper or static document formats were used for the remaining scenarios. Since students experienced both forms of information, student impressions and preferences specifically related the ALP platform could be evaluated. Of the students who responded with a preference, 63% preferred the ALP to the traditional mode of presentation, 86% thought the ALP better assisted their learning, but only 40% found the ALP easier to use. Qualitative responses indicated that students seemed less accepting of flaws or technical 'glitches' in the online platform than when the material was presented in paper based form. In summary although there were mixed responses to which mode of delivery was preferred or easier to use, the overwhealming majority of students felt the ALP assisted their learning better than traditional methods of presenting supplementary information related to a simulated learning environment.

Screenshots from adaptive learning platform. For the slide on the left, students are able to adjust the order of likely diagnoses, predisposing factors, types off interventions, red flags indicating caution in relation to serious pathology, and yellow flags indicating psychosocial factors that may impact on their symptoms. The right-hand slide is an example of where students select which objective assessments

Figure 1.

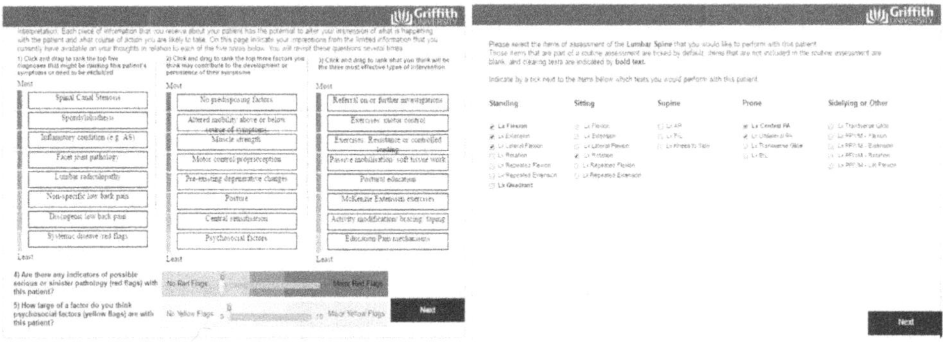

they would perform for a particular region. In this instance the screen is shown for the articular structures of the lumbar spine. Tests that are done routinely are pre-selected, but students can select more or few items.

ISSUES, CONTROVERSIES, PROBLEMS

The two main drivers for computer-based, adaptive, learning environments are increasing efficiency and increasing effectiveness. The initial driver for computer or machine based learning was to increase the efficiency of learning environments. Early machine-based and computer-based lessons required specialized skills to construct and could reach remarkable efficiency when used by a large enough number of users, but were not capable of adaptive responses so maintained a set form regardless of learner input.

The luxury of time that may be needed to achieve the effectiveness of adaptive or individualized learning was illustrated in the introduction by the education of John Stuart Mills. While computer-based lessons evolved into the massive online open courses (MOOCs) in the early twenty-first century, it is only recently that such lessons have been able to include elements of adaptive learning that are necessary for a truly individualized environment. That is, there may have been options of which pathways to take, but once selected, the pathway had an immutable structure. In the last decade platforms that enabled individualized or adaptive computer based learning such as Knewton or SmartSparrow became readily available and the first HarvardX MOOC to use true adaptive learning features only appeared within the last few years.

There is little argument about the potential effectiveness of adaptive ALPs. The difficulties, at least in the first world where accessibility is not an issue, are more related to their efficiency. When is the expenditure of time and resources required to develop courses justified? The development of lessons requires content knowledge, translating the knowledge into a logical structure with clear pathways and branching, and putting the structure into a software platform. The educational design is not a trivial task. In the example given in this chapter, the development was undertaken by educators with up to 30 years of experience who had put a great deal of effort into refining their teaching of similar content. We had not, however reached the level of clarity and specificity needed to translate complex reasoning processes such as those required for clinical practice into the type of algorithms needed for a lesson in an ALP. Firstly it was necessary to understand the structure and potential functionality of the platform. Answers like 'it depends on …' were no longer sufficient. It was necessary to be specific on how an answer was dependent on a range of often interdependent factors. This conceptual work required time, discussion, trial, and error.

Historically, even once the conceptual mind mapping had been accomplished; it would have required specialized programming skills to put the material into a software platform. The content expert needed to understand the structure of the software platform and the programmer needed to understand the structure of the content. Much could be lost in translation between those with different areas of expertise. Several of the adaptive learning platforms that are now available are intended to be usable directly by the content experts. One person being able to do the entire process potentially increases the efficiency by reducing the need for translations. ALPs in their current state however are not necessarily intuitive. They require training and practice, and even then a significant amount of time is necessary to convert the plan into a functioning lesson.

The case study application discussed in this chapter is not a typical application for generic ALPs. There are dedicated software platforms for presenting and working through case studies and some incorporate aspects of adaptive learning, but the authors determined that these would require even more time committed to development than the generic platform that was used. The additional advantage of using a generic platform is that the skills developed could then be applied to lessons other than case studies. In the case described in this chapter, the alternatives were either 1) For the material to be presented such that students were passive recipients of information in a set form which limits their engagement, or 2) for the interactions to be played out in live simulations which is even more time and resource intensive. Although developing the lessons was complex and time consuming, the integration of aspects of each case being presented as a live simulation with others presented in an online ALP enabled students to interact with all aspects of a larger number of cases. Any questions or areas that needed clarification from the ALP were also able to be addressed during the facilitation of the live simulations.

In summary, developing content in ALPs requires time and skill both to re-conceptualize the content and to convert the content into an accessible online form. The point where the investment in development is warranted by the benefits in efficiency and/or effectiveness needs to be considered on a case by case basis.

SOLUTIONS AND RECOMMENDATIONS

ALPs have great potential across a variety of educational settings from MOOCs to small scale clinical reasoning. The exercise of developing content in an ALP requires much greater clarity of process than traditional teaching methods. It is critical to consider the learning objectives, content and audience prior to developing lessons and even then the development of lessons takes large amounts of time. We have not reached what is perhaps the holy grail of computer based learning which would be for an application of artificial intelligence or machine based learning to seek out the knowledge related to the learning objectives, analyze student input and determine the appropriate pathway to best experience for that learner.

CONCLUSION

The application of an ALP has been described that enables students to interactively work through aspects of case presentations in Physiotherapy. The lessons were used to supplement and augment live simulated learning experiences. The development of the module presented a number of challenges, but we feel it provided a superior experience to what would have been possible with other modes of delivery that are currently available. Although progress is being made to make online learning more effective and efficient, there are still challenges in its implementation.

REFERENCES

Benjamin, L. T. (1988). A history of teaching machines. *The American Psychologist*, *43*(9), 703–712. doi:10.1037/0003-066X.43.9.703

Del Mar, C., Doust, J., & Glasziou, P. (2006). *Clinical Thinking: evidence, communication and decision-making*. Malden, MA: BMJ/Blackwell. doi:10.1002/9780470750568

Doody, C., & McAteer, M. (2002). Clinical reasoning of expert and novice physiotherapists in an outpatient orthopaedic setting. *Physiotherapy*, *88*(5), 258–268. doi:10.1016/S0031-9406(05)61417-4

Franzone, J. M., Kennedy, B. C., Merritt, H., Casey, J. T., Austin, M. C., & Daskivich, T. J. (2015). Progressive independence in clinical training: Perspectives of a national, multispecialty panel of residents and fellows. *Journal of Graduate Medical Education*, *7*(4), 700–704. doi:10.4300/JGME-07-04-51 PMID:26692998

Hahne, A. J., Keating, J. L., & Wilson, S. C. (2004). Do within-session changes in pain intensity and range of motion predict between-session changes in patients with low back pain? *The Australian Journal of Physiotherapy*, *50*(1), 17–23. doi:10.1016/S0004-9514(14)60244-0 PMID:14987188

Molnar, A. (1997). Computers in education: A brief history. *The Journal, 24*(11), 63-68.

Rudolph, J. W., Simon, R., Raemer, D. B., & Eppich, W. J. (2008). Debriefing as formative assessment: Closing performance gaps in medical education. *Academic Emergency Medicine*, *15*(11), 1010–1016. doi:10.1111/j.1553-2712.2008.00248.x PMID:18945231

Tuttle, N. (2005). Do changes within a manual therapy treatment session predict between-session changes for patients with cervical spine pain? *The Australian Journal of Physiotherapy*, *51*(1), 43–48. doi:10.1016/S0004-9514(05)70052-0 PMID:15748124

Tuttle, N. (2009). Is It Reasonable to Use an Individual Patient's Progress After Treatment as a Guide to Ongoing Clinical Reasoning? *Journal of Manipulative and Physiological Therapeutics*, *32*(5), 396–403. doi:10.1016/j.jmpt.2009.04.002 PMID:19539124

Watson, K., Wright, A., Morris, N., McMeeken, J., Rivett, D., Blackstock, F., & Watson, G. et al. (2012). Can simulation replace part of clinical time? Two parallel randomised controlled trials. *Medical Education*, *46*(7), 657–667. doi:10.1111/j.1365-2923.2012.04295.x PMID:22646319

WCPT. (2011). *WCPT guideline for the clinical education component of the physical therapist professional entry level programme*. Retrieved from London: www.wcpt.org/guidelines/clinical-education

Chapter 6
Current and Emerging Tools for Flexible Remote Learning

Sapha Mosawy
Griffith University, Australia

ABSTRACT

Distance learning is becoming increasingly common in the higher education sector. Student flexibility and inability of students to access education in remote regions are the main drivers of remote learning. There are many tools available that enable remote learning to reach geographically isolated and remote students as well as to provide extra flexibility to local students. This chapter explores current and emerging tools for flexible remote learning. Specifically, this chapter looks at current and new tools used in remote learning as effective tools for university students as well as graduate continuing learning. The tools, benefits, and models of remote learning are discussed. The objective of the chapter is to discuss the current and emerging tools in remote learning and its importance in emerging technologies and work-integrated learning in allied health.

INTRODUCTION

Remote learning, or distance learning, is becoming an increasingly popular mode of study in many tertiary educational programs including allied health. Remote or distance learning is the delivery of teaching material and the fulfilment of course work from remote locations. This allows students and teachers to interact and communicate without face to face contact. New technologies and tools have made

DOI: 10.4018/978-1-5225-3850-9.ch006

remote learning as an effective and flexible learning environment for students (Thompson, 2016). Remote learning is a mode of study that heavily depends on information and communication technology (ICT). Remote learning is considered as a flexible and interactive learning environment through which students acquire knowledge and complete entire tertiary degrees without having a face to face contact with their teachers. Tools such as virtual classrooms have enabled students and teachers to have a mutual interactive media experience where they can have video conferences, video lessons and other stimulating learning activities.

Information and communication technology has changed significantly over recent decades. The increased application and accessibility of internet based technology has expanded the learning and teaching tools available to universities and education providers. Computers, smart phones and tablets are more powerful, support and contain many different applications that can be used to facilitate learning, their ability to connect teachers and students to each other remotely has allowed students to complete tasks, receive feedback and interact with class mates.

Internet based learning and teaching applications such as Blackboard, Massive Open Online Courses (MOOCs), Moodle and other interactive systems allow universities to reach regional and remote students. Similarly, students who are unable to be physically present in the traditional class room due to employment, family commitments or physical geography will have access to the same teaching experience as the students in the traditional class room. Research studies show that student outcomes were enhanced by the use of learning and teaching tools by providing greater flexibility (Kemp & Livingstone, 2006; Martin, 2008). Furthermore, working allied health professionals completing studies via distance education setting performed significantly better than undergraduate and graduate (Williams, 2006). Universities have recognised the importance of student flexibility and therefore many universities offer courses that are online can be completed via distance education. Furthermore, the advances in internet and its application, it is now possible for allied health professionals to participate and complete continuing professional development without travelling great distances.

This chapter discusses current and emerging tools that are available to teachers and students to support their teaching approaches. Specifically this chapter will look at current and new tools used in remote learning as effective tools for university students as well as graduate continuing learning. The tools, benefits and models of remote learning will be discussed. The objective of the chapter is to discuss the current and emerging tools in remote learning and its importance in emerging technologies and work integrated learning in allied health.

BACKGROUND

Education is a continuing and life long journey, postgraduate training and continuing professional development are necessary to maintain skills and knowledge. Furthermore, access to education and continuing professional development for rural and remote professionals is becoming increasingly difficult due to distance and time constraint. In Australia, health professionals are required to complete continuing professional practice courses and programs on a regular basis, therefore, access to such educational programs for rural and remote professionals is vital, therefore innovative technology is required to deliver education to remote professionals (Sheppard & Mackintosh, 1998). Distance education has provided the needed access and availability to gain education and professional development (Carroll, Booth, Papaioannou, Sutton, & Wong, 2009). There are many other factors that contributed to the increased popularity of distance and remote learning. Educational institutions and universities are challenged with rapidly increasing tuition and operating costs accompanied by reduced funding governments, there are also pressures demanding universities to undertake educational reforms (Olson, 2005). Advocates for educational reform suggest that there is a lack of student engagement from the traditional learning and teaching processes and face to face lecture-based courses fail to inspire student engagement, motivation or critical thinking. Furthermore, it is also suggested that in traditional learning and teaching teachers also lack the motivation to inspire students due to insufficient value placed on teaching and learning and teachers are encouraged to teach course content only, not critical thinking skills.

Advances and expansion in information technology and internet based applications has allowed millions of students and postgraduate professionals to complete higher education studies via distance learning. The internet has become a vital medium for educational institutions to make learning material available for students. Similarly, the internet has given the students greater access to the teaching material; hence, students now enjoy a greater flexibility and autonomy when completing their study tasks. E-learning has been described as a student centred approach due to its design and ability to be interactive, customizable and self-paced.

There are many advantages associated with remote learning. One of the main and important aspects of distance learning is the accessibility and flexibility it provides to students. Remote education provides accessibility and flexibility for students who may not be able to attend a traditional classroom these might include geographically remote students, stay-at-home parents, full time working employees or even members of the military. Because education is delivered via online students are able to work and complete their study at their own place, in other words, students can fit education into their schedule. Flexibility in remote learning program gives the opportunity to student to study and complete tasks without significantly changing their personal life and responsibilities. Students in employment can always plan learning around their working routine and responsibilities, with little effect on personal or professional life. In programs delivered via remote learning, the student is not bound by physical location, but instead, they can complete their course work from just about anywhere, given that they have access to a computer and internet connection. This enables students to work when and where it is more suitable for them without having to significantly alter their busy daily routine to schedule and attend classes. Flexibility and accessibility of education allows students to choose the type of education they require and the education provider that they wish to enrol with.

In addition, distance learning allows people to pursue their choice of education during any time of their life. Because there is no limitation on location or educational institutions, many can live and study from anywhere in the world. However, the most important requirement needed to achieve this is access to a computer and Internet connection at reasonable speed. Continuing professional development is an important feature of many professions particularly in for the allied health professionals. Allied health professionals need continuing professional development to maintain current knowledge and skills, and in some instance they require postgraduate training to acquire or maintain practice registration. Health professionals working in regional and remote locations are constantly challenged by distance and time constrains. Therefore, remote education can provide the required post graduate training and competencies to such professionals without interfering with their employment particularly at times of employee shortages. Furthermore, learning while working is an important feature of allied health industry, therefore, completing an online trading course will provide the necessary hands on skills on the job.

Another advantage of remote and distance education is students who are on very limited income can save money as there is no commuting to and from classes. Furthermore, time will also be saved especially for those students travelling great distances in commuting. Student can utilise this time in worthwhile activities such as employment or time with family. In distance learning, there are no scheduled class times and places, so students can complete their studies at their own pace and suitability. One more advantage is that more knowledge of computer and Internet skills are gained through distance learning. Web based technology is rapidly developing and increasingly incorporated in many industries including allied health industry. Learning remotely will enable students to increase their base knowledge and skills in web based technologies.

Advances in innovative web based technologies and applications allowed remote learning and teaching to be more accessible and flexible. Currently, there are numerous web based tools that universities and education providers use to deliver their teaching materials. These include Blackboard, MOOCs, Moodle, Augmented and virtual reality, gamification of learning and cloud computing.

CURRENT TOOL FOR FLEXIBLE AND REMOTE LEARNING

Blackbaord

Blackboard as a learning management tool has been around for a long time. It is one of most widely used web based platforms for course management and virtual learning. It was developed by Blackboard Inc. Blackboard Learn (previously known as Blackboard Learning System) provides a powerful and flexible learning environment for students. Numerus universities, colleges and educational institutions have adopted Blackboard learn as primary course management system for all students. Distance learning has become an appealing feature for many remote students; with the use of the Blackboard Learning System the teacher can easily provide the course material including lecture notes, audio recordings, learning activities and assessment tasks online. In turn, the student, can review the learning material, reflect and discuss related topics with fellow students and receive feedback from the instructor (Bradford, Porciello, Balkon, & Backus, 2007). The benefits of using a web based course management system such as the Blackboard Learn are briefly discussed below:

Increased Flexibilty

Flexibility achieved for those wishing to study via distance due to the ability of Blackboard to be accessed using the internet at anywhere and anytime. Students are able to acquire all of necessary materials relating to their course including lectures, audio/visual aids, extra reading material and assessment tasks [Bradford et al]. Online submission of assignments can be done as soon as they are completed, the teacher will review the completed task and provide grades and feedback. In addition, the discussion board allows students to interact with each other and with their teacher. This is a great way for students to ask question and reflect on topics and develop their critical thinking processes. The feature of flexibility and accessibility of Blackboard appeals to students the most. In a survey conducted by Duke University in 2004, students were given with ten feature and functions of Blackboard. The students were instructed to rate the features and functions that they found most useful. 85% of students participated in the study indicated that the most useful function of Blackboard was the accessibility to course material (Bradford et al., 2007). Furthermore, a Blackboard Pilot Study of students in courses that were complimented with online access using Blackboard. It was found 61% of the students who responded, suggested that accessibility was the main feature for Blackboard (Bradford et al., 2007). It is clear that web based platforms such as Blackboard gives students great access to study material remotely and hence providing greater flexibility.

Rapid Feedback

Another important feature of Blackboard is that students can receive rapid feedback on their progress and submitted assignments (Moyer, Young II, Weckman, & Cutright, 2015). Using Blackboard there are two ways of provided feedback students. The first is Blackboard generated feedback. Blackboard has the ability to instantly grade submitted assessment tasks, and therefore providing rapid feedback. Instant grading can be given by using Blackboard's Test Manager Feature. This is particularly useful when grading quizzes and multiple choice question (MCQ) exams. If the teacher enters the required answer or feedback options into Blackboard Test Manger, then students can take their tests and have all quizzes and MCQs marked and graded. Student final scores will be available soon after they submit their responses.

The second feedback option is the teacher generated and this is useful when students submit written assignments such as reports and essays. Students can submit their written assignments using Blackboard and track the progress of their feedback. The teacher then accesses the submitted work for grading and feedback. Blackboard Gradebook function allows the teacher to return the assignments to students and grades can be viewed confidentially. Students can take their exams or submit written assignment from anywhere. This is an important feature for geographically isolated students.

Enhanced Time Management and Communication Skills

Communications between students and teachers are easily achieved using Blackboard. There are different ways to communicate on Blackboard; these include announcements, discussion boards, virtual classroom, and e-mail. The teacher can use the announcement function to update students on important activities, once posted the announcements are visible to all students soon after they log on in the Blackboard system. The discussion boards are great for students to communicate and interact with each other. Ii also provides the teacher the ability to facilitate and supervise the discussions. Furthermore, students can post questions or answer question on the Post a Question feature, which allows greater communications amongst students. The virtual classroom is a concurrent learning environment. It allows students to interact using text-based chat and allows live interaction among participants. Finally, teachers can e-mail all students, group of students or individual students regarding updates and activities. This is particularly useful feature especially for students who can't log on in Blackboard system on a regular basis. In addition to enhanced communications. There are several other features enable by Blackboard. These features include time management and organisation, which are useful for students completing course via distance. Students are able to create calendar for individual course in which they are enrolled, hence increasing student efficiency when meeting deadlines.

MOOCs

Approaches to education are rapidly transforming as computers are become more powerful, widespread and affordable (Hew & Cheung, 2014). Through the internet education has become accessible to many students especially in Asia and Africa as well as geographically remote students. Furthermore, many potential students are challenged by increasing costs of traditional university education and lack of flexibility. Therefore, students from different parts of the world and of all ages are enrolling in Massive Open Online Courses (MOOCs) (Armellini & Padilla Rodriguez, 2016).

MOOCs are delivered online for students across the world. Distance learning via MOOCs is one of the approaches aimed at providing education to a diverse range of students. MOOCs as a distance learning tool have evolved into new pedagogical approach to benefit teachers and leaners (Viswanathan, 2012). One of the major features of MOOCs is that it is many of the courses are offered free of charge to students of any age group and location could enrol in the course. It is designed to work on an open networked learning mode. That is it enables learners to connect outside the traditional learning environment, hence providing accessibility and flexibility in gaining new and emergent knowledge. As a learning tool, MOOCs are encouraging connecting learning through construction of networks and discussion groups. Connected learning suggests that learning occurs outside the traditional classrooms and through online networks and exchanges (Onah, Sinclair, Pang, & Jantjies, 2016). Furthermore, the learning process through MOOCs can occur informally by participating in discussion groups, workshops and others. On the other hand, formal learning is achieved via completing e-learning modules and participating in virtual class rooms. This shows very clearly distance learning is becoming more accessible and flexible to many students.

As a pedagogical theory MOOCs fall into the theory of Connectivism. It is has been suggested that Connectivism enhances the learning process by enabling the learner to seek out new information through networks (Crosslin, 2016). Connectivism as a pedagogical theory promotes the inclusion of technology to enhance cognition and knowledge gaining process. In a massive open online course (MOOC) learners are well connected with the teacher as well as other students enrolled in the same course. Therefore, the student acquires knowledge from the teacher, but also through interactions with other students. It has been suggested that learning is greatly enhanced with the help of personal networks and through completion of tasks in a group environment and collaboration (Siemens, 2005).

The effect of MOOCs on learning and teaching processes has always been analysed by researchers. De Waard *et al.* (2011) reported a case study research involving data collection on a six week MobiMOOC course. Respondents to the research survey for the course reported that they felt that they were able empower themselves as they were able to utilise self-organisation and build their own e-learning project. Furthermore, it promoted acquisition of emerging knowledge and personalised learning. In addition, it was reported that students in the course had a common interest in the teaching material and they were more willing to share ideas (De Waard et al., 2011).

There are several benefits from using MOOCs to further develop already acquired knowledge or gain new knowledge. One of the major benefits of MOOCs is low cost education. Indeed, the majority of MOOCs are offered free to students. This is an important feature particularly for those students who cannot afford the cost of attending a course. Furthermore, a large number of MOOCs are developed by major universities and institutions such as MIT. Another benefit of learning through MOOCs is the flexibility and accessibility provided to learners and teachers. Many students are turning to distance education because of their inability to attend a traditional classroom. Furthermore, MOOCs are offered online which means students from around the world can participate to acquire new knowledge. This is particularly important for professionals who have limited time or geographically isolated to continue learning and apply knowledge in their workplace. In addition, learning through MOOCs promotes collaboration and networking which are important for effective learning (Lane, Caird, & Weller, 2014).

Moodle

Modular Object-Oriented Dynamic Learning Environment (Moodle) is an open source web based course management system first released in 2002. Moodle is designed based on student centred pedagogical theories and principles (Crompton, 2014). These pedagogical theories include constructivism and social constructivism, which recognise students as an essential part of the learning experience that the teachers provide and learning is enhanced by social networks and the share of information and ideas. Moodle is now one of the most widely used learning management system worldwide (Mustea, Naaji, & Herman, 2014; Mwalumbwe & Mtebe, 2017). Its popularity has increased to due to its ability to provide an organised and effective platform for web based learning. Moodle enables teachers to construct courses online, in which students can access as virtual classrooms (Martin & Parker, 2014). Similar to Blackboard, Moodle supports online assessment, discussions and forums.

Moodle provides educators the ability to remotely provide and grade assessment tasks, virtual lessons, share documents and information, workshop and discussion boards for learners. All of these features are vital to effectively provide flexibility for remote learners. Moodle has been described as one of the most user-friendly and flexible course management tool, and is especially created to allow education providers to design highly efficient and flexible on-line courses (Martin & Parker, 2014; Yamagata-Lynch, 2014). Moodle is now by a variety of universities, primary and high schools, private education and training organisations, independent teachers and non-profit organisations. The learner-focused strategy to learning is where students construct new knowledge through personalised modification prior knowledge and by taking a more introspective attitude to the knowledge being formulated, and they learn even more by explaining to others what they have learnt. Learner centred approach is particularly effective for remote students as it allows flexibility and students can explore more on the ideas on their own pace (Nguyen & Gu, 2013).

Affordability

Blended learning and distance learning is becoming increasingly an appealing study option from any students (Henry, Pooley, & Omari, 2014). Therefore, universities and education training providers incorporated learning management systems in their systems, and as a consequence, universities and educational institutions are becoming competitive and more efficient in the delivery of their teaching programs. Advances in web based technologies for higher education contributed to the development of integrated web based course management systems that support both the teacher and leaner.

Initial set up cost and ongoing licencing fees to maintain the course management system is an important factor that universities and education providers have to take in to consideration when deciding on which course management system to implement. Currently, there are many providers of course management systems available with different licencing fees (Young, 2008). One clear advantage of Moodle is that it is available free of charge as a web based open source software under the GNU General Public License (Brooks-Young, 2008). Universities, training providers, schools or individuals can download Moodle and implement it to support their teaching processes. Furthermore, organisations with both commercial and non-commercial projects without any licensing fees can adopt Moodle benefiting from the cost savings, flexibility and other advantages of using Moodle.

Highly Flexible and Customizable

The flexibility and customizability of the learning management system play an essential role in delivering an enhanced learning experience to students (Antonenko, Toy, & Niederhauser, 2004). Course management systems have become a technological necessity for delivering education and training to distance student. They allow teachers the ability to design virtual learning environments by creating space and accessibility for learning materials and activities. Furthermore, learning management systems support a wide range of administrative and management tasks required to efficiently manage student progress and achievement. In order to provide the best learning experience for distance learners the course management system must be reliable, scalable and flexible in order to remain up to date in today's evolving learning needs and trends. The technology should be user friendly, compatible with the institution's information technology requirements and teaching objectives. In addition, the chosen course management system must be able support third-party plugin features such as virtual classrooms, blogs and wikis.

Moodle provides a greater flexible tool options to enable universities deliver both blended learning and fully online courses. Moodle users can configure Moodle as per their needs by enabling or disabling core function, and easily integrate what is needed for a course using its range of built-in features and functions, including third party collaborative tools such as blogs, chats, wikis, and discussion forums. Because Moodle is an open source course management system, it can be customized to suit the course's requirement and needs. Its modular set up and interoperable design allows users to design plugins and integrate external applications to achieve specific functionalities. Furthermore, Moodle has been translated into more than 90 languages; therefore, education providers can easily modify their Moodle site to best serve their students. Due to its flexibility and customizability Moodle now has over 100 million users across more than 230 countries with more than 11 million courses (Singh, 2017). This means that blended and distance learning has become more accessible and available to a large number of students worldwide.

EMERGING TOOLS FOR FELXIBLE AND REMOTE LERNING

Augmented Reality

Augmented reality (AR) is an emerging tool that is increasing in popularity within the education sector. AR based applications are described as systems that enable the coexistence of real and virtual worlds in the same space and allowing real time interaction with the user. The ability to combine virtual objects with real life objects provides the users access to meaningful multimedia data that is relevant and can be accurately and immediately used. AR grants the user to sense the real life information via a virtual visualisation. Real life objects that can be incorporated in an AR system may range from text books, animation, video clips and procedures and techniques. The use of AR systems in learning and teaching has been suggested to enhance the learning and teaching processes

AR based applications have been used by educators to enhance and develop students' understanding of learning objective in several felids including science humanities and health and biomedical science. It has been shown that role plays incorporated in AR applications was associated with improved motivation and increased sense of authenticity for students in medical science (Rosenbaum, Klopfer, & Perry, 2007). Furthermore, the use of AR application in learning and teaching has consistently been demonstrated to enhance student motivation and improved student outcomes (Billinghurst & Duenser, 2012; Tarng & Ou, 2012).

An important pedagogical feature of AR based applications is the ability to resize and scale virtual objects, from single molecules to fully grown bodies, allowing students to gain better understand through manipulation the characteristics and relationships of bodies and objects that would be difficult to examine in real life due their size (Johnson et al., 2010). This clear representation of spatial and temporal concepts provides an extra advantage to contextualise the relationship between the virtual object and the real-life environment and hence better student learning outcomes (Sin & Zaman, 2010).

Augmented Reality can play an important role in developing critical reasoning and understanding important concepts for remote learners. Through integration of real life and virtual characteristics of teaching material, AR based systems can provide access to vital teaching resources to off campus students, for example, training on sophisticated laboratory equipment and procedures (Fjeld & Voegtli, 2002).

Emerging AR Tools in for Medical and Allied Health Professionals and Students

Currently, there are a number of different AR based technologies that are used by medical and allied health professionals and students. These include learning human anatomy using augmented reality, AR assisted vein visualisation for phlebotomists and surgical training and assistance.

Learning Human Anatomy Using Augmented Reality

Learning anatomy is very important and fundamental in many medical and health sciences. It is vital that medical and health students and professionals gain advanced understanding of human body structure and function. To enhance student understanding and improve motivation the traditional gross anatomy teaching has changed. Indeed, anatomy teaching nowadays includes plastic models and 2D images of the human body. However, inadequate numbers of cadavers in medical schools, lack of detailed 3D models and the large numbers of students, have contributed to the use of various innovative technologies such as augmented reality (Jamali, Shiratuddin, Wong, & Oskam, 2015). Currently, there are a number of web based interactive AR anatomy applications. Anatomy 4D is one of the most interactive and advanced AR application developed DAQRI (Green, Lea, & McNair, 2014). It provides users a virtual tour of the human body. It can display a 3D computer graphics of the human body and its various organ systems.

AR Assisted Vein Visualisation for Phlebotomists and Nurses

A device that reconstructs 3D images to visualise veins in patients' arms during venipuncture and intravenous injections has been developed to reduce patient anxiety and venipuncture failures and times (Yen & Gorelick, 2013). The technology uses augmented reality to provide fast and accurate 3D images of the vein and skin. This emerging technology is useful and effective when training medical and health students and professionals.

AR Assisted Surgical Training

In many geographically remote locations subspecialty surgical interventions may not be available. Furthermore, further training and development for remote surgeons may be difficult due to time and distance constraints. With advances in technology, hands-on training is now possible with use of AR and telepresence (Dickey et al., 2016). Telepresence utilises non-robotic tools and applications to provide interactive video and audio in which an experienced surgeon provides assistance and training to remote surgeons. Virtual interactive presence and augmented reality (VIPAAR) is one of the companies that developed tools using augmented reality to provide real time and interactive training and assistance for remote surgeons (Davis, Can, Pindrik, Rocque, & Johnston, 2016).

3D Virtual Reality

Virtual reality (VR) is computer based technology that uses headsets and equipment to generate virtual environments representing realistic images, sounds and other emotions replicating a real scenario (Lee & Wong, 2014). VR also provides the user a sense of physical presence within the virtual environment. The use of interactive hardware and software enables the user of to experience an immersive and realistic sensation of a 3D world. Users within VR environment are able to look around, move about and interact with the objects within the virtual world. Sophisticated haptic systems can be embedded within VR technologies to provide tactile sensation and information. These features are particularly useful in training medical and allied health professionals that require hands on experience to develop skills (Mathur, 2015). Furtherer, VR systems can facilitate remote communications which provide a virtual presence through telepresence or the use of a virtual artifact (VA). This is an important feature as it enables education and continued professional development for remote students and graduates.

Using immersive and interactive virtual learning environments for students is an effective learning approach as it provides students with a sense of presence and immersion. Within a VR environment, students particularly in healthcare disciplines are able to explore and interact with their environment from multiple viewpoints including hazardous and unreachable locations. This will stimulate students to experience different scenarios in a virtual environed in ways that would otherwise be unfeasible to achieve in the real world (Hoffman & Vu, 1997). With use of this advanced technology on campus and remote allied health students are able to explore and analyse clinical scenarios and evaluate potential solutions in ways that were not possible before which are necessary to develop their clinical skills and knowledge.

Learning though VR gives the opportunity to strengthen and transform the learning experience of allied health students and professionals through immersion in a non-real environment that closely resembles the real environment (Dalgarno & Lee, 2010). A unique aspect of VR based education is that students can be immersed in different environments without physically leaving their location. This makes the educational experience flexible and effective. Furthermore, VR technology has been shown to be an effective learning tool for students with varying learning needs and styles (Psotka, 1995). It also can facilitate group and team work particularly for students who can't be present in the classroom (Hansen, 2008). Students using VR can actively interact with objects and scenarios which are important to build the skills associated with their profession (Mantovani, Castelnuovo, Gaggioli, & Riva, 2003). It has been demonstrated that VR stimulates active and collaborative learning because other students are participating in the same virtual environment and performing the same tasks, this will enable students to shares ideas and knowledge (Hansen, 2008). Several studies investigated the different features of VR and their potential benefits for teaching and learning have shown positive student outcomes. Mantovani *et al.* (2003) demonstrated that VR is an effective educational tool that provides a rich and interactive learning environment and promotes experiential learning, which allows students and trainees to develop an enhanced understanding.

Another advantage of learning in a VR is that it is cost effective, and at the same time provides stimulated experiences in situations that might not be possible to implement in a real environment setting.

Gamification of Learning

Game-based learning refers to the use of video game elements and design as a tool to provide an effective web-based learning strategy. Games that are designed for education, health care and other industries with the primary objective is other pure entrainment are termed as serious games. It has been shown that employing gamified learning material can provide learners with a learning environment that includes gaming characteristics such as humour, interaction and drama is an effective approach to stimulate students' learning motivation (Su & Cheng, 2015). This learning approach supports the learning process in different domains, cognitive psycho-motor domains. As per the normal video games, the gamified learning materials also include rules and rewards to direct and stimulate learners to think and analyse the scenario to make correct and meaningful decisions (Coller & Scott, 2009). When compared with the traditions web-based learning applications, game-based web education usually provides increased levels of imaginary and more challenging scenarios, and therefore the learning process is more interactive and effective.

There are three main factors that contribute to the effectiveness of this learning strategy. First, feedback and satisfaction, this is an important factor to successfully complete the learning task. Students need to comply with the gaming rules to move from lower to higher levels, and in order to do so they are provided immediate feedback on their performance and the requirements to proceed to the next level. This in turn will provide satisfaction. Second, inquisitiveness, when students successfully complete one level, they tend to be keen to go to the next level. This will provide a sense of adventure and excitement as learns are guided through the game and reflect on their mistakes, increasing their motivation and willingness to go on.

Third, sense of accomplishment, educational games are created with features that enable learners to feel curious and acquire new knowledge and achieve enhanced performance. Once levels are completed the learners can feel sense of accomplishment.

There is clear benefit for using educational games within the health sector. These games provide health professionals the opportunity to play these educational games as many times as they wish or until they become competent, this is important feature that is not possible with real life situations and patents. Some of the currently available games for health professionals training and education include Pulse!! The Virtual Clinical Learning Lab (Dunne & McDonald, 2010), which is a game, set in a hospital environment where participants can practice how to respond to different patient scenarios. Another game that is currently available is (Lamrani, Chraibi, Qassimi, Hafidi, & El Amrani, 2017) which designed to provide training to cardiology and emergency staff in the management of cardiac emergencies.

Learning Through Gesture-Based Computing

Gesture-based technology is an emerging learning tool that has provided new opportunities for the education sector (Shakroum, Wong, & Fung, 2016). Gesture-based technology allows the user to control and interact with a computer devise directly through the use of body gesture such as motions and movements. The body gestures include speech, body motions, finger and eye movements, facial expressions can also be recognised by the gesture-based devices.

Expansions in the development and applications of gesture-based computing in learning and training are continuing with growing number of devices in surgical training, physical therapy and science as well as other disciplines (Shakroum et al., 2016; Wen, Tay, Nguyen, Chng, & Chui, 2014). The use of gesture-based devices in learning allows the students to interact and immerse in a virtual environment and are able to manipulate information intuitively. This is an effective method of delivering teaching materials to students in a highly interactive manner.

Cloud Computing

Cloud computing is an internet based computing service that delivers data storage, software and networking. These computing services are shared with other devices on demand. It is a method for universal and on-demand access to a shared group of configurable computer networks, servers, data storage and applications which can be promptly activated and released with little management effort. There are several benefits of using cloud computing to deliver services; these include cost saving on infrastructure, purchasing servers and ongoing fees (users only pay for what they use), reduced maintenance and management of computing services and improved performance of the network applications (Weber, 2013).

There are three different types of services provided by cloud computing:

1. **Software as a Service (SaaS):** This service allows a cloud computing provider to host applications and network service and distribute them to customers over the Internet. This type of service allows the applications to be accessible anytime and anywhere.
2. **Platform as a Service (PaaS):** Internet based application building tools and platforms are provided by a cloud computing provider which allows the user to build, run, and maintain applications without the need of building and

maintaining the complex infrastructure typically required when developing and running an application.

3. **Infrastructure as a Service (IaaS):** This cloud computing service allows users to rent virtual computing resources such as processors and data storage over the internet. These virtual resources can then be used to run the users' existing computing systems and applications. This an on-demand service and users only pay for what they use.

Although cloud computing has been extensively used by Google and Microsoft and others to provide computing and data storage services, it is an emerging technology within the education sector. Cloud computing can potential play an essential role in the delivery of remote and flexible learning to students. With increase in on-line delivery of course, cloud computing can provide the necessary means to facilitate effective learning environment for students.

CONCLUSION

The number of courses provide as an e-learning is on the rise. Better student flexibility and technological advances in the internet based applications provided as foundation for development of educational tools to facilitated remoted and distance learning. Currently, there is a wide range of tools available that allow education and training to reach geographically isolated and remote learners as well as providing extra flexibility to local students. In this chapter key current and emerging tools for flexible remote learning were discussed. It is anticipated that as the internet based technology progresses, there will be new tools to facilitate on-line learning.

REFERENCES

Antonenko, P., Toy, S., & Niederhauser, D. (2004). *Modular Object-Oriented Dynamic Learning Environment: What Open Source Has to Offer.* Association for Educational Communications and Technology.

Armellini, A., & Padilla Rodriguez, B. C. (2016). Are Massive Open Online Courses (MOOCs) pedagogically innovative? *Journal of Interactive Online Learning*, *14*(1), 17–28.

Bradford, P., Porciello, M., Balkon, N., & Backus, D. (2007). The Blackboard learning system: The be all and end all in educational instruction? *Journal of Educational Technology Systems*, *35*(3), 301–314. doi:10.2190/X137-X73L-5261-5656

Brooks-Young, S. (2008). Got moodle? The free, open source program enjoys great appeal among K-12 teachers, as it allows them to get the upper hand on course management and assessment. *T.H.E. Journal*, *35*(4), 28.

Carroll, C., Booth, A., Papaioannou, D., Sutton, A., & Wong, R. (2009). UK health-care professionals' experience of on-line learning techniques: A systematic review of qualitative data. *The Journal of Continuing Education in the Health Professions*, *29*(4), 235–241. doi:10.1002/chp.20041 PMID:19998474

Coller, B. D., & Scott, M. J. (2009). Effectiveness of using a video game to teach a course in mechanical engineering. *Computers & Education*, *53*(3), 900–912. doi:10.1016/j.compedu.2009.05.012

Crompton, H. (2014). A diachronic overview of technology contributing to mobile learning: A shift towards student-centred pedagogies. *Increasing Access, 7*.

Crosslin, M. (2016). From Instructivism to Connectivism: Theoretical Underpinnings of MOOCs. *Current Issues in Emerging eLearning, 3*(1), 6.

Dalgarno, B., & Lee, M. J. (2010). What are the learning affordances of 3-D virtual environments? *British Journal of Educational Technology*, *41*(1), 10–32. doi:10.1111/j.1467-8535.2009.01038.x

Davis, M. C., Can, D. D., Pindrik, J., Rocque, B. G., & Johnston, J. M. (2016). Virtual interactive presence in global surgical education: International collaboration through augmented reality. *World Neurosurgery*, *86*, 103–111. doi:10.1016/j.wneu.2015.08.053 PMID:26342783

De Waard, I., Abajian, S., Gallagher, M. S., Hogue, R., Keskin, N., Koutropoulos, A., & Rodriguez, O. C. (2011). Using mLearning and MOOCs to understand chaos, emergence, and complexity in education. *The International Review of Research in Open and Distributed Learning*, *12*(7), 94–115. doi:10.19173/irrodl.v12i7.1046

Dickey, R. M., Srikishen, N., Lipshultz, L. I., Spiess, P. E., Carrion, R. E., & Hakky, T. S. (2016). Augmented reality assisted surgery: A urologic training tool. *Asian Journal of Andrology*, *18*(5), 732. doi:10.4103/1008-682X.166436 PMID:26620455

Dunne, J. R., & McDonald, C. L. (2010). Pulse!!: A model for research and development of virtual-reality learning in military medical education and training. *Military Medicine*, *175*(7Suppl), 25–27. doi:10.7205/MILMED-D-10-00158 PMID:23634475

Green, M., Lea, J. H., & McNair, C. L. (2014). Reality check: Augmented reality for school libraries. *Teacher Librarian*, *41*(5), 28.

Hansen, M. M. (2008). Versatile, Immersive, Creative and Dynamic Virtual 3-D Healthcare Learning Environments: A Review of the Literature. *Journal of Medical Internet Research*, *10*(3), e26. doi:10.2196/jmir.1051 PMID:18762473

Henry, M., Pooley, J. A., & Omari, M. (2014). *Student motivations for studying online: A qualitative study*. Academic Press.

Hew, K. F., & Cheung, W. S. (2014). Students' and instructors' use of massive open online courses (MOOCs): Motivations and challenges. *Educational Research Review*, *12*, 45–58. doi:10.1016/j.edurev.2014.05.001

Hoffman, H., & Vu, D. (1997). Virtual reality: Teaching tool of the twenty-first century? *Academic Medicine*, *72*(12), 1076–1081. doi:10.1097/00001888-199712000-00018 PMID:9435714

Jamali, S. S., Shiratuddin, M. F., Wong, K. W., & Oskam, C. L. (2015). Utilising Mobile-Augmented Reality for Learning Human Anatomy. *Procedia: Social and Behavioral Sciences*, *197*, 659–668. doi:10.1016/j.sbspro.2015.07.054

Kemp, J., & Livingstone, D. (2006). Putting a Second Life "metaverse" skin on learning management systems. *Proceedings of the Second Life education workshop at the Second Life community convention.*

Lamrani, R., Chraibi, S., Qassimi, S., Hafidi, M., & El Amrani, A. (2017). *Serious Game to Enhance and Promote Youth Entrepreneurship. In Europe and MENA Cooperation Advances in Information and Communication Technologies* (pp. 77–85). Springer. doi:10.1007/978-3-319-46568-5_8

Lane, A., Caird, S., & Weller, M. (2014). The potential social, economic and environmental benefits of MOOCs: Operational and historical comparisons with a massive 'closed online'course. *Open Praxis*, *6*(2), 115–123. doi:10.5944/openpraxis.6.2.113

Lee, E. A.-L., & Wong, K. W. (2014). Learning with desktop virtual reality: Low spatial ability learners are more positively affected. *Computers & Education*, *79*, 49–58. doi:10.1016/j.compedu.2014.07.010

Mantovani, F., Castelnuovo, G., Gaggioli, A., & Riva, G. (2003). Virtual reality training for health-care professionals. *Cyberpsychology & Behavior*, *6*(4), 389–395. doi:10.1089/109493103322278772 PMID:14511451

Martin, F. (2008). Blackboard as the learning management system of a computer literacy course. *Journal of Online Learning and Teaching / MERLOT*, *4*(2), 138–145.

Martin, F., & Parker, M. A. (2014). Use of Synchronous Virtual Classrooms: Why, Who, and How? *Journal of Online Learning and Teaching / MERLOT*, *10*(2), 192.

Mathur, A. S. (2015). *Low cost virtual reality for medical training*. Paper presented at the Virtual Reality (VR). doi:10.1109/VR.2015.7223437

Moyer, A. C., Young, W. A. II, Weckman, G. R., & Cutright, K. (2015). Rubrics on the Fly: Improving Efficiency and Consistency with a Rapid Grading and Feedback System. *Journal of Teaching and Learning with Technology*, *4*(2), 6–29. doi:10.14434/jotlt.v4n2.13473

Mustea, A., Naaji, A., & Herman, C. (2014). *Using Moodle for the development of Massive Open Online Courses*. Paper presented at the The International Scientific Conference eLearning and Software for Education.

Mwalumbwe, I., & Mtebe, J. S. (2017). Using Learning Analytics to Predict Students' Performance in Moodle Learning Management Systems: A case of Mbeya University of Science and Technology. *The Electronic Journal on Information Systems in Developing Countries*.

Nguyen, L. T. C., & Gu, Y. (2013). Strategy-based instruction: A learner-focused approach to developing learner autonomy. *Language Teaching Research*, *17*(1), 9–30. doi:10.1177/1362168812457528

Olson, P. W. (2005). Significant success factors in distance education. *International Journal of Case Method Research & Application*, *17*(2), 235–245.

Onah, D. F., Sinclair, J., Pang, E. L., & Jantjies, M. (2016). Exploring the multi-dimensional attainment of self-regulatory learning skills in educational contexts: A comparative study. *EDULEARN16 Proceedings*, 1-10.

Psotka, J. (1995). Immersive training systems: Virtual reality and education and training. *Instructional Science*, *23*(5), 405–431. doi:10.1007/BF00896880

Shakroum, M. A., Wong, K. W., & Fung, C. (2016). The effectiveness of the Gesture-Based learning system (GBLS) and its impact on learning experience. *Journal of Information Technology Education: Research*, *15*, 191–210.

Sheppard, L., & Mackintosh, S. (1998). Technology in education: What is appropriate for rural and remote allied health professionals? *The Australian Journal of Rural Health*, *6*(4), 189–193. doi:10.1111/j.1440-1584.1998.tb00311.x PMID:9919075

Siemens, G. (2005). Connectivism: Learning as network-creation. *ASTD Learning News, 10*(1).

Singh, J. (2017). *Moodle Stats – Moodle surpasses the 100 million users mark and India rises in the top 10 Moodle countries list #moodlestats*. Retrieved 06/04, 2017, from http://www.moodleworld.com/moodle-stats-moodle-surpasses-the-100-million-users-mark-and-india-rises-in-the-top-10-moodle-countries-list-moodlestats/

Su, C. H., & Cheng, C. H. (2015). A mobile gamification learning system for improving the learning motivation and achievements. *Journal of Computer Assisted Learning*, *31*(3), 268–286. doi:10.1111/jcal.12088

Thompson, C. J. (2016). Disruptive innovation: The rise of distance education. *Clinical Nurse Specialist CNS*, *30*(4), 238–241. doi:10.1097/NUR.0000000000000213 PMID:27309788

Viswanathan, R. (2012). Teaching and Learning through MOOC. *Frontiers of Language and Teaching*, *3*(1), 32–40.

Weber, A. S. (2013). *Cloud computing in education. In Ubiquitous and mobile learning in the digital age* (pp. 19–36). Springer. doi:10.1007/978-1-4614-3329-3_2

Wen, R., Tay, W.-L., Nguyen, B. P., Chng, C.-B., & Chui, C.-K. (2014). Hand gesture guided robot-assisted surgery based on a direct augmented reality interface. *Computer Methods and Programs in Biomedicine*, *116*(2), 68–80. doi:10.1016/j.cmpb.2013.12.018 PMID:24438993

Williams, S. L. (2006). The effectiveness of distance education in allied health science programs: A meta-analysis of outcomes. *American Journal of Distance Education*, *20*(3), 127–141. doi:10.1207/s15389286ajde2003_2

Yamagata-Lynch, L. C. (2014). Blending online asynchronous and synchronous learning. *The International Review of Research in Open and Distributed Learning*, *15*(2). doi:10.19173/irrodl.v15i2.1778

Yen, K., & Gorelick, M. H. (2013). New Biomedical Devices That Use Near-Infrared Technology to Assist With Phlebotomy and Vascular Access. *Pediatric Emergency Care*, *29*(3), 383–385. doi:10.1097/PEC.0b013e31828680f9 PMID:23462399

Young, J. R. (2008). Blackboard customers consider alternatives. *The Chronicle of Higher Education*, *55*(3), A1.

Chapter 7
Integration of E-Learning Technologies:
RPi, E-Portfolio, and Virtual Reality in Medical Laboratory Science

Indu Singh
Griffith University, Australia

Avinash Kundur
Griffith University, Australia

Yun-Mi Nguy
Griffith University, Australia

ABSTRACT

Increasing automation along with other recent advancements in the field of pathology has highlighted the importance of integrating e-learning technologies within the program Medical Laboratory Science (MLS). E-learning tools such as 3D virtual pathology laboratory, e-portfolio using Pebble Pad, and Raspberry Pi (RPi) have been added to the MLS program at Griffith University, Gold Coast Campus (GUGC). Incorporation of these e-learning tools has the ability to potentially improve learning outcomes and increase the chances of employability by aiding in the production of work-ready graduates. The aim of this chapter is to highlight the recent developments, issues, and possible solutions along with future directions in the development and integration of these e-learning tools in MLS.

DOI: 10.4018/978-1-5225-3850-9.ch007

INTRODUCTION

Industrial automation has had a global impact on clinical laboratories and biopharmaceutical Science. The adaptation of total laboratory automation (TLA) and advancing technology alongside innovative information software, has not only changed the working environment for technicians and scientists but has also transformed the way students are being trained and educated (Sédille-Mostafaie, Engler, Lutz, & Korte, 2013). This chapter will discuss current implementation of technologies in health science education. It will also consider the future directions of the application of upcoming technologies in tertiary education. Industry demands for universally adaptive multi-skilled work ready graduates, which has challenged the need to educate our future health professionals to meet the demands of this global workforce. Recent advancements through applications of e-learning tools and 3D modeling have opened the gateway to potentially improve student engagement, accessibility and learning outcomes.

Alongside inclusive 24 hours access to classroom material, additional benefits also include the support of undergraduate employability through vertical and horizontal scaffolding, thereby linking core courses continually across year levels. Web-based electronic learning (e-learning) tools such as simulated virtual labs, demonstration videos and mobile micro-computing using Raspberry Pi are increasingly becoming a part of modern educational systems that can break down many traditional access barriers to learning resources. Access to current and expensive resources without the heavy financial burden, can provide an interactive learning environment for students to gain a wide variety of practical experiences within educational budgetary constraints.

The end product of the tertiary education system is to produce highly employable graduates. Integrating technology-based blended e-learning tools into various teaching modules can assist students in meeting the growing demands of an industry, which heavily relies on automation. Implementation of these techniques at GUGC, can demonstrate how information science and technology can be used in standardizing tertiary health education to produce graduates who are; better prepared, require less on the job training, are more globally aware and adaptable, and are equipped to further their own career development through self-directed life-long learning.

This chapter will describe an array of mixed models of e-learning tools being implemented and trialed in the MLS program at GUGC. It will discuss the benefits of some of the innovative ways of "taking the classroom to students" by enhancing flexible learning through use of virtual reality 3D pathology made available to personal handheld devices. It will also share information about how e-portfolios are created by student for staff to monitor individual student progress both on and off campus and how the implementation of Raspberry Pi2 systems in collaboration with Pebble Pad personal leaning system can be a solution to low cost computing in teaching laboratories.

BACKGROUND

Preparing students for the workforce has increasingly become an important aspect in tertiary education. Blending academic content of a program with work experiences to enhance student experiences have become an important part of university education (Radloff & Coates, 2010). The Australasian Survey of Student Engagement (AUSSE) by Radloff & Coates (2010), have shown a collection data from first- year and later-year students highlighting critical aspects of student learning and development. In the above-mentioned report, several findings demonstrated the significance of student participation in work-integrated learning in order for them to be career ready. Although the academics within the university value the importance of work-integrated learning, the amount of exposure to clinical workplace environments among students during their four-year period was limited. At Griffith University, the School of Medical Science established the Medical Laboratory Science (MLS) degree in 2012 and has been successful in increasing student exposure to work integrated e-learning tools and assessments to the existing courses of the program. For example, as course criteria, students are required to complete a fourth year clinical placement in order to successfully attain the degree. However, with an increase in student enrollments, finding affordable clinical placements and standardizing student clinical work experience has evolved into one of the biggest challenges that teaching teams have had to address. Introducing blended e-learning techniques such as 3D virtual laboratories, e-portfolios and micro-computer Raspberry Pi's in Physical Containment level 2 (PC2) laboratories may be one of the most effective ways to close the gap and enhance student work integrated experiences for MLS students. In order to encourage student engagement and promote self-education the MLS program encourages the use of these work-integrated learning tools to produce competent and trained health professionals for future generations to come.

CURRENT E-LEARNING TECHNOLOGIES IN MEDICAL LABORATORY SCIENCE

3D Virtual Reality Pathology

Virtual Reality (VR) simulates environments which are presented in two or three dimensional (2D or 3D) audio and visual representation to create an immersive experience (Gaba, 2004). Modern approaches to teaching through the use of VR simulation can provide artificial cases to students for discussion and management without risking quality assurance of patient samples and reduce disruption of services to health institutions. Available computer technology allows the use of dynamic platforms to bring a new dimension in teaching, which can allow for collaborative and problem-based learning to make teaching more efficient (Le Beux & Fieschi, 2007). In an article by Locatis (2008) a virtual computer lab for distance biomedical education identified that the use of 3D molecular visualization software was necessary in teaching technologies and methods where the content of a certain course changes frequently (Locatis, Vega, Bhagwat, Liu, & Conde, 2008). The 3D molecular visualization software allows training students on complex computer applications at a distance in real time, in the presence of an instructor to monitor student's progress. Simulation may not only be used as a training tool, it can provide indirect ways to improve safety, facilitate recruitment and retention of skilled personnel, and improving quality and risk management activities (Gaba, 2004; Locatis et al., 2008).

Developed in conjunction with Gold Coast University Hospital (GCUH), the 3D VR laboratory aims to give students and hospital staff a simulated laboratory experience mimicking the pathology industry with its daily use of analyzers and streamline processes. Simulation of analytical testing, troubleshooting and performing routine maintenance on analyzers are just a few techniques that can be virtually assimilated to real time working processes. Benefits to re-creating a 3D virtual lab environment include enhancing accessibility to training hospital staff and MLS students without physically interrupting services in the main laboratory and reducing the risk of biological exposure when entering into a PC2 contained laboratory. Similarly, hands on practical experience in a virtual lab may enhance work-integrated experiences that allow students to visualize a lab setting within the first few years of their course. The 3D virtual laboratory can also be used as an introductory video, which can show the standard protocols that the students have to follow in a hospital pathology laboratory, before going for their fourth year clinical placement. This technology can improve the transition of students and new staff into the working industry by ensuring students and staffs are competently trained in specific training modules before entering into the facility, ultimately reducing the workload on the hospital staff. Similarly, completion of this training module can be added to a student's resume to reflect competencies in assimilated experiences.

Standardization of training can also be achieved, as all students will be exposed to the same analyzer, completing training competencies in the maintenance and handling of equipment and understanding concepts and methods of sample processing. Troubleshooting without physically dismantling the analyzer or resolving issues that arrive in real world time would be demonstrated when required. Inclusively, having a video library showcasing the techniques required to troubleshoot some of the most common errors displayed by an analyzer can not only be beneficial to the students and to new staff but also to the existing staff of a hospital laboratory. The development of 3D virtual laboratory can also promote building an association between the industry and tertiary institutions, which can close the gap between students and professionals, and help institutions in setting a standard of teaching that produces graduates who are updated with the most recent advancements within current laboratory practices.

Pathology laboratories today face increasing pressure to streamline operations due to increasing workload and the need to decrease expenditure. However, for many smaller laboratories, such as tertiary facilities, TLA can often be too expensive due to the prize of the analyser and its associated expenses such as laboratory renovation costs (Sédille-Mostafaie et al., 2013). Allowing universities to share resources and reduce implementation costs of analyzers would be economical for training purposes. Training large number of staff and students using the 3D virtual laboratories can significantly reduce the number of staff resources that are usually invested by the hospital staff in laboratory training. Re-creating a workplace using VR systems may also assist in rural rotational staff members that need additional training prior to their deployment to the rural labs where training and supervision of staff can be limited.

E-Portfolios

The Radloff and Coates (2009) Student Engagement Questionnaire (SEQ) highlighted five new items to measure the areas, in which students were considered as career ready, one of these items included whether students have an up-to date resume (Radloff & Coates, 2009). The electronic based portfolio is a recording of various skills and techniques that a student has accumulated not only during his time in the university but also after graduation. E-portfolio has developed as an effective alternative that may soon replace the traditional paper based resume. At Griffith University, e-portfolio allows students to engage in self-learning and development as future medical scientists. An e-portfolio provides an online personal space where students can collect digital resources, by blending a series of information with literacy, technology to show evidence of their experiences in achieving their course outcomes (Reese & Levy, 2009). Simultaneously it allows the student to move beyond the learning outcomes and inherently link their understanding to the bigger picture of what they have learnt and to be proactive in reflecting upon academic and professional goals (Hallam & Creagh, 2010; Reese & Levy, 2009). Bloom (2013) highlights a series of projects where the use of e-portfolios have facilitated in the growth, development and enrichment of teaching and learning where students engage in such activities as reflection and long-term career planning (Blom, Rowley, Bennett, Hitchcock, & Dunbar-Hall, 2013).

Similarly, Reese and Levy (2009) regard the implementation of e-portfolios to be advantageous in documenting real world learning experiences where each student is accountable for their own education. In the MLS program, students for the first time will be using Pebble Pad to record their assessments and self-reflections in their individualized e-portfolios. Pebble pad is a personalized learning and assessment system used in many tertiary institutional courses to enhance student-learning experiences and encapsulate a lifelong holistic learning experience. Application of Pebble Pad from first year through to forth year allows the student to present a timeline showcasing self-reflections, accumulation of resources and competent training skills, which together will help the students to create a resume that can be updated in real-time through their years of studying. Furthermore, Pebble Pad acts an effective medium to allow individuals from the industry, whom are usually considered as future employers, to be able to access the training modules completed by the student, and in turn positively influence the employability of a student.

Via the use of the Pebble Pad program, a collection of case studies from a number of core and elective disciplines of pathology, practical competencies and external association meetings will provide a comprehensive display of academic and work related experiences. Having a sound knowledge of all the core and elective disciplines in pathology is essential for an MLS graduate to provide diagnosis of a patient. For example, in order to confirm the provisional diagnosis of a patient, a blood sample usually undergoes analysis in different departments of a pathological laboratory such as Heamatology, Biochemistry and Microbiology. Using Pebble Pad has enabled students and staff to link case studies under all disciplines in pathology. Using the case study as an example, academics from different pathology discipline courses can help students correlate results, and build on understanding pathogenesis of diseases. Horizontal and vertical platforming to connect and build knowledge will deepen the links and communication between courses and how disciplines interlink through a number of clinical presentations. From first year subjects applying core basic biology, chemistry and health science into selective and specialized disciplines can vertically allow students to develop their knowledge and build upon concepts and principles. By interconnecting cases throughout different pathology disciplines, this can horizontally provide a scaffold of intertwined pathogenesis and the concept that students need to look at the bigger picture.

Raspberry Pi

Since the early 1990s, integration of multimedia laboratories and computerized laboratories have been the way of the future for clinical pathologies (Sédille-Mostafaie et al., 2013). Mimicking laboratories found across many health industries instigate the need to simulate these facilities to students, in order to enhance the learning experience and provide educational resources that allow the students to access to the latest information within the laboratory setting. However, upgrading these teaching facilities into computerized labs that are PC2 certified, can be very expensive as the number of working stations in a teaching lab can be far greater than a pathology lab (Sédille-Mostafaie et al., 2013). With Griffith facilities offering an intake of forty-five students per year, there is a need to uniformly provide resources individually to each student to standardize the learning facility. The introduction of RPi may be the economical answer to implementing computerized labs at minimal costs.

The Raspberry Pi is a family of credit card sized SBC (single Board computers) with open-ended versatility, that can run a number of different operating systems such as Raspbian, Ubuntu Mate and other Linux OS distributions (Ioannou, Ioannidis, Papadopoulos, & Tapeinos, 2014). Recent advances in information technology would allow dedicated single purpose applications to be compiled with tools like Ultibo to individualize the needs of each teaching facility just by swapping the MicroSD card (Ioannou et al., 2014). Furthermore these RPi can be linked to an old DVI monitors or Television sets with a HDMI port for graphical output. Recent development of RPi touch screen monitors have shown to have several advantages due to its compact size, easy usage and increased versatility. The RPi offers a cheaper alternative in low socio-economical as well as in developed societies, using which students can familiarize themselves with computers and programs that are associated with MLS. Around the world especially in third worlds countries, these mini computers have been the answer to educationally advancing students into the technological world (Ali, Vlaskamp, Eddin, Falconer, & Oram, 2013).

At Griffith University, RPi could potentially offer the same educational step into advancing the teaching labs to being computerized labs. Replacing manual counters with electronic cell counters is one of the primary uses of the RPi. Upgrading the laboratories using RPi can be economically beneficial as the lab can potentially purchase two RPi along with the monitors for the price of one manual metal 8-chamber cell counter that is traditionally used to perform white cell count differentials.

Other than running cell counter programs, the secondary function of the RPi is to eventually run Pebble Pad so that the student can access their e-portfolio and regularly update case studies that are presented in their practical laboratories. Updating practical cases in the lab and manually inserting results can provide the students and their potential employers in future a recording of all the cases that the student has reviewed in a period of 4 years, which can significantly benefit the student by acting as a detailed and updated version of his resume. Linking RPi to the Internet can allow students to access lecture notes, blackboard profile and online journal articles to incorporate resources that connect to the laboratory teachings. Finally, RPi can act as a platform to run integrated lessons for Histology and Haematology microscopic tutorials by showing live view of microscopic images on individual screens, which are controlled by the main user. This format can open discussions about clinical cases and provide an interactive lesson for students.

Issues, Controversies, Problems

3D virtual laboratories can be considered as one of the most effective ways of introducing and inducting students and new staff to automation in pathology laboratories across educational institutions and health industries, without investing capital in establishing a fully functional lab. The 3D virtual laboratory that has been developed for the MLS program at Griffith University shows the journey of a patient sample (e.g., blood, urine or tissue section) in a pathology lab from the specimen reception through to the analyzer of the respective department and showing processes such as running the samples, releasing the results and troubleshooting. In the past few years, pathology laboratories have undergone significant automation in various departments such as Heamatology, Transfusion Science and Microbiology. Previously, students may not have been exposed to these recent advancements in process or equipment that can be found in a number of industry and research pathology laboratories. 3D virtual labs offer consistent exposure and standardized work-integrated learning for all students. Introduction into the pathology environment can be initiated from first year entry through to final year students by exposing students to various levels of training from basic laboratory introduction to complex analytical procedures and troubleshooting methods based on their year of study.

The teaching team the Griffith University faced several challenges during the development of 3D virtual laboratories. Accumulating financial resources for developing the 3D virtual lab was one of the first challenges the teaching team had encountered. Filming the different departments of a laboratory for developing the 3D virtual reality labs was a time consuming and expensive process. Furthermore, once the videos were complete, smart devices along with portable headsets were necessary for viewing the videos. Gaining access to these resources such as smart devices and portable headsets can be a significant challenge in low socio-economic regions. The development of these videos was collaborative project between Griffith

University, School of Medical Science and Gold Coast University Hospital (GCUH), involved several teams such as academics from the university, medical scientists from the pathology lab and the filming crew. Successful initiation and implementation of 3D virtual laboratories require these teams to actively communicate and collaborate to constantly monitor factors such as availability, cost and management, without any disruption to the patients' diagnostic flow.

The level of automation and the kind of equipment used in a pathological laboratory is greatly dependent on factors such as location, workload, patient turnover and manufacturers the laboratory were affiliated with. The pathology laboratory at the Gold Coast University Hospital (GCUH) is one of the largest pathology labs in the Gold Coast region, with significantly high amount of automation to cope with the workload and patient turnover. However, 3D virtual pathology filmed at the university hospital pathology lab may not resemble other private laboratories, which may use analyzers from different manufacturers, or small regional laboratories, where the rate of automation may be limited. Therefore, one of the major issues with the 3D virtual pathological lab is that the video does not provide students with theoretical knowledge about the analyzers developed by other manufactures that are currently being used in different laboratories. Hence, it is essential that 3D virtual pathology is used to complement the laboratory skills and lectures that provide theoretical background to the students, which takes us back to traditional teaching methods.

Self-reflective learning and sharing educational teachings are gaining traction in tertiary education. Engaging students in active learning and incorporating multimedia technology is key in teaching students to share their work not only during their stay at the university but also as alumni. Initiating e-portfolios in tertiary universities however was not an easy task. The slow adoption of e-portfolios from senior directors and gaining the support on how e-portfolios could support the universities missions, had to be driven from the ground up. Cost considerations included costs in resources, time and role change, requirements for allocation of resources via each faculty, enterprise IT to develop hardware, software and technical support (Reese & Levy, 2009). Initially use of an in-house built self-reflective program for fourth year MLS clinical placement students identified a series of issues that were also reflective in Blom (2013) (Blom et al., 2013). These included difficulties in maintaining the in-house system, where university networks were unable to allow bi-directional flow of information between the students and the staff. Accessibility and transfer of information to industry professions, linking other resources was difficult and proposed a number of issues for postgraduate students entering into the work force. Secondly, the cross platform and browser issues including coding inconsistencies, associability issues, ownership and long-term storage were also a problem for Griffith students. The application was self-limiting to the period of use and could not be transferable for individual portfolio usage.

RPi were initially suggested as a cost effective alternative in providing students with electronic cell counters that can replace several pieces of equipment. RPi versatility and wide range of medical application has opened doors to the potential future of computerized MLS labs at Griffith University. RPi may allow students to access their e-portfolios and enable them to journal their case studies in practical labs, as well as horizontally and vertically linking several pathology disciplines when considering course structure and outcomes. RPi and Pebble Pad may allow students to work on a clinical case that is spread across a number of disciplines, mimicking real world cases where a patient is treated and managed holistically.

Implementation of RPi is a slow process as there was a need to fully develop applications that can support the RPi operating system. Even though these systems are affordable, maintenance and running costs could be expensive and time consuming. Specialized collaboration between engineering support staff and technical staff of the MLS program in ensuring these applications are running optimally, which would be one the most significant challenges that will be faced by the teaching team at MLS. Supporting RPi units to have Internet connection and ensuring that all 45 units run without lag or technical glitches will need regular connection monitoring. In addition other factors such as connecting the RPi to the server, renovating the lab infrastructure to support additional Ethernet ports and monitors in the lab may significantly elevate the cost of installing these units.

SOLUTIONS AND RECOMMENDATIONS

Various strategies were employed by the teaching team at Griffith University to overcome the issues that were raised during the development and implementation of technologies such as 3D virtual laboratory, e-portfolio and RPi. First and foremost, the issue to which funding the development of 3D virtual pathology lab could be solved was by making this assignment a collaborative project between the University and the Health industry. Furthermore, the cost of production can be further reduced by collaborating with the manufacturer of the analyzers used in the pathology lab. This can be beneficial to the manufacturer as well, as they can share this training video with the existing and possible future customers. Designing the virtual videos based on the industry requirements can significantly improve student outcomes, as graduates ready for the workforce would need minimal training. When designing these videos the academic staff has to ensure that the virtual pathology lab teaches students the different operational skills and methods that they need to be proficient in, but also in trouble shooting an error displayed by the analyzer and reflecting on their work to improve themselves. At Griffith University, the academic staff have created personalized 3D videos of equipment maintenance and common errors simulated with assessment embedded in the video to provide students similar training as they will receive upon job recruitment. Once the student has complete the assessment this innovative model can then saved by students on their e-portfolio with trainer's feedback and endorsement of their skills.

Recommendations for e-portfolio practice researched by Hallam and Creagh (2010), highlighted that in order for e-portfolio practice to be advantageous, government departments responsible for education should engage with industry, professional and employer bodies to see the potential of e-portfolios being used a way to articulate employability skills (Hallam & Creagh, 2010). Secondly, government policy should also recognize e-portfolio as a strategy in building relationships between higher and tertiary education in supporting the individual's lifelong learning needs and the potential for career progression. In order to potentiate the value of e-portfolio and its use in education and industry, different stakeholders (government department, policies and institutional policies) need to start incorporating the use of e-portfolio and communicate the benefits of e-portfolio practice. Although the benefits of e-portfolio are significant, a recent study has reported that without proper guidance, students have faced technological and logistical challenges when using e-portfolios (Birks, Hartin, Woods, Emmanuel, & Hitchins, 2016). Continuous support and encouragement from the education institution are crucial for successful integration of e-portfolios with the respective programs (Posey, Plack, & Snyder, 2015; Slade, Murfin, & Readman, 2013). Implementation of Pebble Pad was to be particularly beneficial for students as it provides an excellent interface for students to record their work over a period of time during their stay at the university and to update their e-portfolios in real-time. Computerization of MLS labs by installing RPi would greatly complement Pebble Pad, as the students can upload their practical activities and academic achievements during their laboratory sessions, thereby saving time.

FUTURE RESEARCH DIRECTIONS

Even though there have been significant increases in the introduction of e-learning technologies within the MLS program, it is still only in its early stage of development. Future research has to be conducted to tailor these e-learning technologies to meet the needs and improve the learning outcomes of each student. The 3D virtual laboratory could significantly expand to include training modules for multiple disciplines and techniques that are not just limited to analyzers. These 3D virtual pathology labs can be used to establish benchmarks and criteria for competency based performance assessment using simulation on students and hospital staff. Use of simulation for testing a number of new analytical devices before deployment of new analytical prototypes can be a direction towards which these technologies are heading towards (Gaba, 2004).

The latest updates in Pebble Pad include access to new resources and several other multimedia resources that promote self-education. Sharing these resources with industry and standardizing training modules between industry and tertiary institutions can significantly improve the quality of work ready graduates. Encouraging employees and MLS alumni to continue building their e-portfolios for professional development and self-education can also help the academic and hospital staff by sharing any interesting case studies that are usually rare. Governing bodies and leaders in health care education and training have to recognize the potential of e-portfolios being used in the system to train professionals and maintain their continuing professional development training records.

Connecting RPi to the Internet and developing applications that would allow students to access cell image software and current student systems such as e-portfolios would be a big step in modernizing practical laboratories. The use of digital touch screen monitors to combat lab space shortage will also be an effective solution in computerizing MLS labs at minimal costs. Encouraging university to invest in IT facilities and staff that can provide help with the setup, maintenance and updating these technologies would be beneficial, as upon successful implementation of RPi, these technologies can be applied to other programs within health science. Once these systems are in place, student evaluations via surveys can be implemented to evaluate how these work-integrated tools assist in student's career readiness.

CONCLUSION

In conclusion, several universities have shown to invest a significant amount of resources for the integration of e-leaning technologies within the programs associated with Health Science. However, these technologies are still in their early stages of development and require significant contributions from the industry and academic staff for further development. At Griffith University, several new e-technologies such as 3D virtual pathology laboratory, e-portfolio using Pebble Pad and RPi have been have been implemented to enhance work-integrated learning, student experience and positively influence employability for students studying Medical Laboratory Science. Integration of these e-learning tools has shown to positively influence the learning and teaching outcomes for MLS students. However, there are certain challenges that are associated with the developments of these e-learning tools such as funding and standardization of training protocols. In future, industry advisory boards and surveys such as student evaluations should be used to accumulate data on these e-learning tools in order to improve and standardize these technologies.

REFERENCES

Ali, M., Vlaskamp, J. H. A., Eddin, N. N., Falconer, B., & Oram, C. (2013). *Technical development and socioeconomic implications of the Raspberry Pi as a learning tool in developing countries*. Paper presented at the Computer Science and Electronic Engineering Conference (CEEC), 2013 5th. doi:10.1109/CEEC.2013.6659454

Birks, M., Hartin, P., Woods, C., Emmanuel, E., & Hitchins, M. (2016). Students' perceptions of the use of eportfolios in nursing and midwifery education. *Nurse Education in Practice*, *18*, 46–51. doi:10.1016/j.nepr.2016.03.003 PMID:27235565

Blom, D., Rowley, J., Bennett, D., Hitchcock, M., & Dunbar-Hall, P. (2013). Two-way impact: Institutional e-learning policy/educator practices in creative arts through ePortfolio creation. *Proceedings of the 12th European conference on e-learning*.

Gaba, D. M. (2004). The future vision of simulation in health care. *Quality & Safety in Health Care*, *13*(suppl 1), i2–i10. doi:10.1136/qshc.2004.009878 PMID:15465951

Hallam, G., & Creagh, T. (2010). ePortfolio use by university students in Australia: A review of the Australian ePortfolio Project. *Higher Education Research & Development*, *29*(2), 179–193. doi:10.1080/07294360903510582

Ioannou, N. K., Ioannidis, G. S., Papadopoulos, G. D., & Tapeinos, A. E. (2014). *A novel educational platform, based on the Raspberry-Pi: Optimised to assist the teaching and learning of younger students*. Paper presented at the Interactive Collaborative Learning (ICL), 2014 International Conference on.

Le Beux, P., & Fieschi, M. (2007). *Virtual biomedical universities and e-learning*. Elsevier.

Locatis, C., Vega, A., Bhagwat, M., Liu, W.-L., & Conde, J. (2008). A virtual computer lab for distance biomedical technology education. *BMC Medical Education*, *8*(1), 12. doi:10.1186/1472-6920-8-12 PMID:18366629

Posey, L., Plack, M. M., & Snyder, R. (2015). Developing a Pathway for an Institution Wide ePortfolio Program. *International Journal of ePortfolio*, *5*(1), 75-92.

Radloff, A., & Coates, H. (2009). *Australasian Student Engagement Survey 2009 institution report*. Academic Press.

Radloff, A., & Coates, H. (2010). *Doing more for learning: enhancing engagement and outcomes: Australasian Survey of Student Engagement: Australasian Student Engagement Report*. Academic Press.

Reese, M., & Levy, R. (2009). *Assessing the future: E-portfolio trends, uses, and options in higher education*. Academic Press.

Sédille-Mostafaie, N., Engler, H., Lutz, S., & Korte, W. (2013). Advancing haemostasis automation–successful implementation of robotic centrifugation and sample processing in a tertiary service hospital. *Clinical Chemistry and Laboratory Medicine*, *51*(6), 1273–1278. doi:10.1515/cclm-2012-0625 PMID:23241682

Slade, C., Murfin, K., & Readman, K. (2013). Evaluating Processes and Platforms for Potential ePortfolio Use: The Role of the Middle Agent. *International Journal of ePortfolio, 3*(2), 177-188.

KEY TERMS AND DEFINITIONS

Cell Differentiation Counters: A counting tool used to count and tally different types of leukocytes.

E-Portfolio: A collection of electronic evidence assembled and managed by a user, usually on the web. They are becoming standard practice for academics, students, and professionals and typically include examples of skills and achievements, as well as a reflective blog element.

Medical Laboratory Science: A four-year undergraduate course in the field of medical science diagnostics and pathology.

Raspberry Pi: A credit-card-sized computer that uses Linux operating system.

Self-Directed Learning: Individuals perform their own study in an un-facilitated environment.

Simulations: A program or external setting that mimics an event or process, where participants can re-enact the process outside of a real-time event.

Tertiary Education: All post-secondary school education including but not limited to universities.

Chapter 8
Virtual Microscopy in Haematology and Histopathology Education:
Virtual Microscopy in Science Education

Vinod Gopalan
Griffith University, Australia

Abishek B. Santhakumar
Charles Sturt University, Australia

Indu Singh
Griffith University, Australia

ABSTRACT

Virtual microscopy is a method by which real-time microscopic illustrations get transmitted digitally via computer networks. There is increasing evidence to suggest that virtual microscopy combined with other didactic methods in teaching make significant improvements in student interaction and curiosity in histopathology and haematology teaching. The introduction of virtual microscopy has opened up a big arena in the field of e-learning in histopathology and haematology curriculum. Case studies prove the technological benefits of virtual microscopy in interacting off-campus students and educators. Recent technological advances have improved the use of virtual microscopy and enabled them to complement students learning in class room as well as for routine diagnostics. In this chapter, the authors discuss the significance, usefulness, and limitations of virtual microscopy in education. In addition, the chapter has provided several technical considerations to develop a friendly web-based virtual microscopy tool in teaching.

DOI: 10.4018/978-1-5225-3850-9.ch008

INTRODUCTION

Due to the rapid transformation in university curricula, it's has been a colossal challenge to engage students solely by conventional face-to-face teaching. Integration of traditional teaching methods with digital, online or virtual modes of learning has emerged over last decade as one of the mainstream teaching tools in multiple disciplines especially teaching haematology and histopathology subjects. Digital microscopy tools combined with other didactic methods in teaching shown to have a significant role in improving student interaction and curiosity in teaching (Diaz-Perez et al., 2014).

This chapter will discuss the incorporation and use of virtual microscopy as a simulation based educational tool that could be optimised for enhanced student learning in haematology and histopathology teaching. The innovative ways of merging this technology with other technological mediums at Australian Universities will be the focus of this chapter allowing students are learning both off campus and on campus to complement their classroom directed morphology learning with self-directed learning.

BACKGROUND

Virtual Microscopy and Digitalisation in Haematology

Diagnosis of haematological diseases using blood film morphology microscopy and blood cell count analysis is a crucial skill for students under training to become medical laboratory scientists. Use of virtual slides in haematology teaching is instrumental in mimicking everyday laboratory activities of medical laboratory scientists in the haematology department. The concept of multiple microscopic fields of view and virtual/digital slides was first described in 1985 and later expanded during the early 1990s (Silage & Gil, 1985; Westerkamp & Gahm, 1993). A virtual slide is a large digital image of a section of the blood film to be examined. In the past, digital images of specific areas in a blood film have been used in the training and identification of pathological abnormalities. The virtual slide is a collection or in other words a 'real-time' virtual picture of the whole blood film to be examined (Figure 1). It consists of several high resolution/power microscopic images of areas of blood films stitched together using an image processing software. There are several advantages of using virtual slides in training and education over traditional blood slides:

- Virtual slides are easy to store, annotate, file or retrieve.
- Virtual slides can be easily duplicated, shared and integrated into online teaching modules.
- Virtual slides do not deteriorate over time.
- One-of-a-kind blood slides can be stored and circulated more efficiently.
- Virtual slides closely emulates the pan and zoom function of traditional microscopy.
- Quicker slide viewing related to no requirement of adjustment of focus, lighting or condenser adjustment.
- Rapid access to the next slide in the slide box consequently increasing blood slide study turn-around time.
- Promotes group discussion as the inter-connected computer screens may serve as a multi-head/instructor microscope.
- Side-by-side student access to annotations, clinical case description, haematological parameters.
- Quicker access to any macroscopic and microscopic area of the blood film.

There are several technical considerations in order to develop a web-based virtual microscopy tool in teaching: (a) digital information from numerous fields of view in high resolution and power needs to be acquired to create a large unified mosaic of a virtual slide; (b) information from the virtual slide requires conversion to a file format that can allow the x-y axis pan and zoom function; (c) merge the resulting product into a software and database that will support annotations.

Virtual microscopy is also an effective way to integrate and implement e-learning in the curriculum. Considering the current impulsion in the use of technology in teaching, virtual labs and microscopy have been a practical consideration. Virtual microscopy has been well acknowledged and received by educators and students (Heidger et al., 2002). In a study performed at the University of South Carolina, students found it very easy to navigate within the slide when compared to traditional microscopy (Lee, 2005). Virtual microscopy also enhances the ability of the educator to point out specific lesions and morphological changes in the blood slide to effectively engage the students and improves the student's overall learning experience and ability to grasp information from the virtual slide presented. A study conducted by Brueggeman et al., also supported this evidence by demonstrating that undergraduate level distance education students performed significantly better in the haematology morphology assessment using virtual microscopy in comparison to when they used traditional microscopy (Brueggeman, Swinehart, Yue, Conway-Klaassen, & Wiesner, 2012).

Another key advantage of the use of virtual microscopy in haematology teaching is the ability to provide identical assessment slides for all the students during morphology assessments. It is almost impossible to provide identical blood slides for the whole cohort of students taking a blood film morphology assessment. This issue could be overcome by utilising the same virtual slide across the student cohort. This not only minimises the morphological variation in blood slides but also aids in providing accurate feedback from the assessor.

In the recent times, there has been a steady increase in the number of students enrolling into haematology programs on a part-time basis. Due to the nature of their enrolment, round-the-clock access to traditional microscopes and blood slides has been a challenging ordeal. Virtual microscopy has been very successful in providing the round-the-clock access to a collection of blood film slides and databases with pre-loaded clinical information and cases thereby promoting self-study and resourceful revision material in preparation for assessments. Furthermore, these virtual slides on web-based interfaces have also been instrumental in improving the ease-of-access in smart devices such as tablets and smartphones.

Virtual slides have also been increasingly used in synergy with other innovative technological platforms in haematology teaching. One of which is the use of blood cell counting applications available for Android and iOS devices. The traditional approach in blood cell counting in haematology morphology was the use of hand-held clickers or tally counters with reliability, specificity and precision being the associated drawbacks with such instruments. The smartphone applications have improved user-friendly, visually engaging, reliable and precise functionality. The blood cell counting smart applications, a) utilizes visual representation of blood cells enhancing student experience and counting accuracy b) provides an option for amending the counted blood cell hence reducing the necessity to restart the cell counting c) delivers audible instructions during counting and d) offers diverse selections for counting rare cell structures thus augmenting counting specificity. This approach also gives the opportunity for students to provide real-time feedback to the educator hence encouraging an active learning environment.

In addition to the use of virtual microscopy in tertiary education, they have been increasing introduced into self-assessment and continuing education programs in commercial/national pathology laboratories. For instance, the Royal College of Pathologists Australasia conducts quality assurance programs (RCPAQAP) nationally and internationally to monitor the quality of laboratory services offered and to ensure they meet accreditation standards. They utilise virtual microscopy to assess the haematological morphological competence of practising medical scientists to ensure the pathology provider maintains quality requirements. In 2005, a pilot study was conducted with the UK National External Quality Assessment Scheme for General haematology participants (N=166) to assess the use of digital virtual slides in the quality assessment of haematology morphology (Burthem et al., 2005). The results revealed significant concordance of morphological observations were made using digital slides compared to their glass slide counterparts. The feedback from participant's also strongly supported the use of digital microscopy in haematology for education and assessment purposes.

Several automated digital imaging systems have been introduced in recent years to improve turnaround time and proficiency in examining peripheral blood smears in haematology laboratories.

Live digital imaging systems such as CellaVision came into the market for more than 15 years ago. It automatically locates and then captures digital images of cells from barcoded slides. Software extracts cellular features from the images to deliver a pre-classification/ pre-characterization of cells that is presented to the technologist for review and verification. Structured interfaces, intelligent functionalities and embedded tools help speed up the review and verification process while promoting analysis accuracy and consistency. Remote access functionality facilitates sharing

Figure 1. This is a simple example of a virtual microscopy platform (Best Network, Slice) demonstrating a haematology blood film at a 40X objective. The web-based software/database allows the educator to add layers and annotate the virtual slide. The image presents an annotation of the neutrophil using a pin location icon. The top right corner of the image also displays a pan and zoom function, in addition, to move to any particular area of the virtual blood film.

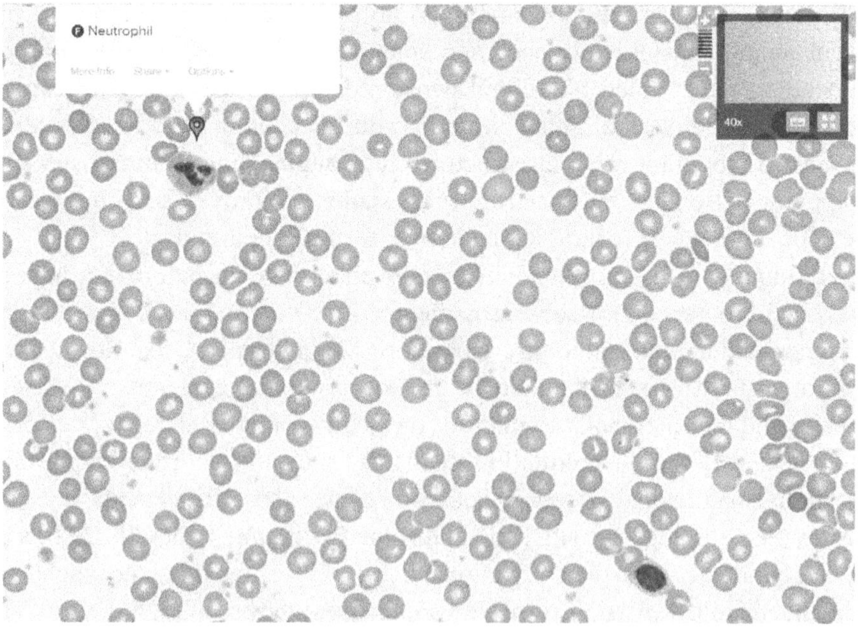

of cell images for collaboration and consultation, from any computer or site within a network.

EasyCell assistant uses image-processing and pattern-recognition technologies to automate white cell differential counting. EasyCell automatically locates white cells on a blood smear, preclassifies the cells, and then presents them to a technologist for review on an LCD display. The haematology system typically reduces sample review times by 50% over the manual differentiation method using a microscope while helping the technologist achieve improved efficiency, accuracy, and precision. Additionally, EasyCell presents images of red cells and platelets for the performance of red cell morphology and platelet estimate.

Recent technological advances have improved the whole slide imaging (WSI) scanner quality and reduced the cost of storage, thereby enabling the deployment of digital pathology for routine diagnostics.

The performance of modern haematology analysers is suboptimal in identifying specific blast cells, whereas a manual review is still required in the presence of immature granulocyte flags or abnormal white blood cell distribution. The Beckman Coulter HematoFlow analyser is a promising new technique, but cytology remains the gold standard because to date it is the only modality to reach a definitive diagnosis in many cases. Automated microscopy count shows good correlation with the reference manual microscopy count and may replace the regular microscope in high-volume haematology laboratories and adult samples. Automated microscopy analysers can provide accurate WBC differential counts, which may replace manual microscopy, but should not replace the eye of the cytologist.

Virtual Microscopy in Histopathology

A huge technical advancement in the acquisition of virtual slides had occurred in the early 2000s when Aperio (www.aperio.com) released a linear scanner that can quickly acquire digital stripes across the whole slide. Another commercial platform, Dmetrix (www.dmetrix.net/), have introduced an array microscope that could acquire rapid simultaneous digital images of the whole slide by multiple microlenses (Weinstein et al., 2004). These microscopy tools generally referred as digital or virtual microscopy, aids in the demonstration of microscopic pathology using live digital pathology slides without accessing a teaching laboratory physically with a microscope.

This digital imaging system also has excellent use in the demonstration of histology and pathology slides via on-line access to students for self-study during on and off campus (Lam et al., 2005; Marchevsky et al., 2003; Hays et al., 2005; Weisnstein et al., 2009; Dee. 2009; Hamilton et al., 2012). This can be assessed on their electronic gadgets and on handheld devices such as smartphones at any time.

Another key feature of virtual microscopy is its pan-optical zoom and annotation options (Figure 2) which mimic a live objective view through a light microscope.

The recent modifications in the virtual microscope software have allowed academics to track student participation, create self-study modules and to set up these modules for distance learning. After the investment in these digital microscope stages (Aperio or Dmetrix), there is a huge economic saving on the financial and administrative cost to run these virtual microscopy sessions. Importantly, the ethical/biological risks, as well as health and safety concerns associated with using patient-derived tissue materials and microscopes, can be avoided during digital microscopy based laboratory training (Gabril and Yousef, 2010; Holland and Bosch, 2006). In addition to histopathology, virtual microscopy implementation can host multiple venues for health education, small and large group teachings, problem-based curricula (Kumar et al., 2006), specialised fields such as cytology (Stewart et al., 2008), and veterinary (Simms et al., 2007) and for staff education and evaluations (Bennett, 2006). Furthermore, it helps to train students to get acquainted with future digital diagnostic modes such as telepathology where long-distance interaction and consultation with multiple clinicians are possible at the same time (Leifer, 2015; Weinstein et al., 2004).

Aperio and Digital Microscopy in Histopathology: A Case Study

In order to analyse the effectiveness of digital microscopy, we have conducted a study to evaluate its impact on medical student's pathology learning experience. Approximately 272 medical students were participated in this study and were invited to complete questionnaires rating the value of their learning experiences of the whole year after the completion of their final practical session. A paired t-test has noted 53% positive correlation for the overall responses between virtual microscopy-guided pathology modules and practical sessions indicating its use in better preparing students for these sessions ($p < 0.001$). Qualitative feedbacks have also suggested that the virtual microscopy sessions along with clinical scenario based learning were extremely useful for students' learning in pathology.

On the other hand, no significant differences in students' overall learning experience were noted between digital pathology modules and conventional teaching methods (pathology/histology lectures and practical sessions) (Table 1). Scoville and Trent have previously demonstrated analogous findings where they noted that first-year medical students learned equally well in virtual or light microscopy slides (Scoville and Trent, 2007). Also, Koch et al's study could find no difference in diagnostic interpretations between virtual slides and glass microscopy slides despite having candidate's preference for the virtual slides (Koch et al., 2009).

Figure 2. Visual representation of live virtual microscopy session using Aperio Scanscope. A- Arteriovenous malformation in the brain without annotation; B- Demonstration of the flexibility of the software to annotate the features in different representation styles. Hyalinization of the blood vessel is highlighted in a circle. Tortuous and malformed blood vessels are indicated by arrows during the live lecture sessions.

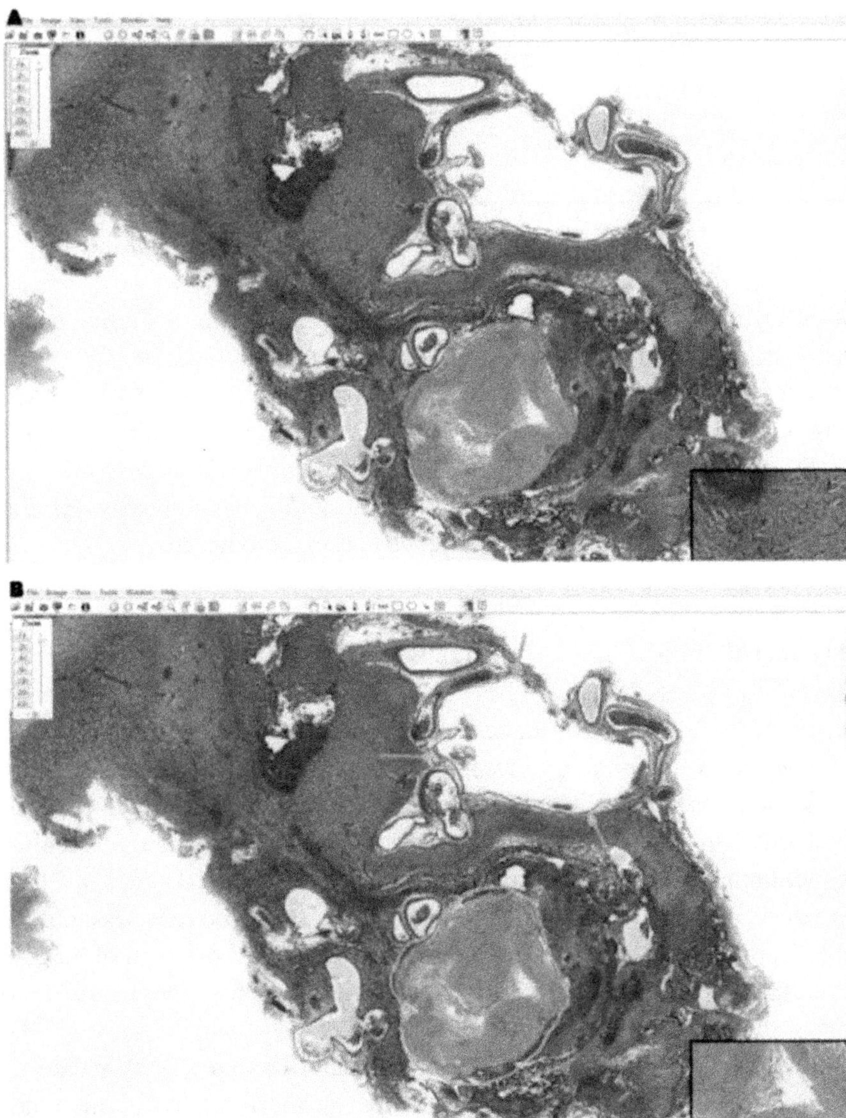

Table 1. Students learning experience with virtual microscopy sessions

Question	Total/Missing	Student rating (1 = strongly disagree, 5 = strongly agree) 1	2	3	4	5	Mean/Median
Pathology Lectures							
Delivery	268/4	0	0	16	114	138	4.46 (± 0.61)/5
Clinical Integration	268/4	4	16	84	108	56	3.73 (± 0.91)/4
Overall	272/0	0	1	14	125	128	4.42 (± 0.61)/4
Virtual Microscopy Lectures							
Innovation	246/26	0	2	16	80	149	4.53 (± 0.64)/5
Delivery	247/25	0	2	14	77	154	4.55 (± 0.64)/5
Clinical Integration	246/26	0	1	24	82	139	4.46 (± 0.69)/5
Overall	245/27	0	0	16	81	148	4.54 (± 0.62)/5

Based on own and others findings, we believe that these digital pathology resources are suing virtual microscopy act as a valuable resource for improving students' learning experience. However, they make little or no effect on students' learning outcome or diagnostic skills. Thus, the traditional teaching methods and their priorities in pathology should be maintained, while the digital microscopy-based approaches should be complemented these traditional methods for a productive outcome both in a better learning experience and in the outcome.

VIRTUAL MICROSCOPY IN EDUCATION: BOON OR BANE?

In spite of the tremendous advantages and feasibility of using virtual microscopy in haematology and histopathology education, there are several disadvantages associated with it. Students or trainees who familiarise or favour the use of digital microscopy, do not learn to use the traditional microscope proficiently. Though teaching and quality assurance programs are progressing to the use of digital slides, the students training to become medical laboratory scientists are required to assess glass slides prepared from patient samples. The inexperience in the preparation of blood films and tissues samples and manually focusing traditional microscopes hands-on would become a challenge.

Digital slides at a lower magnification do not retain the same clarity and resolution as a glass slide when viewed under a microscope. Furthermore, 100X oil immersion magnification, to assess intricate inclusions in blood cells, does not zoom into the cells as effectively as the traditional microscope. Lastly, refractive cells do not refract well in virtual slides hence making it difficult to distinguish them.

Another major concern around teaching morphological features to students on an online web-based platform is internet speed. Due to the large size associated with each virtual slide, the time taken in the acquisition of the slide and transmission speed to the interface is usually delayed in lower internet speeds. This is especially true of students studying a program via distance education, especially in regional areas, where high-speed Internet might not be accessible. In addition to the above drawback, the amount of time taken by slide scanners to scan specific areas of blood films and histological slides have been arguable. Different models of slide scanners have varying throughputs and speed and have been associated with a high cost. Besides, compatibility of web browsers to the database and web-based virtual slides have also been a concerning issue.

Virtual microscopy alone does not provide a realistic initial learning experience for students or novice trainees. On the other hand, based on overload of information and limited resources classroom time, there is a lack of sufficient supervision to provide the morphology training for students to be work ready at graduation after four years full-time study.

There is also fear of students' self-directed learning through distance or virtual microscopic training only, providing them inaccurate learning outcome. Morphology can be very subjective, and there are no black and white answers when identifying the diagnostic features on the blood films or histological slides.

FUTURE OPPORTUNITIES

It is apparent that commercial entities and new developing technologies, both hardware, and software, will continue to influence and impact the development of virtual microscopy in teaching. However, file formats and compatibility with web browsers are a stagnant concern. This has consequently provoked a sagacity of negativity around the use of technology for both educators and students. This diminutive issue around technical anomalies in virtual microscopy warrants intervention.

Mixed mode teaching with imaging by Aperio used for classroom microscopy under the direct supervision of fully trained and experienced morphologist could prove beneficial. Virtual microscopy should complement the self-study and it should have the options to email questions related to annotations and a 24 hrs access to virtual images of the same blood films or tissue slides that the students use for learning in the classroom.

In the recent years, a steady increase has been observed in the number of educational institutions implementing the technological intervention, especially virtual microscopy. More specifically in histopathology and haematology teaching, educators strive to develop and implement new or current institutional databases. In certain scenarios, educators even consider adapting expensive commercially available tissue and blood slide databases. A central nationally recommended standardised blood film and tissue pathology slide database linked to a simple, user-friendly web browsing interface developed purely based on contributions from educators, medical scientists and clinicians, and which could be adapted at no cost by educators or accreditation/assessment bodies would be hugely beneficial to tertiary education teaching.

REFERENCES

Bennett, B. (2006). Certification from the American Board of Pathology: Getting it and keeping it. *Human Pathology*, *37*(8), 978–981. doi:10.1016/j.humpath.2006.02.023 PMID:16867858

Brueggeman, M. S., Swinehart, C., Yue, M. J., Conway-Klaassen, J. M., & Wiesner, S. M. (2012). Implementing virtual microscopy improves outcomes in a hematology morphology course. *Clinical Laboratory Science*, *25*, 149. PMID:22953514

Burthem, J., Brereton, M., Ardern, J., Hickman, L., Seal, L., Serrant, A., & De la Salle, B. et al. (2005). The use of digital 'virtual slides' in the quality assessment of haematological morphology: Results of a pilot exercise involving UK NEQAS (H) participants. *British Journal of Haematology*, *130*(2), 293–296. doi:10.1111/j.1365-2141.2005.05597.x PMID:16029459

Dee, F. R. (2009). Virtual microscopy in pathology education. *Human Pathology*, *40*(8), 1112–1121. doi:10.1016/j.humpath.2009.04.010 PMID:19540551

Diaz-Perez, J. A., Raju, S., & Echeverri, J. H. (2014). Evaluation of a teaching strategy based on integration of clinical subjects, virtual autopsy, pathology museum, and digital microscopy for medical students. *Journal of Pathology Informatics*, *5*(1), 25. doi:10.4103/2153-3539.137729 PMID:25191624

Gabril, M. Y., & Yousef, G. M. (2010). Informatics for practicing anatomical pathologists: Marking a new era in pathology practice. *Modern Pathology*, *23*(3), 349–358. doi:10.1038/modpathol.2009.190 PMID:20081805

Hamilton, P. W., Wang, Y., & McCullough, S. J. (2012). Virtual microscopy and digital pathology in training and education. *APMIS*, *120*(4), 305–315. doi:10.1111/j.1600-0463.2011.02869.x PMID:22429213

Hays, R., Veitch, J., & Lam, A. (2005). Teaching clinical pathology by flexible delivery in rural sites. *The Australian Journal of Rural Health*, *13*(4), 232–235. doi:10.1111/j.1440-1584.2005.00707.x PMID:16048465

Heidger, P. M., Dee, F., Consoer, D., Leaven, T., Duncan, J., & Kreiter, C. (2002). Integrated approach to teaching and testing in histology with real and virtual imaging. *The Anatomical Record*, *269*(2), 107–112. doi:10.1002/ar.10078 PMID:12001217

Holland, L., & Bosch, B. (2006). Medical students' perceptions of pathology and the effect of the second-year pathology course. *Human Pathology*, *37*(1), 1–8. doi:10.1016/j.humpath.2005.10.004 PMID:16360409

Koch, L. H., Lampros, J. N., Delong, L. K., Chen, S. C., Woosley, J. T., & Hood, A. F. (2009). Randomized comparison of virtual microscopy and traditional glass microscopy in diagnostic accuracy among dermatology and pathology residents. *Human Pathology*, *40*(5), 662–667. doi:10.1016/j.humpath.2008.10.009 PMID:19144382

Kumar, R. K., Freeman, B., Velan, G. M., & De Permentier, P. J. (2006). Integrating histology and histopathology teaching in practical classes using virtual slides. *Anatomical Record. Part B, New Anatomist*, *289*(4), 128–133. doi:10.1002/ar.b.20105 PMID:16865702

Lam, A. K., Veitch, J., & Hays, R. (2005). Resuscitating the teaching of anatomical pathology in undergraduate medical education: Web-based innovative clinicopathological cases. *Pathology*, *37*(5), 360–363. doi:10.1080/00313020500253331 PMID:16194846

Lee, S. H. (2005). Virtual microscopy: Applications to hematology education and training. *Hematology*, *10*(supl), 151–153. doi:10.1080/10245330512331390249 PMID:16188659

Leifer, Z. (2015). The use of virtual microscopy and a wiki in pathology education: Tracking student use, involvement, and response. *Journal of Pathology Informatics*, *6*(1), 30. doi:10.4103/2153-3539.158063 PMID:26110097

Marchevsky, A. M., Relan, A., & Baillie, S. (2003). Self-instructional "virtual pathology" laboratories using web-based technology enhance medical school teaching of pathology. *Human Pathology*, *34*(5), 423–429. doi:10.1016/S0046-8177(03)00089-3 PMID:12792914

Scoville, S. A., & Trent, D. B. (2007). Traditional and virtual microscopy compared experimentally in a classroom setting. *Clinical Anatomy (New York, N.Y.)*, *20*(5), 565–570. doi:10.1002/ca.20440 PMID:17109440

Silage, D. A., & Gil, J. (1985). Digital image tiles: A method for the processing of large sections. *Journal of Microscopy*, *138*(2), 221–227. doi:10.1111/j.1365-2818.1985.tb02615.x PMID:3894672

Simms, M. H., Mendis-Handagama, C., & Moore, R. N. (2007). Virtual microscopy in a veterinary curriculum. *Journal of Veterinary Medical Education*, *34*(4), 416–422. doi:10.3138/jvme.34.4.416 PMID:18287467

Stewart, J., Bevans-Williams, K., Bhattacharya, A., Ye, C., Miyazaki, K., & Kurtycz, D. (2008). Virtual microscopy: An educator's tool for the enhancement of cytotechnology student's locator skills. *Diagnostic Cytopathology*, *36*(6), 363–368. doi:10.1002/dc.20821 PMID:18478604

Weinstein, R. S., Descour, M. R., Liang, C., Barker, G., Scott, K. M., Richter, L., & Bartels, P. H. et al. (2004). An array microscope for ultrarapid virtual slide processing and telepathology. Design, fabrication, and validation study. *Human Pathology*, *35*(11), 1303–1314. doi:10.1016/j.humpath.2004.09.002 PMID:15668886

Westerkamp, D., & Gahm, T. (1993). Non-distorted assemblage of the digital images of adjacent fields in histological sections. *Analytical Cellular Pathology*, *5*, 235–247. PMID:8363984

Chapter 9
Technology Associated With Dental Prosthetics and Learning Experiences:
Collaborative Initiative, Australian and Norwegian

Jane Lesleigh Evans
Griffith University, Australia

Trude Myhrer
Oslo and Akershus University College, Norway

ABSTRACT

Design and manufacturing of dental restorations has evolved to embrace digital technology. So too has the paradigm of learning and teaching dental prosthetics. Once a didactic teacher-driven process, it has become student-focused, reliant on collaboration and directed toward employability. This chapter describes the stages, processes, and experiences of developing a collaborative partnership to "internationalize" dental technologist curricula which led to a model for developing shared digital resources and enhanced work-integrated learning. The discussion is supported by reflection of dental technology student learning experiences from Oslo and Akershus University College and Griffith University. Issues, controversies, and problems are explored through a descriptive analysis of experiences that aim to encourage other academics to rethink curriculum design, delivery, and assessment to create international partnerships. International collaboration in higher education can provide academics with a platform to share digital resources and create flexible, transferable qualifications.

DOI: 10.4018/978-1-5225-3850-9.ch009

INTRODUCTION

This chapter takes the reader on a journey through the globalization of dentistry, the evolution of digital prosthetics culminating in an example of how dental technology education can evolve in the digital era. It will highlight the benefits that an international collaboration can create. The primary focus is to establish an understanding for the use of the flipped classroom as a teaching method through an international collaboration. In a flipped classroom, students prepare learning material (both theoretical and practical) before they attend physical classes, thus, enabling enhanced collaboration between students and academics to resolve issues related to prosthetic cases. Developing demonstrations for practical use in dental technology will support the teaching teams and provide flexible learning opportunities. To succeed with this flipped classroom approach as a teaching method, it is helpful to embrace the PICA model, which includes four key elements: presentation, interaction, collaboration and analysis. These will be elaborated on throughout the chapter.

The intent of the international collaboration described in this chapter is to ensure qualifications are relevant, transparent, and transportable. To achieve this, curricula was mapped, assessment moderated and student exchange experienced - all were consistent with contemporary dental technology practices. The stages and experiences of developing a collaborative partnership to 'internationalize' dental technology curricula has raised motivation and a desire to develop and share digital resources, and enhance opportunities for work integrated learning. This is a distinct advantage for the students and teaching team which promotes engagement and continued learning.

To achieve a successful international collaboration, a reliable open, online platform is necessary. One such example is Open EdX using a mobile application, and platform to meet a wide variety of requirements. This enables program designers to collaborate and develop accessible course content. The international program development team, situated in Norway, aims to develop courses collaboratively that can serve students all over the world thus enhancing consistency and transportability of qualifications. The project has been going for a number of years beyond this dental technology venture, and continues to grow.

Overview of Internationalization in This Project

Internationalization in the context of this study refers to the development of a curriculum that: spans international boundaries, fosters personal development through international exchanges, cultivates world standards of contemporary standards in dental technology and promotes sharing of knowledge. The purpose is to enable qualifications to be transparent, tractable and transferable. Students and academic staff experience shared affiliations that promote connectedness and collaboration.

Context: Description of Collaboration Between Griffith University Australia and Oslo and Akershus University College Norway Dental Technology Programs

The collaboration commenced in 2011 when the previous Head of Department for Radiography and Dental Technology programs at Oslo and Akershus University College of Applied Sciences (HiOA) Norway, invited the dental technology Program Director from Griffith University (Griffith) Australia, to visit Oslo to investigate opportunities for collaboration. During this time, the team alliance sprouted with a study to compare Interprofessional Education (IPE) between the programs of study (Evans et al., 2015). The next year, program directors established a Memorandum of Understanding (MOU) to enable the sharing of curricula, and discover different approaches to learning and teaching. After mapping and auditing of curricula, a pilot study was conducted to moderate assessment. This enabled all students at each location to complete the same practical tests across five areas of dental technology. In 2013, the process of assessment moderation was refined and calibration of markers was achieved from site visits and online discussions (Myhrer et al., 2015). Furthermore, some minor changes were implemented to curricula and the learning, teaching and assessment strategies were viewed as congruent and worthy of an exchange agreement. The student exchange opportunity was created in Semester 5 for Oslo students and Trimester 1 final year for Griffith students, and staff exchanges recommended. The goal was to increase consistency, transparency and portability of dental technology education, and the collaboration continues.

Computer Assisted Design and Computer Assisted Manufacture (CAD CAM)

Studying dental technology requires insight into Computer Assisted Design and Computer Assisted Manufacture (CAD CAM). Therefore, the use of digital resources in the learning environment is not an alien experience to students. The dental technology programs at both universities value the need to develop core practical skills and theoretical knowledge and address the need for dental services provision in their respective communities (Myhrer et al., 2015). This means that the two programs are not exactly alike, but qualitatively comparable. The majority of technical procedures are consistent, and therefore digital resources are considered useful for both programs.

Objectives

1. Outline the phases in international collaboration and provide an example of a flipped classroom module through a systematic process using the PICA-model (presentation, interaction, collaboration and analysis) that may be replicated by other educators.
2. Discuss the interaction and collaboration using the PICA framework (Høivik, 2016).
3. Highlight considerations for the future. Dental procedures are suitable for digitalization into an audio visual format due to the uniqueness and quality standardized requirements. However it is not without shortcomings.

BACKGROUND

This section provides broad definitions and literature in regard to the evolution of dental education in a digital era, the relationship of globalization and influence of internationalization of curricula.

Evolution of Dental Education to Respond to the Digital Transformation of Dentistry

Prosthetic design and manufacturing has changed over the past four decades due to the expansion of digital dentistry such as: intra oral scanners, digital impressions and Computer Aided Design/Computer Aided Manufacturing (CAD/CAM) systems (vanNoort, 2012). The availability of digital technology has transformed the way oral prosthesis are designed and produced by dental technologists in dental laboratories (Miyazaki, Hotta, Kunii, Kuriyama, & Tamaki, 2009). These advancements are dynamic and influence the way dental education is delivered (van der Zande, Gorter, & Wismeijer, 2013). These trends suggest that graduating dental technologists and dentists will be required to adapt to the digital changes in order to maintain efficiency and productivity in professional practice (Reifeis, Kirkup, Willis, & Browning, 2014). It is therefore expected that dental curricula should enable the current and future generations of dental professionals with the techniques and knowledge for preparedness of the digital era.

It is known that aesthetics contributes to the overall health of individuals (Goldstein, 1998). Therefore, as dental technology education providers, there is a distinct need to prepare graduates to consult with clinicians to meet the needs of the patient. Individuals expect to be able to change or alter their appearance (Rountree &

Davis, 2011) or they fear the facial changes that come with aging (Henderson-King & Henderson-King, 2005). Through the internet and World Wide Web, patients have access to more health care information and are often aware of the variety of treatment available world-wide (Donaldson et al., 2007; Harorli & Harorli, 2014). Whether, that particular approach of treatment is suitable for the patient or circumstance is arguable. None the less, patients will often seek out practitioners who can deliver aesthetic goals to match expectations, and not always close to home (Ahmad, 2010; Donaldson et al., 2007).

Globalization of the Dental Market and the Influence This Has on Education, Significance of Internationalization and Collaboration

The evolution of the internet and the various social networking platforms means the world is a much smaller place (Friedman, 2006). Combined with communication technology and improved shipping networks, access to medical devices and oral health care has spread to countries with lower labour costs (Avery, 2012). This popular trend is termed globalization which "is a broad term referring to the increasing connectivity, integration, and interdependence of economies, societies, technologies, cultures, and political and ecological spheres across the world (Donaldson et al., 2007p. 408). The Merriam-Webster (2017) online dictionary states that Globaliszation is "the development of an increasingly integrated global economy marked especially by free trade, free flow of capital, and the tapping of cheaper foreign labor markets" (https://www.merriam-webster.com/dictionary/globalization). Over the years, globalization of the dental professions has gained momentum in Australia, Norway, United States, and other developed countries whereby indirect dental restorations (oral prosthesis such as crowns and bridge) are manufactured in countries with lower labour costs (Avery, 2012; Zheng, Yue, Zhou, & Yu, 2013).

The consequence of globalization of the dental technology profession means more work is going off-shore to be completed by mostly unqualified dental technologists who operate on a production line and complete only one component of the process (Chaoyi, Liwei, Li, Min, & Haiyang, 2012). Often to lower standards using less qualified dental technologists (Chaoyi et al., 2012; Zheng et al., 2013), this initial outflow of work may not be sustainable and/or desirable. Consequently, education providers need to prepare graduates for these changes. In Australia and Norway, employers are seeking graduates with the knowledge and skills in digital processes who can organise work flow and communicate to provide the attention and services demanded by clinicians, specialists and patients.

Internationalization of Curricula and Transportability of Qualifications

Knight most recently defines internationalization as "the process of integrating an international, intercultural, or global dimension into the purpose, functions or delivery of postsecondary education" (2015, p.2). The elements, such as rationales, benefits, outcomes, participants, activities, and/or stakeholders may vary. The meaning or term 'internationalization', and connotations surrounding the use of the word, varies between academics, institutions and countries (Knight, 2008). The *Bradley Report* acknowledged the importance of international education as an export endeavor which "*increases Australia's skills base, greater global awareness among Australian graduates, increased international research collaboration and improved international business and diplomatic relationships*" (2008, p.213). However, in this chapter internationalization focusses on dental technology students gaining a global perspective so they can contribute to oral health care on an international platform rather than in isolation. This focus is perhaps in line with Sanderson's (2008) use of the term *"cosmopolitanism" which* seeks to expand the individual's personal and professional outlook with the goal of fostering acceptance of cultural differences, developing an appreciation of how personal and social worldviews develop and are upheld across cultures (Sanderson, 2008). It is proposed that where students are equipped with greater insight and understanding, students and staff are better equipped to function effectively across diverse cultural contexts, in other words, to become international or global citizens, capable of contributing in a range of contexts (Leask, 2009). Internationalization becomes a mechanism to increase knowledge transfer that enables opportunities to explore the role of different learning environments and context through the use of open *e-learning* which co-exists alongside the current curricula (Yang, 2002). Internationalization in this context aims to enrich the university experience and to lead to changes in knowledge, attitudes, and behaviours of all those involved in the learning process (Barker, 2011, p.4).

Paradigm of Dental Education

The General Assembly of the Association of Dental Education in Europe in 2010 urged dental schools around the globe to engage in e-learning' strategies to bring flexibility to curricula and share resources between institutions (Manogue et al., 2011). Two years earlier attempts were made to encourage dental educators to embrace the ideals of information technology to assist with education of dental students (Mattheos et al., 2008). However, dental education seems to be slow to reform and embrace new learning frameworks to enhance critical analysis through utilization of computer based and web based information technology (Buchanan, 2004; Donaldson et al., 2007). Or perhaps dental educators struggle with the "adoption of emerging technologies and the incorporation of these technologies into the educational process" (Stein, Eisenberg, O'Donnell, & Spallek, 2014, p.520). In contrast, Problem Based Learning (PBL) has been used frequently among dental schools and is reported to be 'enjoyable and nurturing' for students (Townsend & Winning, 2011). However, PBL has shown to have high financial costs of "implementation and maintenance, and a concern that students may not develop sufficient cognitive scaffolding in the basic sciences" (Townsend & Winning, 2011 p. 193). Although in the past, dental education on the whole has been slow to take up the inclusion of technology in education to share resources or promote collaboration (Donaldson et al., 2007), there has been more recent progress. Bridges and colleagues (2014) reviewed a blended digital learning approach and found that creating "online student learning communities through a blended approach to learning stimulated motivation and intellectual engagement" (p. 170). Another example is the Harvard School of Dental Medicine, which has adopted the "flipped classroom as a blended learning model in which students access foundational content online before class time, enabling the instructor to engage students in group discussions and educationally purposeful interactive and collaborative activities during class"(Park & Howell, 2015, p.563). Thereby, lower level learning on the Blooms taxonomy of cognition is achieved independently and higher level analysis and collaboration is experienced with guidance from the teaching team and peers (Anderson & Krathwohl, 2001). This appears to have synergies with IPL and creating communities of practice (Stephenson et al., 2016; Wenger, Dermott, & Snyder, 2002). Both of which are embedded in the Griffith dental technology curriculum (Evans, Henderson, & Johnson, 2010, 2012).

Recently, the digital application of prosthetic restorations has been trialed in a number of dental specialty curricula throughout the United States (Fernandez, Nimmo, & Behar-Horenstein, 2016; Reifeis et al., 2014) along with computer assisted learning/computer assisted simulation (CAL) (Kwon et al., 2015). "In the CAL/CAS framework digital evaluation and feedback are generated based on comparison of scanned student work to a scanned gold standard" (Kwon et al., 2015, p.1093). However, Kwon and colleagues (2015) concluded that technology-assisted learning did little to improve performance or self-evaluation skills. However, Rice and McKendree (2014) remind us of the following; "technologies are tools, not teachers" (p, 161). Rather,

[T]echnology has the potential to enhance learning but needs to be integrated into educational processes, related to learning aims and outcomes, connected to reflective practice and linked to learner needs and preferences. The technology itself should not be viewed in isolation. (Bullock & deJong, 2014, p. 149)

Although these studies have been applied to dentistry education, there is limited evidence to consider the inclusion of digital resources or learning in dental technology education throughout the world. There are only a small number of studies reporting on dental technology education world-wide, which provides an incentive for this international alliance to evolve.

INTERNATIONAL COLLABORATION EMBRACING PICA AND WIL MODELS

Internationalization of the curricula that leads to shared resources goes through a variety of stages. As described in the early section of this chapter, it is essential to develop a cohesive partnership with collaborators. The following three stages have been used to establish the collaboration in this project (Figure 1).

- **Establishment Phase:**
    - Finding suitable collaborators.
    - Mapping curricula (relevance, purpose, blended learning, WIL assessment consistency, constructive alignment and other relevant areas of interest to the collaborators and stakeholder groups).
    - Congruence (equivalence) and a willingness to change and adapt.
- **Shared Goals:** Program learning outcomes and graduate capabilities.
- **Focused Outcome:** Requirements, sharing digital resources, student/staff exchange, WIL

A collaboration between international academic partners requires shared goals and intentions. Individuals' contribution, commitment and dedication to group goals enables good collaboration, if there is a willingness to evolve and change

Figure 1. Framework for international collaborations

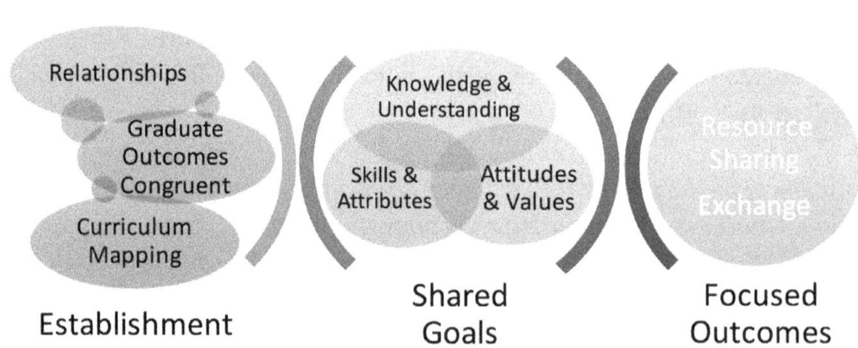

through the process. Program outcomes need to be consistent or capable of achieving congruence and consistency. Assessment moderation and calibration is essential to establish early in the process, as it is known that assessment motivates students' learning (Newble & Jaeger, 1983). Joint and digitally supported blended courses may improve international cooperation in the academic field. New tools, techniques and behaviors in this field require efficient learning and teaching methods. The e-learning dimension is not only limited to learning skills. E-learning challenges the educational thinking and practices in many dimensions and in different areas.

Planned Framework

- Develop structured processes for simultaneous internationalization.
- Develop and publish courses in the blended mode which support online and in-situ/same-time (streamed) and time-shifted venues for international cooperation in education using a blended mode/flipped classroom approach.
- Develop and describe efficient production models for joint development of multi-linguistic online teaching and learning resources (learning outcome consistent, digital resources and textbooks).
- Lay the foundation for interchangeable courses and affiliated degrees.

Integration of Electronic Resources in Learning and Teaching

Through international collaboration and aspirations to improve student engagement, augment critical thinking opportunities and increase employability rates, the authors embraced the notion of the 'flipped' classroom as a mechanism to achieve these goals. With an international collaboration and student exchange program already in place, it was logical to continue to develop shared digital resources to support student learning and transition.

The global institutions of higher education have developed within disparate contexts for several decades or more. They are not naturally aligned to each other's 'modus operandi'. When they exchange students, the transaction costs therefore tend to be high. This is the case not only for the institutions as such, but also for students. Therefore, joint and digitally supported blended courses may ameliorate this situation. A substantial part of the work happens in time-shifted mode with pre-made online courses and real-time face-to-face sessions. The latter is partly organized at localized venues in seminar and workshops and partly as virtual online seminars. (Høivik, 2016)

Digital Resources in Regard to This Project

The term digital resources in this chapter specifically focuses on audio visual learning used in conjunction with open source learning management systems or local online learning management systems. This topic is covered in other chapters so will not be elaborated on here, but rather provide some guidance to what audio visual learning entails – the following taken from the seminal text An Encyclopedia of the Science of Learning (Seel, 2011) provides a comprehensive description.

Audio-visual (AV) learning is a type of learning which is described by delivery and the use of instructional content that involves sound (auditory stimuli) and sight (visual stimuli). AV learning takes place when the instructional process is accompanied by AV learning aids such as handouts, flip charts, transparencies, whiteboards, illustrations, still and motion pictures, slide shows, television, videos, audiotapes, records, projectors, computer graphics, multimedia, physical objects, and 3D models. AV learning can appear when an instructor's verbal presentation is reinforced with a series of images or slides or as a self-standing instructional practice consisting of an instructional movie or virtual reality simulation. (Podolskiy, 2012, p.384)

Flipped Classroom Project: Applying the PICA Model

Design of a flipped classroom module comprises four key elements: presentation, interaction, collaboration and analysis. Designed somewhat differently than traditional courses, the modules are designed and inspired from MOOC's (massive open online courses). The modules are primarily characterized by participation and engagement opportunities for students. Furthermore, they are characterized by their flexible nature and open source availability, offering a range of digital learning resources from videos to traditional scientific articles, that optimally become publically available. However in the Australian and Norwegian context, consideration needs to be given to copyright laws. An integral component of the project is the practical use and testing of digital approaches and online activities as learning methods. This project aims to customize courses and workshops related to the profession. Online learning portfolios can store a collection of students' completed projects to assist them in providing evidence for employers. Meta data generated from online student participation will be generated automatically through Open Edx,(https://www.edx.org/) including: time spent reviewing videos, clicks, use of the digital resources and number of attempt at quizzes or self-tests. Together with real-time meetings and interviews with/between students or student groups, analysis will be made to improve the module of study and provide academics with an overview of the status and learning outcomes achieved by students.

Eventually the emphasis will be created around a specific patient cases to enhance authenticity and engagement of students. A complete module will be developed to include the following items:

- Presentation of materials (texts, videos, animations, slideshows).
- Interaction in pedagogically planned activities (quizzes, self-tests, reflection).
- Collaboration through real time social interactions (dynamic face-to-face workshops, events, practicum, use of social media, international exchange and comparative investigation).
- Analysis and collection of metadata (for teachers and research use).

A Trial in Dental Technology: Description of the 2016 Experience of a Student Led Digital Learning Project

In 2016, four dental technology exchange students from Griffith participated in the prosthetics course at HiOA from January to June. During this time, the students were exposed to WIL opportunities through external placements and onsite learning and practice. All students were provided with the theoretical material for the course, and were assigned an academic teacher to coach and mentor them to stimulate learning (Bergmann & Sams, 2013). Together with the assigned teacher and the production team, the exchange students collaborated to plan, design, and finally develop a video suitable for education in fixed prosthetics across the dental technology programs. During the planning phase the group cohesively discussed content and main focus areas, highlighting particular sections in the production process to promote learning. When students collaborated with the teacher in this way they displayed a deeper understanding and knowledge of the themes and appeared to consider the practical process more pragmatically. The students prepared the stages of the procedures to be filmed over two weeks to ensure succinct delivery. They selected appropriate phases that would maximize participant's interest. During the project, students were extremely focused on the varying stages and were determined to achieve a high level of accuracy and precision. The film was designed to be only 3-7 minutes, as student attention declines after 10 minutes (Hartley & Cameron, 1967; MacManaway, 1970), and the transcript and voice-over was produced in English and Norwegian. This was a pilot exercise for use in e-learning sessions as part of the advancement to the flipped classroom model. The audiovisual material will continue to be part of the presentation material in the four-item unit (presentational materials; texts, videos, animations, slideshows). The audiovisual can be viewed at: https://www.youtube.com/watch?v=bdTrdHdhaz8&list=PLgTQSl0KxseqiduFWNc5eP2YQ4-H1DQi7&index=1

The first key element in the flipped classroom concept is the presentation of a theme. This could be done through digital resources such as audiovisual learning materials, which is accompanied by a digital interactive learning manual, an e-book, and/or specific literature for the students to read prior to viewing the audiovisual. It is essential for the teaching team to provide prompts throughout to guide and direct students' 'self-study'. The second key element is the pedagogically planned interaction. What activity will the students interact with to enhance their level of understanding and synthesis of learning material? It may be centered around measurable activities (assessment) that promote learning and require student to move from novice to expert over time, or at least, from knowing to doing (Miller, 1990). It requires questions or activities that challenge students' thinking and highlight the most important aspects of the presentation (audiovisual) that relates to common themes. If electronic quizzes are used, detailed preparation is essential to guide and invigorate pedagogically programmed interaction (PPI). The third key element requires 'real time' social interaction and may be the most critical to reinforce learning (Hoivik, Cong, Haihuang, & Xiaochun, 2015). Increasing teacher-student and student-student contact is ideal best practice in higher education (Chickering & Gamson, 1997). The digital module alone will not provide the desired learning outcomes or influence, therefore a face-to-face interaction with the teacher and other students is required (Chickering & Ehrmann, 1986; Rice & McKendree, 2014). Therefore, after taking part in the online e-learning material by studying the advised literature, reading the recommended readings in the flipped classroom module, viewing the video and completing the self-test, students join the teaching team on campus. Seminars or group-meetings at this stage gain the full attention of all participants. Experiences from HiOA revealed that students have acquired background knowledge and are ready to engage in deeper learning, resulting in constructive discussions for all members. At this point, there is often a need for an activity, dynamic workshop or practicums to reinforce the learning. The forth, and final key element analysis, is imperative for teachers and researchers to delve behind the assessment scores or results to see what students really do with the digital learning material during the duration of the module. Exploring the meta data behind students' online engagement in the module will provide insights into their e-learning habits (time spent on task, activity across days, preparedness and common faults). From this point, the teaching team has the opportunity to reflect on the four elements in the module and formulate changes to increase student participation, engagement, experience and learning.

To embrace the ideals of internationalization 'at home', students from HiOA and Griffith will complete the same first and second elements and then complete the third element through an online discussions or blog posts. Using active learning like this can develop a deeper understanding for the themes. Blended learning, combining online and face-to-face teaching, is the most common approach to e-learning in

undergraduate medical education (Rice & McKendree, 2014) and is certainly appropriate for dental technology education. The flipped classroom approach compels students to be more active, and well-designed learning activities generate better understanding and increase student performance (Freeman et al., 2014).

Work Integrated Learning Ideals

Work integrated learning (WIL), from Groenwalds' (2004) point of view is "a structured strategy integrating classroom studies with learning through productive work experiences in a field related to a student's academic or career goals" (p.17). WIL relates to the explicit development of skills and capabilities within the professional context and relies on positive experiences and interactions (Cooper, Orrell, & Bowden, 2010). WIL is woven throughout both Oslo and Griffith curricula and occurs on and off campus whereby students integrate academic and practical knowledge to achieve authentic work-based learning in a work based context (Lanning, Wetzel, Baines, & Byrne, 2012). Students' success in WIL is often dependent on their engagement with the theoretical and contextual knowledge that underpins the profession. Criterion referenced assessment for all procedures were established with National and Internationally stakeholders (Myhrer et al., 2015). The Criterion referenced assessment is used to compare the individual's performance with specified principles and standards (Brown & Knight, 1994). Academics, examiners, and markers use the criteria as a framework to provide constructive verbal and written feedback, to acknowledge areas of success and recommend improvements (Nicol, 2010). Students utilize the criteria, initially, to evaluate their progress on simulated cases, and then finally, in authentic patient cases. The ideals of WIL appear to have congruence with the flipped classroom approach. WIL is known to develop students' professional identity (Campbell, Herrington, & Verenikina, 2009), provide genuine opportunity for reflection and transformation (Billett, 2010) and promote work readiness (Murphy & Calway, 2008). Anecdotal evidence from employers of Oslo and Griffith dental technology graduates have been positive, and the majority of graduates are sought by employers upon graduation.

WIL Opportunities During a Student Exchange

A common theme around the dental technology programs at HiOA and Griffith is the inclusion of Work Integrated Learning (WIL), albeit, to varying degrees (Myhrer et al., 2015). The inclusion of WIL seeks to develop skills and capabilities in an authentic learning environment to enhance formal learning and productive practice (Cooper et al., 2010) with the intention that graduates are capable and ready for the world of work. The HiOA program provides an opportunity for students on exchange to attend a dental laboratory one day per week during the spring semester. In 2016, four final year Griffith exchange students learnt contemporary practices in fixed prosthetics along-side suitable qualified professionals. Students were exposed to varying business models and complexity of cases that differed from those previously experienced. Students created reflective case studies that displayed enhanced scholarship and practical application of skills. Although the context was different from what students were familiar with, their confidence and skills grew.

In 2017, a HiOA exchange student will experience a 12-week trimester of WIL on campus at Griffith. Along with final dental technology students, they collaborate with dentistry and dental prosthetists students in Team Based Treatment Planning (TBTP), whereby students learn teamwork, peer learning and evidence-based treatment planning strategies (Storrs, Alexander, Sun, Kroon, & Evans, 2015). Students cooperate on specific cases and provide comprehensive treatment for patients under their care. This is part of a Capstone experience (Professional Practice), whereby students integrate the knowledge and skills gained over the past five semesters into a final semester course (Holdsworth, Watty, & Davies, 2009). By integrating and applying knowledge and skills gained earlier in the program, it provides students with a ‘safe environment’ (Lee, 2013) to complete patient cases with support from the teaching team. Although this experience is on-campus, the work flow is similar to that of a commercial dental laboratory albeit on a larger scale and the teaching team includes practitioners from local laboratories.

Despite the differing WIL experiences, both complement the other and act as an incentive for future exchange opportunities. Both revolve around ‘real-time’ ‘real-life’ authentic learning scenarios which enhance teamwork and collaboration (Evans et al., 2012). In future, a formal buddy system in the host University will provide practical guidance and support to the exchange student.

Technology an Imperative for Dental Technologists’ Employability

Due to the continued advancement of CAD/CAM technologies and 3D printing, dentistry is no longer a static profession. Rather, it is in a period of significant change, many procedures can be completed using digital technology, and for those not using digital technology there is a machine that is equally as complex to operate (Miyazaki et al., 2009). It is envisaged that advancements will continue into the future and thus require modification to dental education to embrace interactive learning strategies (van der Zande et al., 2013). Consequently, graduating dentists and dental technologists will be required to adapt to the current digital changes in order to maintain efficiency and productivity in professional practice (Reifeis et al., 2014). It is therefore expected that the current dental curricula should enable the current and future generations of dental professionals with the techniques and knowledge for preparedness in the digital era.

Employability has been recognized as a measure of the success of higher education (Stwine & Alves, 2010). Employability skills have been defined as "a set of achievements, understandings and personal attributes that make individuals more likely to gain employment and be successful in their chosen occupations" (Knight & Yorke, 2004, p.22). There is limited evidence surrounding the dental technology graduates' employability or readiness to practice. Dental Technology programs of study require students to perform, within the laboratory setting, the range of dental technology procedures based on artistry, sound scientific evidence, and ethical practice. Students and graduates need to exhibit the skills, professional attitudes and behaviors required to facilitate effective and appropriate interaction with members of the dental care team. Registration authorities and employers expect dental technology graduates to be adequately prepared for their role, act in a professional manner, display adequate technical and organizational skills and a comprehensive knowledge base with skills across all parameters of oral prosthetics including digital applications.

The HiOA and Griffith dental technology programs focus on craftsmanship and technological expertise; and rely on a combination of theoretical knowledge and critical thinking to develop sense of design and colour. With the global economically changes, employers of dental technology graduates no longer have time or resources to provide 'on-the-job-training'. Dental Technologists must be prepared for the world of work on graduation: mentally and physically. The dental technologists will more than likely be required to make decisions about material selection and design that are legally assigned or the responsibility of the dentist (Carr & Brown, 2011). However, communication and teamwork between the dentist and dental technologists remains far from ideal (Berry, Nesbit, Saberi, & Petridis, 2014; Berry, Nesbit, Saeri, & Petridis, 2014). This means it is even more important to ensure dental technology graduates are ready for the responsibilities that they face in contemporary work places. However, there also needs to be an awareness around what is an acceptable standard for a graduate.

There are a variety of views concerning dentistry graduates' readiness to practice, particularly around prosthetics (Arena, Kruger, Holley, Millar, & Tennant, 2007; Brand, Kamell, Kharbanda, & Dozic, 2013). However there is an overarching acceptance that the graduate is perceived as a '*safe beginner*' (Ali, Tredwin, Kay, Slade, & Pooler, 2014), so maybe dental technology graduates could be viewed similarly. For example, dentistry graduates are viewed as:

... 'safe beginners', capable of carrying out patient assessment and treatment planning, perform routine, straightforward dental procedures safely, provide holistic care,

communicate effectively, demonstrate professionalism and team-working skills, recognize their limits and know when to seek help. (Ali et al., 2014)

Similarly, dental technology graduates may need to be viewed as a:

...*greenhorn artist*, [inexperienced artist] capable of functioning efficiently as part of the oral health care team to design and safely fabricate a variety of routine prosthetic cases as prescribed by clinicians, communicate effectively, demonstrate professionalism and team work skills, recognize their limitations and seek guidance when needed as shown in Figure 2.

Issues, Controversies, Problems

There is no doubt that developing a collaborative partnership to 'internationalize' dental technology curricula and share digital resources is not without its challenges. There are no suitable models to replicate nor is there one suitable system to adopt. Both institutions vary in terms of cultural perspectives, funding, functioning and accessing resources. Differing online platforms are advocated at each location and access to different networks varies. In an already busy work schedule academics

Figure 2. Proposed key attributes of dental technology graduate preparedness (Adapted from Ali et al., 2014)

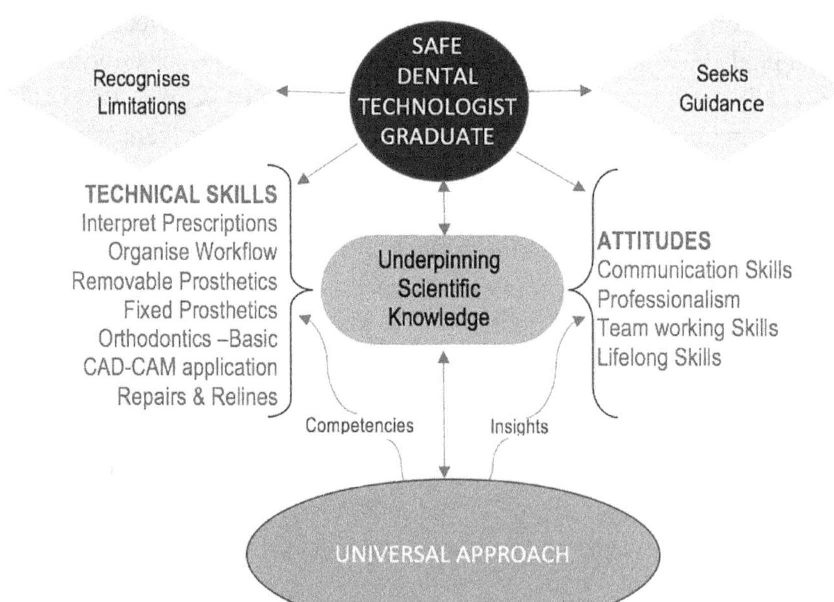

and teaching teams struggle to find the time for preparation and development of resources. Copyright laws and sharing resources between institutions varies broadly which often stifles the project.

Globalization has changed the way dental technologists function (Avery, 2012). A more dynamic approach is needed to meet the needs of the clinicians and public. Therefore, graduates need to be prepared for the fluctuating nuances of the profession. Dental technology education needs to respond to these changes. Inclusion of CAD CAM and 3D printing are now essential components, no longer a luxury. Rather they are a core element of the curriculum. Although both institutions have embraced technology in prosthetic production, not all academics and teaching teams are fluent and responsive to the change. Some lack the specialist knowledge and skills to teach the specific digital techniques. Likewise, the CAD/CAM equipment between universities differs, where one system is open and the other uses a network restricting resource sharing. This becomes problematic when aiming to share digital prosthetic cases.

Logistics and planning of an international collaboration has many challenges, such as time zone differences, language constraints and distance between locations. Similarly, the responsibilities of collaborators need to be explicitly planned and coordinated to ensure all team members are responsive to the project. Coordination of what, when, how and where needs to be considered. If not, then what is actually achievable may differ from the perception of the collaborators.

Preparing the pilot video demonstrated that planning, designing and producing audio visual resources requires time and resources. However, students' learning increases when they are directly involved in the process. The advantages were twofold. It not only deepened current students' knowledge but provided learning resources appropriate for future students of dental technology. Although, to date, the pilot has not proceeded past this stage, the intention is to continue with it into the flipped classroom unit. It is also envisaged that the inclusion of subtitles will improve access to students and allow it to be played as students are practicing technical skills in the prosthetic laboratory.

Although there are several issues and complexities to deal with, the awareness of these areas helps the project evolve. The collaboration will continue to grow and discover solutions so that students have a positive learning experience that leads to employment.

SOLUTIONS AND RECOMMENDATIONS

The preceding section focused on the issues and problems that emerge from an international collaboration and sharing of electronic resources. This section counters that view point with some useful solutions and suggestions to progress the project. Consideration was given earlier to the PICA model for designing the flipped classroom module. Particular attention was given to the third element, collaboration, as being critical for success. Collaboration through social interaction, face-to-face discussions and engagement not only enhances the flipped classroom but strengthens the connectedness and alliance of the project team. Staff international exchanges bring opportunities to revitalize teaching methods and scholarly endeavors. Face to face cooperation is essential to establish the foundations for a successful collaboration. However, it also requires consistent revision of expectations to ensure there are no misunderstandings. Ideally the individual collaborators goals and values around work practices, curricula, resources and assessment are similar so the overarching direction is clear. The institutional nuances may differ but the intent of the individuals is clear and they can adapt to the different contexts to meet specific requirements.

Fundamentally the inclusion of others in the project will aim to enhance the longevity of the project and share responsibilities and outcomes. Not only does engagement with others spread the workload, it has the potential to bring a range of specialties in specific areas. Not only profession specific members need be involved, but also education designers, blended learning advisors, production crews and external professionals. This would not only bring specialized expertise but it could potentially bring a broad perspective.

It appears that digital resources are easy to develop and share online all over the world. Voice-over techniques can be applied to videos to prepare audiovisual resources for a variety of languages. Similarly, subtitles can be added in both English and Norwegian languages to reduce the need for sound and/or reiterate the spoken word. Not everything needs to be perfect to work. Partners from different countries can work collaboratively to develop joint online courses and can use the product as 'internationalization at home', or to encourage student and teacher exchanges.

In future, a formal buddy system in the host University will provide practical guidance and support to the exchange student. However, the more shared digital resources that are used between the institutions the more familiar the student is likely to feel in the learning environment and with the teaching team. Equally, the teaching team need to engage formally with their local profession to ensure curriculum is meeting market demands. Engagement with the profession brings opportunities for WIL and thus enhances the curriculum and opportunities for graduates in terms of employment.

The ongoing collaboration and aspiration to continually improve means solutions will always be found. Consequently, the opportunities for research are vast. It is only limited by the logistics and tight daily time schedules.

FUTURE RESEARCH DIRECTIONS

From this chapter, it is clear to see that limited attention has previously focused on researching into dental technology education, let alone the inclusion of digital technology to promote learning or internationalization. However, with the emerging global trend of digital prosthetics and the continued commitment to collaboration, this project will transform over time, as it has since 2011. Commencing with a project to moderate assessment, it is evident that the dedication to collaborate and research is strong and there are clear aims to focus on. Although time lines are yet to be established for this project, the PICA framework provides some guiding principles to direct the project. Therefore, the team will continue to create digital resources that can be shared and find opportunities for face to face engagement. Sometimes it is not the outcome but the 'journey' where the learning and experiences emerge.

There are several opportunities to engage in formal research around the project, however first the team will need to monitor and evaluate the project and outcomes relating to the curricula. Through a deeper analysis of students' experiences of the flipped classroom, there will be evidence to maintain or adjust the project as needed. A pre-and-post survey with students enrolled in the flipped classroom module could be completed to ascertain cognition and interactions. These findings would provide conclusive evidence which is currently lacking (O'Flaherty & Phillips, 2015).

For a protracted analysis of the inclusion of the flipped classroom, a longitudinal case study of students/staff who take part in the international exchange would be worthwhile for tracking their employment and occupational experiences. Similarly, an evaluation of employment outcomes for exchange students verse non-exchange students could be applied over a shorter time frame. Therefore, there is plenty of scope across the project.

CONCLUSION

The paradigm of learning and teaching, in dental technology, as a didactic teacher driven process in static surroundings has no doubt been transformed in the two institutions. The broader focus is on student engagement in learning and directed towards employment. Employment for the digital era and to cope with the added responsibilities and demands. Internationalization has contributed to the continued advancement between HiOA and Griffith, by providing opportunities to not only benchmark curriculum, moderate assessment but to share digital resources. Through the development of a flipped classroom module, a systematic process was created and evaluated for continued development. The flipped classroom project has evolved into a formidable venture that is already leading to flexible delivery and transferable qualifications between our institutions. The exchange program has offered rich opportunities beyond that of dental technology, however requires further research to draw such conclusions. It appears that this is the beginning of the next phase to enhance students' experiences and strengthen collaboration.

Although this chapter is centered around the field of dental technology there are synergies with other professional programs, such as Nursing, Allied Health or even Engineering. Processes and phases of curricula and learning may be consistent across programs. However, attitudes, values and beliefs may differ between academics, teaching teams and students. Establishing robust partnerships with like-minded academics is based on shared values and beliefs which provides stable foundations from which to collaborate.

ACKNOWLEDGMENT

This project was partially supported by the International Joint Course Development (IN:Code) Project, HiOA. We are grateful for the contribution and inspiration provided by Professor Helge Høivik. Our thanks extend to the students who participated enthusiastically in this project. We are thankful to our colleagues for their commitment and contribution to dental technologists' education. We also appreciate the continued support and assistance from production teams and blended learning advisors and are grateful to those who assisted with editing and moderation of this paper.

REFERENCES

Ahmad, I. (2010). Risk management in clinical practice. Part 5. Ethical considerations for dental enhancement procedures. *British Dental Journal*, *209*(5), 207–214. doi:10.1038/sj.bdj.2010.769 PMID:20829856

Ali, K., Tredwin, C., Kay, E. J., Slade, A., & Pooler, J. (2014). Preparedness of dental graduates for foundation training: A qualitative study. *British Dental Journal*, *217*(3), 145–149. doi:10.1038/sj.bdj.2014.648 PMID:25104700

Anderson, L. W., & Krathwohl, D. R. (Eds.). (2001). *A taxonomy for teaching, learning and assessing: A revision of Bloom's taxonomy of educational objectives*. New York: Longman.

Arena, G., Kruger, E., Holley, D., Millar, S., & Tennant, M. (2007). Western Australian dental graduates' perceptions of preparedness to practice: A five-year follow-up. *Journal of Dental Education, 71*(9), 1217–1222. PMID:17761629

Avery, D. (2012). The globalization of the dental laboratory industry. *Journal of Esthetic and Restorative Dentistry, 24*(2), 79–82. doi:10.1111/j.1708-8240.2012.00507.x PMID:22524712

Barker, M. (2011). *The GIHE Good Practice Guide to Internationalising the Curriculum*. Retrieved from https://www.griffith.edu.au/__data/assets/pdf_file/0006/345291/Internationalising-the-Curriculum.pdf

Bergmann, J., & Sams, A. (2013). Flip your students' learning. *Educational Leadership, 70*(6), 16–20.

Berry, J., Nesbit, M., Saberi, S., & Petridis, H. (2014). Communication methods & production techniques in fixed prosthodontics fabrication: A UK based survey. Part 2: Production techniques. *British Dental Journal, 217*(6), E13. doi:10.1038/sj.bdj.2014.644 PMID:25257017

Berry, J., Nesbit, M., Saeri, S., & Petridis, H. (2014). Communication methods and production techniques in fixed prosthesis fabrication: A UK based survey. Part 1: Communication methods. *British Dental Journal, 217*(6 (E12)). doi:10.1038/sj.bdj.2014.643

Billett, S. (Ed.). (2010). *Learning Through Practice*. Dordrecht, The Netherlands: Springer. doi:10.1007/978-90-481-3939-2

Bradley, D., Noonan, P., Nugent, H., & Scales, B. (2008). *Review of higher education: Final report*. Retrieved from http://www.voced.edu.au/content/ngv%3A32134

Brand, H. S., Kamell, H., Kharbanda, A. K., & Dozic, A. (2013). Students' Perceptions of Materials and Techniques Used at European Dental Schools in the Education of Fixed Prosthodontics. *Journal of Dental Education, 77*(9), 1140–1146. PMID:24002851

Bridges, S., Chang, J. W. W. W., Chu, C. H., & Gardener, K. (2014). Blended learning in situated contexts: 3-year evaluation of an online peer review project. *European Journal of Dental Education, 18*(3), 170–179. doi:10.1111/eje.12082 PMID:24460682

Brown, S., & Knight, P. (1994). *Assessing learning in higher education*. London: Kogan Page.

Buchanan, J. A. (2004). Use of simulation technology in dental education. *Journal of Dental Education, 68*(12), 1258–1265. PMID:15576814

Bullock, A., & deJong, P. G. (2014). Technology-enhanced learning. In T. Swanwick (Ed.), *Understanding medical education: Evidence, theory and practice* (2nd ed.; pp. 149–160). Oxford, UK: John Wiley & Sons.

Campbell, M., Herrington, A., & Verenikina, I. (2009). Journeying from college to work: The changing identity of early-career policep. *The Journal of Cooperative Education and Internships, 43*(1), 55–64.

Carr, A. B., & Brown, D. T. (2011). Work authorizations for removable partial dentures. In A. B. Carr & D. T. Brown (Eds.), *McCracken's removable partial prosthodontics* (12th ed.; pp. 284–288). St. Louis, MO: Mosby. doi:10.1016/B978-0-323-06990-8.00019-1

Chaoyi, M., Liwei, Z., Li, Y., Min, Z., & Haiyang, Y. (2012). Current status, crisis and trends in Chinese dental technicians. *International Dental Journal, 62*(2), 79–83. doi:10.1111/j.1875-595X.2011.00093.x PMID:22420476

Chickering, A. W., & Ehrmann, S. (1986). *Implementing the seven prinicples: Technology as a lever.* American Association of Higher Education. Retrieved from https://case.edu/ucite/media/caseedu/ucite/documents/seven_principles.pdf

Chickering, A. W., & Gamson, Z. F. (1997). Seven prinicples of good practice in undergraduate education. *AAHE Bulletin*, 3–7. Retrieved from https://eric.ed.gov/?id=ED282491

Cooper, L., Orrell, J., & Bowden, M. (2010). *Work-integrated Learning: A guide to effective practice*. New York: Taylor and Francis.

Donaldson, M. E., Gadbury-Amyot, C. C., Khajotia, S. S., Natterstad, A., Norton, N., Zubiaurre, L. A., & Turner, S. P. (2007). Dental education in a flat world: Advocating for increased global collaboration and standardization. *Journal of Dental Education, 72*(4), 408–421. PMID:18381847

Evans, J. L., Henderson, A., Haugen, H., Myhrer, T., Nordin-Ivanow, K., Maryan, C., & Johnson, N. W. et al. (2015). The value of interprofessional education: A comparative study of dental technology students' perceptions across four countries. *British Dental Journal, 218*(8), 481–487. doi:10.1038/sj.bdj.2015.296 PMID:25908364

Evans, J. L., Henderson, A. J., & Johnson, N. W. (2010). The future of education and training in dental technology: Designing a dental curriculum that facilitates teamwork across the oral health professions. *British Dental Journal*, *208*(5), 227–230. doi:10.1038/sj.bdj.2010.208 PMID:20228758

Evans, J. L., Henderson, A. J., & Johnson, N. W. (2012). Interprofessional learning enhances knowledge of roles but is less able to shift attitudes: A case study from dental education. *European Journal of Dental Education*, *16*(4), 239–245. doi:10.1111/j.1600-0579.2012.00749.x PMID:23050506

Fernandez, M., Nimmo, A., & Behar-Horenstein, L. (2016). Digital denture fabrication in pre- and postdoctoral education: A Survey of U.S. dental schools. *Journal of Prosthodontics*, *25*(1), 83–90. doi:10.1111/jopr.12287 PMID:26098406

Freeman, S., Eddy, S. L., McDonough, M., Smith, M. K., Okoroafor, N., Jordt, H., & Wenderoth, M. P. (2014). Active learning increases student performance in science, engineering, and mathematics. *Proceedings of the National Academy of Sciences of the United States of America*, *111*(23), 8410–8415. doi:10.1073/pnas.1319030111 PMID:24821756

Friedman, T. L. (2006). *The world is flat: a brief history of the twenty first century*. New York: Farrar, Straus & Giroux.

Goldstein, R. E. (1998). *Esthetics in Dentistry* (2nd ed.). Ontario, Canada: D C Decker.

Groenewald, T. (2004). Toward a Definition for Cooperative Education. In R. K. Coll & C. Eames (Eds.), International Handbook for Cooperative Education: An International Perspective of the Theory, Research, and Practice of Work-Integrated Learning (pp. 17-25). Boston: World Association for Cooperative Education.

Harorli, O., & Harorli, H. E. (2014). Evaluation of internet search trends of some common oral problems, 2004 to 2014. *Community Dental Health*, *31*, 188–192. PMID:25300156

Hartley, J., & Cameron, A. (1967). Some observations on the effeciency of lecturing. *Educational Review*, *20*(1), 30–37. doi:10.1080/0013191670200103

Henderson-King, D., & Henderson-King, E. (2005). Acceptance of cosmetic surgery: Scale development and validation. *Body Image*, *2*(2), 137–149. doi:10.1016/j.bodyim.2005.03.003 PMID:18089182

Høivik, H. (2016). *Introduction to the IN:Code Project 2016-2017*. Paper presented at the International Joint Course Development (IN:Code) Oslo and Akershus University of Applied Sciences, Norway.

Hoivik, H., Cong, J. B., Haihuang, F., & Xiaochun, W. (2015). Teaching and learning in the digital age. In H. Holvik (Ed.), *Experiential approaches to learning design in Norway and China* (pp. s107–s128). Capital Normal University Press.

Holdsworth, A., Watty, K., & Davies, M. (2009). *Developing capstone experiences*. Melbourne Centre for Study of Higher Education, University of Melbourne.

Knight, J. (2008). The internationalization of higher education: Are we on the right track? *Academic Matters: The Journal of Higher Education*, *52*, 5–9.

Knight, J. (2015). Updated internationalisation definition. *Industry and Higher Education*, *33*, 2–3.

Knight, P., & Yorke, M. (2004). *Learning, curriculum and employability in higher education*. London: Routledge.

Kwon, S. R., Hernández, M., Blanchette, D. R., Lam, M. T., Gratton, D. G., & Aquilino, S. A. (2015). Effect of computer-assisted learning on students' dental anatomy waxing performance. *Journal of Dental Education*, *79*(9), 1093–1100. PMID:26329034

Lanning, S. K., Wetzel, A. P., Baines, M., & Byrne, B. E. (2012). Evaluation of a revised curriculum: A four year qualitative study of student perceptions. *Journal of Dental Education*, *76*(10), 1323–1333. PMID:23066131

Leask, B. (2009). Using formal and informal curricula to improve interactions between home and international students. *Journal of Studies in International Education*, *13*(2), 205–221. doi:10.1177/1028315308329786

Lee, N. (2013). *Learning to fly: Capstones and the transformation of student experience*. Paper presented at the Griffith University Learning and Teaching Conference: Capstones: The time is now! Brisbane, Australia.

MacManaway, L. A. (1970). Teaching methods in higher educaion - innovation and research. *Higher Education Quarterly*, *24*(3), 321–329. doi:10.1111/j.1468-2273.1970.tb00346.x

Manogue, M., McLoughlin, J., Christensen, C., Delap, E., Lindh, C., Schoonheim-Klein, M., & Plasschaert, A. (2011). Curriculum structure, content, learning and assessment in Euorpean undergraduate dental education - update 2010. *European Journal of Dental Education*, *15*(3), 133–141. doi:10.1111/j.1600-0579.2011.00699.x PMID:21762317

Mattheos, N., Stefanovic, N., Apse, P., Attstrom, R., Buchanan, J., Brown, P., & Walmsley, A. D. et al. (2008). Potential of information technology in dental education. *European Journal of Dental Education*, *12*(s1S1), 85–91. doi:10.1111/j.1600-0579.2007.00483.x PMID:18289271

Merriam-Webster On-line Dictionary. (2017). *Globalization*. Retrieved from https://www.merriam-webster.com/dictionary/globalization

Miller, G. E. (1990). The assessment of clinical skills/competence/performance. *Journal of Academic Medicine*, *65*(9), S63–S67. doi:10.1097/00001888-199009000-00045 PMID:2400509

Miyazaki, T., Hotta, Y., Kunii, J., Kuriyama, S., & Tamaki, Y. (2009). A review of dental CAD/CAM: Current status and future perspectives from 20 years ofexperience. *Dental Materials Journal*, *28*(1), 44–56. doi:10.4012/dmj.28.44 PMID:19280967

Murphy, G., & Calway, B. (2008). Professional development for professional: Beyond sufficiency learning. *Australian Journal of Adult Learning*, *48*(3), 424–444.

Myhrer, T., Evans, J. L., Haugen, H., Gorman, C., Kavanagh, Y., & Cameron, A. (2015). Exploring the consistency, transparency and portability of dental technology education: Benchmarking across Norway, Ireland and Australia. *European Journal of Dental Education*. doi:10.1111/eje.12160 PMID:26147858

Newble, D. I., & Jaeger, K. (1983). The effect of assessments and examinations on the learning of medical students. *Medical Education*, *17*(3), 165–171. doi:10.1111/j.1365-2923.1983.tb00657.x PMID:6865814

Nicol, D. (2010). Improving written feedback processes in mass higher education. *Assessment in Higher Education*, *35*(5), 501–517. doi:10.1080/02602931003786559

O'Flaherty, J., & Phillips, C. (2015). The use of flipped classrooms in higher education: A scoping review. *Internet and Higher Education*, *25*, 85–95. doi:10.1016/j.iheduc.2015.02.002

Park, S. E., & Howell, T. H. (2015). Implemenation of a flipped classroom educational model in a predoctoral dental course. *Journal of Dental Education*, *79*(5), 563–570. PMID:25941150

Podolskiy, O. (2012). Audio-visual (AV) learning. In N. Seel (Ed.), *Encyclopedia of the Sciences of Learning* (pp. 384–386). New York: Springer.

Reifeis, P. E., Kirkup, M. L., Willis, L. H., & Browning, W. D. (2014). Introducing CAD/CAM into a predoctoral dental curriculum: A case study. *Journal of Dental Education, 78*(10), 1432–1441. PMID:25281677

Rice, S., & McKendree, J. (2014). e-learning. In T. Swanwick (Ed.), Understanding medical education: Evidence, theory and practice (2nd ed.; pp. 161-173). Oxford, UK: Wiley & Sons.

Rountree, M. L., & Davis, L. (2011). A dimensional qualitative research approach to understanding medically unnecessary aesthetic surgery. *Psychology and Marketing, 28*(10), 1027–1043. doi:10.1002/mar.20426

Sanderson, G. (2008). A foundation for the Internationalization of the academic self. *Journal of Studies in International Education, 12*(3), 276–307. doi:10.1177/1028315307299420

Seel, N. M. (Ed.). (2011). *Encyclopedia of the Sciences of Learning*. New York: Springer.

Stein, C. D., Eisenberg, E. S., O'Donnell, J. A., & Spallek, H. (2014). What dental educators need to understand about emerging technologies to incorporate them effectively into the educational process. *Journal of Dental Education, 78*(4), 520–529. PMID:24706681

Stephenson, C. R., Wang, A. T., Szostek, J. H., Bonnes, S. L., Ratelle, J. T., Mahapatra, S., & Wittich, C. M. et al. (2016). Flipping the continuing medical education classroom: Validating a measure of attendees' perceptions. *The Journal of Continuing Education in the Health Professions, 36*(4), 256–262. doi:10.1097/CEH.0000000000000113 PMID:28350306

Storrs, M. J., Alexander, H. G. I., Sun, J., Kroon, J., & Evans, J. L. (2015). Measuring teams-based interprofessional education outcomes in cinical dentistry: Psychometric evaluation of a new scale at an Australian dental school. *Journal of Dental Education, 79*(3), 249–258. PMID:25729018

Stwine, E. E., & Alves, M. G. (2010). Higher education and the employability of graduates. *European Educational Research Journal, 9*(1), 32–44. doi:10.2304/eerj.2010.9.1.32

Townsend, G., & Winning, T. (2011). Research in PBL - where to from here for dentistry? *European Journal of Dental Education, 15*(3), 193–198. doi:10.1111/j.1600-0579.2010.00655.x PMID:21762325 van der Zande, M. M., Gorter, R. C., & Wismeijer, D. (2013). Dental practioners and a digital future: An inital exploration of barriers and incentives to adopting digital technologies. *British Dental Journal*, *215*(11E21), 1–5. doi:10.1038/sj.bdj.2013.1146 PMID:24309814

vanNoort, R. (2012). The future of dental device is digital. *Dental Materials*, *28*(1), 3–12. doi:10.1016/j.dental.2011.10.014 PMID:22119539

Wenger, E., Dermott, R. M., & Snyder, W. M. (2002). *Cultivating communities of practice: A guide to managing knowledge*. Boston: Harvard Business School.

Yang, R. (2002). University internationalisation: Its meaning, rationales and implications. *Intercultural Education*, *13*(1), 81–95. doi:10.1080/14675980120112968

Zheng, L., Yue, L., Zhou, M., & Yu, H. (2013). Dental laboratory technology education in China: Current situation and challenges. *Journal of Dental Education*, *77*(3), 345–347. PMID:23486899

Chapter 10
Simulated Learning Environments to Prepare for Clinical Placements:
Transition to Placement (T2P)

Neil Tuttle
Griffith University, Australia

E-Liisa Laakso
Griffith University, Australia

ABSTRACT

Students commencing clinical placements often have difficulty applying their knowledge to produce meaningful clinical interactions. Patient-centred simulation can provide a bridge to clinical practice but can be expensive. This chapter describes the development and evaluation of a simulated environment integrating patient-centred simulation with an online adaptive learning platform to assist students to transition from classroom to placement. Student confidence increased significantly from pre- to post-simulation in all 12 areas that were surveyed from 3.4/6 (2.9–4.2) to 3.9/6 (3.7-4.5). Ninety-one percent of students felt better prepared for placement. The activity was not assessable and students rated this aspect highly for engagement and efficacy of learning. Student marks on their subsequent clinical placement were significantly higher for professional behavior, communication, and evidence-based practice compared with previous cohorts of students who had not undertaken a similar program.

DOI: 10.4018/978-1-5225-3850-9.ch010

INTRODUCTION

Work integrated learning is a mandatory component of physiotherapy education and primarily occurs during clinical placements where students undertake live patient care in a real-life setting. There are increasing numbers of physiotherapists being trained and there are often not sufficient clinical placements to meet the placement needs. Simulated learning environments and simulation-based learning are being used in several ways to address this shortage. Simulation-based learning has been used to either replace or supplement clinical placement time thereby reducing the demand on limited placement capacity. An example of how simulated learning environments can benefit student preparation for practice is described in detail in this chapter. The authors contend that students who are better prepared beforehand are more productive when they reach a clinical placement, thereby making them more attractive to the placement provider and perceived as less of a burden by clinical educators and clinical placement facilities.

BACKGROUND: THE ROLE OF CLINICAL PLACEMENTS

In Australia, physiotherapy is a registered profession under the Australian Health Practitioner Regulation Agency (AHPRA). To become qualified and registrable, an individual must undertake physiotherapy studies within a university-based program of physiotherapy studies accredited by the Australian Physiotherapy Council (APC). The APC undertakes the task of accrediting entry-level physiotherapy programs on behalf of the Physiotherapy Board of Australia which is supported by AHPRA.

The enormous growth in Physiotherapy programs in Australia is illustrated by an increase from six entry-level physiotherapy programs in 1998 to 29 in 2017. Each physiotherapy program has at its core, a curriculum reflective of contemporary Western physiotherapy. Integral to the curricula are clinical placements wherein physiotherapy students, apply their knowledge and skills in clinical settings under the supervision of registered physiotherapists. Typically such placements are of five weeks duration (or in multiples of five weeks) across a range of areas of practice either incorporated into the program structure such that a placement immediately follows a period of theoretical and practical learning (integrated model); or follow directly after each other once the bulk of theoretical and practical learning has been completed (immersive model). Each model has its benefits and challenges but these placements are required to include exposure to people of all ages in a range of specified areas of practice (Australian Health Practitioner Regulation Agency, 2015).

In order to assure public safety, the APC accreditation standard requires students:

- "Achieve the relevant competencies before providing supervised patient care as part of the (university) program" of studies, and
- "Are supervised by suitably qualified and registered physiotherapy and health practitioners during clinical education". (Australian Physiotherapy Council, 2015).

The APC accreditation standards are designed to link to the physiotherapy binational practice thresholds (Australian Physiotherapy Council, 2015). The threshold statements are a reference point of threshold competence in the context of physiotherapy practice in Australia and New Zealand. The threshold statements are used to assess "student's performance in the context of a clinical placement or simulated setting for education purposes."

A range of key competencies are listed within the binational threshold statements. Of relevance to this chapter, is the role domain of 'physiotherapy practitioner', and specifically the key competencies that registered physiotherapists in Australia and New Zealand are able to:

- Plan and implement an efficient, effective, culturally responsive and client-centred physiotherapy assessment; and
- Involve the client and relevant others in the planning and implementation of safe and effective physiotherapy using evidence-based practice to inform decision-making.

The enabling components that inform the above competencies describe the elements that physiotherapy programs seek to instill in their students in order for them to become registrable for practice. The expectation is that students reach a threshold level of competency by the end of each clinical placement as measured by the Assessment of Physiotherapy Practice (APP), a reliable tool widely used in Australian and New Zealand clinical placement settings to assess physiotherapy students (Dalton, Davidson, & Keating, 2012).

Until recently, the main responsibility for educating and assessing physiotherapy students in clinical placements has fallen to the government-funded public hospital system. Griffith University data from 2015 demonstrated approximately 70% of placements were in the Queensland Department of Health (Queensland Health) facilities and only 15% were located in private hospital and private practice settings. This trend is consistent with other Australian universities (Buchanan, Jenkins, & Scott, 2014).

As "the employment based element of health professional education has struggled to cope with (a range of) pressures" (Buchanan et al., 2014) universities have been exploring alternatives for clinical education. For example, Griffith University is increasingly placing students in private practice settings, community, aged care, schools and other non-traditional settings. However, there is increased competition from existing and new university providers for these placements putting sustainability of placement supply at risk. There is also an increasing trend of behaviours that would appear to run counter to the 'vocational ethic' described by Buchanan et al,(2014) such as offers of payments to placement providers beyond established agreements and requests for payments for student placements at rates well above the historical industry norm.

Coupled with the increase in student numbers is a change in hospital-based patient care (A. Wright et al., 2015). Increased in-patient acuity, reduced length of stay and the shift of rehabilitation services to home and community settings has placed a different emphasis on where and how students need to be prepared for practice. Constrained health budgets may also contribute to a reduction in clinical placements from the increasing the difficulty of finding sufficient staff to undertake clinical education (Stillman, Burpeau-Di Gregorio, Nicholson, Sabers, & Stillman, 1983).

All of these factors contribute to systems-wide strains across the higher education and clinical provider settings and highlights the need for technology-based alternatives. In the case of physiotherapy, simulation-based learning in entry-level programs has become one such alternative.

SIMULATION AND CLINICAL EXPERIENTIAL LEARNING

The authors describe simulation-based learning in the context of the definition provided by Gaba (2004), who states that "simulation is a technique – not a technology – to replace or amplify real experiences with guided experiences that evoke or replicate substantial aspects of the real world in a fully interactive manner".

Whatever the setting or method, the notion of 'deliberate practice' is a goal of simulation-based learning (Mori, Carnahan, & Herold, 2015) providing the learner with an opportunity to refine their skills and make mistakes in a supportive and safe environment without fear of personal failure or risk of patient harm. The benefits of simulation-based learning are multifaceted and include reduced training time, improved clinical and communication skills, and increased confidence (A. Wright, Moss, Watson, & Rue, 2016). Simulation-based learning has been used in various ways but for physiotherapy clinical education it is generally used to supplement traditional learning, replace clinical learning, in preparation for clinical placement experiences, remediate or premediate student performance, or in the later stages assist mastery of complexity. The authors have used simulation-based learning in each of these ways.

The next sections describe applications of simulation-based learning that the authors have utilized, and refer to the relative strengths and weaknesses of each approach.

Supplementary Applications of Simulation-Based Learning

Simulation-based learning can be used to supplement clinical learning by providing experiences that are difficult to access such as paediatric care (S. Wright, Mandrusiak, Ramsbotham, Hayles, & Kelly, 2014); providing a greater variety of cases not available in all practice settings; or, where the inherent risks to patients might be high (such as in a critical or intensive care environment) (Ohtake, Lazarus, Schillo, & Rosen, 2013))

Often this type of supplemental activity involves high fidelity, computer-operated mannequin with monitoring attachments and lines portraying the simulated patient. The patient may have unremarkable responses in a simulation modeling routine care, or alternatively responses requiring urgent attention. The scenario (or parts thereof) can be repeated allowing students to achieve success.

A major drawback of high fidelity simulations is the cost including initial infrastructure, on-going maintenance and replacement of equipment, and professional resources. As a result of costs, high fidelity simulations are likely to remain in the domain of supplemental simulation activities occurring while students are on placement, in pre-clinical preparation or in post-registration professional development.

In a study wherein simulation-based learning was interspersed throughout a cardiopulmonary clinical placement, the simulation groups demonstrated significantly better evaluations than control groups (Blackstock et al., 2013). Student confidence was also significant higher in students after cardiopulmonary simulations (regardless of the simulation model) than students who did not experience the simulation. These results underline the value of supplemental simulations in specific areas of physiotherapy practice such as intensive care settings which have a high burden of care and expensive monitoring technologies.

Supplemental simulations can take a number of other forms depending on the circumstances required by the education or health care facility. These forms of simulation are, as described below, more typically used for other purposes.

Simulation-Based Learning as a Replacement for Clinical Learning

An Australian partnership of seven universities, conducted a multi-centre randomized controlled trial comparing clinical placements that included 20% to 25% of the placement time as simulation-based learning with traditional placements found the inclusion of simulation did not affect student learning outcomes (Watson et al., 2012). These findings demonstrated that there are simulation-based modes of learning may address some of the inter-sectoral strains discussed at the start of this chapter. As a result, many universities use simulation-based learning to replace a proportion of clinical placements.

The above trial was expanded in a partnership of the majority of Australian physiotherapy programs. This nationwide project trialed three models of simulation in an effort to clarify a range of factors including timing of simulations and costs versus benefits and efficacy (S. Wright et al., 2014). The aim was "to embed simulation training into pre-registration physiotherapy clinical units across Australia in a manner that could be sustained beyond the life of the project".

The outcomes of the nationwide project positively demonstrated that simulations can be resourced and modeled in a number of ways at varying costs, with and without technology and without detriment to the physiotherapy learner. The following summarises the quantitative outcomes of the project (S. Wright et al., 2014) in which replacement of clinical placement time utilising various models was evaluated in different ways.

- **Overall Evaluation:**
    - Staff and students indicated that simulation-based learning was valuable in developing clinical skills, and assessment and communication skills.
- **Student Evaluation:**
    - As noted in other research, of the simulation strategies employed in the project, working with peers and the ability to take 'time-out' in a scenario were considered highly for clinical learning.
    - Cardiopulmonary physiotherapy simulation was rated significantly higher than the other core practice areas for both value for clinical learning and usefulness (in linking theory to practice).
    - Student ratings of the benefits of making mistakes in a protective environment were rated most highly by those undertaking simulations once a week over five weeks.
    - Self-rated student confidence in communication, assessment/analysis and treatment skills increased significantly in all clinical practice areas although awareness of hazards and limitations in a clinical scenario

delivered using a mobile smart device did not increase to the same amount. The least amount of improvement in confidence was in students who undertook five days of simulation in the first week of a five week placement.

- **Simulation Facilitator Evaluation:**
    - Simulation facilitators reported that students who undertook simulation-based learning across all practice areas were generally more competent clinically than comparable students.
    - On the matter of communications skills, simulation facilitators felt that those students who undertook simulation-based learning prior to immersion in consecutive (back-to-back) clinical placements had lower skills than those who undertook simulations either integrated throughout a traditional placement or in the first week of a traditional placement.
- **Clinical Placement Outcomes:**
    - The Professional and Clinical Skills domains of the APP tool were significantly lower at the end of 5 days of simulation in the students who undertook simulation-based learning prior to immersion in consecutive (back-to-back) clinical placement simulations, compared to integrated simulation-based learning throughout a traditional placement or in the first week of a traditional placement.
    - When overall APP scores were compared between students who experienced simulation-based learning and those who had not, a significant group difference was found for the Professional Skills domain but not for the Clinical Skills domain. The report's authors note however, that the maximum percentage difference in grade was relatively inconsequential.

Specific to Griffith University, was feedback from our clinical partners who did not wish to have simulations impacting on existing five week placements. As clinical placements in Queensland are aligned across all universities that offer physiotherapy programs, the starting and finishing times for placements could not be altered without significant impact on clinical placement providers.

It is interesting to note that students rated the cardiopulmonary scenarios highest for clinical learning and its usefulness in linking theory to practice. As noted earlier, cardiopulmonary physiotherapy is most likely to be influenced by technology especially in critical care settings and as a result this area of simulation-based learning is most likely to include high fidelity technologies. As technology factors were not evaluated as part of the nationwide project, it is not possible to comment on what aspects of the cardiopulmonary simulation-based learning might have contributed to this outcome. Nor was it possible to know the degree to which psychological fidelity needs to be developed prior to gaining the most from a simulation experience at any level of engineering or technological fidelity.

One of the questions that could not be answered from the data collected in the nationwide project was whether the students who undertook simulation-based learning were better prepared or had greater readiness for the subsequent clinical placement experience and, therefore if they added greater value for longer over the duration of a traditional clinical placement. This aspect is important to interrogate as it may assist in establishing the added value of simulation-based learning in improving patient outcomes and increasing occasions of service in a clinical setting.

Furthermore, the nationwide project did not specifically measure the impact on the development of clinical reasoning. Clinical reasoning is a complex cognitive process that is not easily observed until a deliberative action or explanation of ones thinking and decision-making takes place. Clinical reasoning is challenging to teach and learn and usually evolves as an iterative process over the entirety of a program of theoretical learning, developing further during pre-clinical studies and as part of the exposure of students to patients in clinical settings. Although capable of being described (e.g. (Edwards, Jones, Carr, Braunack-Mayer, & Jensen, 2004)), measurement of the hypothetico-deductive processes and narrative elements of clinical reasoning development and progress is difficult and few have been able to do so as a discreet entity separate to the totality of the clinical engagement. As it plays such a critical part in the outcomes of interactions between physiotherapists and patients, clinical reasoning requires purposeful attention in simulation-based learning. It is unclear if this has been the case in physiotherapy simulations previously.

Simulation-Based Learning as Preparation for Clinical Placements

In a systematic review of using simulation in preparation or as a substitute for clinical placement, Larue et al (2015) noted that "". The data from the Australian project presented in the previous section (A. Wright et al., 2016) sheds some light on the value of simulation-based learning as preparation for clinical placements. It was clear that by temporally positioning the simulation experience as close as possible to the clinical placement (either in the first week of a five week placement or throughout a five week placement) students performed better on assessment of communications skills, and professional and clinical skills.

The proximity of the simulations experience to a traditional placement setting is an unexpected finding from the nationwide project yet one that makes sense intuitively. The value of placing tasks requiring motor learning in to close proximity (but not too close) to the application of the skill is well-known (Wolpert et al, 2001) and the theory supports content sequencing and timing elements in traditional forms of pedagogy. It would appear to be a critical factor also in its value to the development of students' clinical competencies and needs to be taken in to account as part of a whole-of-program approach including those that utilize simulation-based learning.

Simulation-Based Learning as Pre-Mediation or Remediation

The authors enacted simulations as a method of pre-mediation and remediation of weaker students as part of both Griffith University's involvement in the nationwide study described earlier (Wright et al, 2016) and the STEPS study described below.

As a remediation strategy, some students who had not passed a clinical placement, undertook a simulation-based learning setting in order to strengthen areas of weakness. This remediation strategy, particularly with students whose first language was not English, provided the students with an opportunity to improve their clinical, professional and communications skills prior to undertaking a supplementary or repeat placement. By utilizing simulation-based learning in this way, we were able to provide additional (surrogate) clinical time and support for the students without impacting on existing goodwill with clinical education providers. An added bonus was that we were able to more closely supervise the weaker students and identify students who might be unlikely to pass a repeat placement. This was indeed the case with one student who, after discussion with academic staff and simulation facilitators, took a leave of absence from studies thus saving the unnecessary expense of a repeat placement.

Our success in using simulation-based learning as a remediation model provided us with the confidence to utilize a similar strategy to pre-mediate other students. We identified students with demonstrated weaknesses in a given practice area and offered them the extra-curricular opportunity to undertake simulation sessions. Generally these students were achieving low Pass grades through the written and spoken assessment items often without coming to the specific notice of academic staff; and also in practical vivas used as a hurdle assessment prior to all clinical placements undertaken by Griffith Physiotherapy students. Whether a student passes or fails a clinical placement cannot necessarily be attributed to any specific factor but probably the most common deficit is in clinical reasoning. If students who are weak in this area can be identified early they may be able to be assisted through simulation to increase their chances of being successful in subsequent clinical placements. The authors have found this to be a particularly valuable application of simulation-based learning.

The insights provided by these experiences were extremely valuable. As we later set out to use the results of the nationwide project and the STEPS project to develop a structure of simulations that would integrate with the existing physiotherapy program at Griffith University, we realized that by making only minor changes to the simulation models used in each project we should be able to create additional value. That is, if we could better prepare our students for clinical placements by providing a transitional bridge between their on-campus theoretical and practical learning and their five week clinical placement, the students should start the subsequent placement at a higher capability level. By doing so, we hypothesised that we would be relieving the clinical educators of the burden of constant supervision in the first week of a placement, and leveraging the opportunities that this presents by having the students operating at a level equivalent to week two instead of week one of a traditional five week placement. The program that was developed as a result of this realization became known as Transition to Placement (T2P), a formalized part of the first year Master of Physiotherapy curriculum which is described in greater detail later in this chapter.

Other Forms of Simulations Used in Physiotherapy

A range of technologies has been used as stand-alone or hybridized forms of simulation-based learning. These include part-task training models of spines to develop manual therapy skills (Australian Physiotherapy Council, 2015); device simulators such as therapeutic ultrasound (Gann, Rogers, & Dudley, 2002); manual hyperinflation simulators (Hila, Ellis, & Holmes, 2002); baby and infant simulators (Hassam & Williams, 2003); and computer-based games and virtual worlds (Sabus, Sabata, & Antonacci, 2011).

The majority of these studies have found that while short-term skills development improved, longer-term recall or retention of skills was best when the simulation was placed firmly in the clinical context. To aid recall and increase authenticity, the authors consider that task-simulators should be utilised as part of hybrid models of simulation-based learning.

Hybrid Simulation Models

We refer to simulation-based learning when co-mingled with different simulation strategies as a hybrid model of simulation. Others have referred to the adjunctive use of simulations and cohabitation of simulations and clinical experiences (Larue, Pepin, & Allard, 2015) for optimizing learning. Hybrid simulations and mixing of learning methods allows the educator to harness the best aspects of a range of approaches and methods to achieve outcomes that may be difficult or more costly to do in any other way. We have used high fidelity mannequins as part of hybrid simulation wherein the mannequin supplements the broader and more complex aspects of the simulation learning environment.

Another way in which we have hybridized simulation-based learning is through pre-briefing and de-briefing of students as individuals and groups before and after interactions with simulated patients or simulation sessions. Such briefing sessions are not simply about the simulation experience itself but about what the students have learned – about themselves and the case characteristics and how they might use that knowledge to perform better in future patient engagement. This approach permits the students to learn from their peers, to receive timely and specific feedback on performance from the simulation facilitator, and to practice a technique or approach to management in a timely way but outside of the simulation scenario. Such opportunities combine the best aspects of peer learning, timely feedback and practice-based learning specific to the student's learning style and is likely to contribute to the students' development of clinical reasoning and prepare them better for subsequent clinical placement settings. The opportunity to de-brief in itself simulates the conversations that would ideally be had in a traditional placement setting with the clinical educator or supervisor. Much of Griffith Physiotherapy's simulation-based learning would now best be described as being hybridized, as the case below demonstrates.

A CASE STUDY

The project that is the subject of this section is one module of simulated learning that takes place immediately prior to a clinical placement and is intended to act as a transition from the on-campus content in musculoskeletal physiotherapy to the relevant five week clinical placement. This and similar modules in the Physiotherapy program at Griffith University are referred to as transitions to placement (T2P) and have resulted from of a series of evolutionary iterations over a five year period between 2011 and 2016. Each developmental stage of simulation-based learning had specific drivers, strengths and weaknesses and informed each subsequent stage. Here we provide a brief description of the evolution of the simulation strategy to place the project in an appropriate context followed by a description of the structure of the project and its evaluation.

STEPS Version One

In response to a looming crisis in clinical placement capacity across most health professions (described earlier in this chapter), the Government of Australia (through Health Workforce Australia) supported a number of initiatives with the primary aim of increasing the quality and quantity of clinical education. One project supported by this initiative was the Simulated Telemedicine Environment Project for Students

(STEPS) which started in 2012. The Physiotherapy component of the STEPS addressed three issues in physiotherapy clinical education:

1. An overall lack of sufficient physiotherapy clinical placement capacity.
2. A critical shortage of clinical education placements in rural and remote locations.
3. Technology-assisted occasions of service using, for example, telerehabilitation.

Telerehabilitation was an emerging area of practice at the time yet few students were experiencing the management of clients in this type of environment during their clinical placements.

The STEPS Version One project intended to address the above issues by enabling students to gain experiences that might not otherwise have been possible in all placements, provide supplementary simulated learning environments even if the student was at rural or remote placement sites, provide student-free 'respite' time for clinical educators, or to ensure students could be gainfully occupied if clinical educators were not available full time. Students who were on clinical placement remained in their clinical placements at remote locations and accessed an on-campus simulated learning environment, via a teleconferencing platform. Two half-days per week (approximately 20% of their five week full-time musculoskeletal clinical placement) were dedicated to this project.

Students assessed and managed, simulated patients using scenarios based on what would occur in a telerehabilitation environment. Students worked in groups of four with each student alternating between live interactions, pre-recorded videos of some aspects of the assessment, peer interaction and debriefing with the clinical facilitator. The intention of the specific scenarios was to improve new graduate outcomes. To that end we determined: 1) which aspects of professional behaviour resulted in complaints to the Physiotherapy Board of Australia; 2) what type of incidents, injury or negligence resulted in claims to professional indemnity insurers; and 3) the perceptions from employers regarding areas in which the clinical practice of new graduates could be improved.

Student confidence improved and they perceived that the sessions were useful (Bialocerkowski & Tuttle, 2013) but the program was not popular with either students or clinical educators largely due to a range of technical issues with the videoconferencing platforms. Connectivity was limited by internet bandwidth and by firewalls at either the university or remote health service provider. Many students also thought they would rather be seeing 'real' patients during the simulation time. Participation was voluntary for the clinical placement facilities and each facility selected their preferred times for the students to be involved in the project. Nonetheless clinical educators found it difficult to fit in with the scheduled times and felt the simulations took too much time away from the students' clinical experience.

STEPS Version Two

Based on the outcomes of STEPS Version One, we thought that students would benefit from developing the skills targeted in the STEPS program earlier in their program. The next iteration of the STEPS program used a similar structure but took place during the students' first full clinical placement where they worked with in-patients receiving orthopaedic surgery. A videoconferencing platform was again used to model remote provision of service. The structure of the STEPS Version Two responded to concerns raised about the STEPS Version One and halved the time that students were involved to one half-day per week. To make them simpler and more relevant, case scenarios were modeled on the first physiotherapy follow-up contact that a patient living in a remote location (without access to a physiotherapist) would require after discharge from a metropolitan hospital. Technical issues were reduced but still caused significant difficulties (N. A. Tuttle & Bialocerkowski, 2014). There were positive outcomes particularly in student communication skills (N. Tuttle, Waite, & Bialocerkowksi, 2015), but both students and clinical educators felt the sessions would have been better conducted at times other than during clinical placement. Several clinical educators also failed to see the relevance of an outpatient follow-up treatment to an in-patient clinical placement.

STEPS Version Three

The circumstances in which STEPS Version Three developed had several differences to the earlier iterations. The funding body no longer required telemedicine to be used in the majority of the modules and external funding was expected to reduce or disappear entirely with time. The project therefore needed to be sustainable within the university budget envelope if it was to continue. With these considerations in mind, and combined with feedback from the previous versions, we revised the timing, intention and structure of the simulated learning environments.

In spite of the intention of previous iterations of STEPS to benefit the clinical placement and the clinical educators, the feedback received from clinical educators and students was that simulation-based clinical learning was not perceived as a benefit to the facility. Both students and clinical educators suggested that the simulated learning environments conducted within the STEPS project were effective but the timing would have been better if the activities occurred prior to clinical placements. In line with this feedback STEPS Version Three was scheduled to occur outside of clinical placement times and it became more similar to activities undertaken in the nationwide simulation-based learning project (A. Wright et al., 2016) described earlier in this chapter.

Although the costs of running a week of simulation were significantly greater than the equivalent on-campus content, several factors contribute to the sustainability of the initiative. The costs per student were less than when the same amount of simulation was delivered while students were on clinical placement because staffing could be used more efficiently. There were also a number of indirect savings resulting from the program. We had noted that savings could be made if students were better prepared for clinical placement. We were of the belief that improved student preparation would result in fewer students needing to repeat their placements due to failure. Some of the resources developed for the simulation modules, particularly those that enabled students to perform some aspects of clinical reasoning independently, were potentially capable of reducing face to face teaching time.

Transition to Placement (T2P) modules (as they became known) were instituted immediately prior to the two main clinical placements (orthopaedic in-patients and musculoskeletal out-patients) that are undertaken by Physiotherapy students at Griffith University in their penultimate year. The following section describes the structure of the T2P module occurring before the musculoskeletal placement.

Transition to Placement (T2P)

Physiotherapy students at Griffith University undertake the five-week ambulatory (out-patients) musculoskeletal clinical placement between the end of the first year and the start of second year of a two year graduate-entry Master degree program. During clinical placements, students work initially under a close level of supervision by clinical educators which is progressively withdrawn over the course of the placement as student competence increases and as students become more independent and capable of taking an increased patient load.

The week prior to the musculoskeletal placement had historically been taken up with study time and assessment (including written assessment, and viva examinations). Based on knowledge of temporal spacing of learning and based on the feedback received from earlier versions of the STEPS project, we decided that the week immediately before the musculoskeletal placement would be the optimal time for simulation-based learning in preparation for the musculoskeletal placement. As we did not want students to be pre-occupied with pre-placement assessment, the students' schedules were revised so that some clinical reasoning content was removed from the academic component of the semester and time allocated for studying prior to assessment was reduced slightly. Assessments were moved forward chronologically to the penultimate week prior to placement thus leaving one week free for simulation-based learning intended as a transition to placement (T2P).

The intention of the STEPS Version Three (T2P) was adjusted to more closely meet the immediate needs of the students whilst still meeting the requirements set by the Physiotherapy Board of Australia and the APC. In previous iterations of STEPS, students were on clinical placements where support is provided by their clinical educators to prepare them for the time when they are independent practitioners, but in those earlier iterations, the simulations were conducted as if the learners were independent practitioners without support from clinical educators during the patient interactions. In T2P, students were at the threshold of a clinical placement, so the level of competence that was at the edge of their expertise (Jenny W Rudolph, Raemer, & Simon, 2014) was being on clinical placement rather than being independent practitioners. The clinical scenarios used in T2P were modeled on what would occur during a clinical placement rather than, as we had previously done, being modeled on when the students would be independent practitioners one year later at the end of their physiotherapy studies.

For T2P, students worked together in groups of four for a total of 20 hours over five days. For three hours on each of the five days students participated in live patient-focused simulations with the remainder of the time spent on related independent activities within their groups.

All simulation facilitators had a minimum of two days of specific training in being a simulation educator (Nestel & Bearman, 2014). Simulation facilitators were drawn from academic teaching staff, university-based coordinators of clinical placements, and clinical educators. The diversity of facilitators was considered important both for the students and staff. On one hand it is a useful recalibration of practice for the educators from both sides of the academic / clinical divide to ensure a consistency between teaching and practice. Also, having facilitators who students see both on-campus and in clinical settings can highlight to students the links and consistencies between classroom and clinical practice.

The content of the T2P simulation scenarios were adjusted to fit with adjustments in timing and intention of the simulations in three ways. First, rather than the students performing as independent practitioners as in our previous iterations, the expectations of the students were modeled on what the student would be doing the following week when they were on clinical placement. That is, they were in the role of students and with access to a clinical educator played by the simulation facilitator. As would occur in their upcoming placement they had discussions with their clinical educator particularly at transition points between elements of the simulation session or when a teaching moment was indicated from the interaction between the student and simulated patient. Secondly, the clinical task requirements were structured so that students were working at the edge of their expertise (Nestel & Bearman, 2014; Jenny W Rudolph et al., 2014), a threshold which was expected to change and evolve over the course of the T2P week. The focus of each day changed with the intention of chasing the moving edge of the students' expertise. Thirdly, an online adaptive learning platform was used to simulate some aspects of the case scenarios.

Previously we provided scenario-related background or follow-up information that was not part of the live simulation to students in non-interactive formats such as text, image and/or video. The use of the adaptive learning platform meant that students were actively engaged with all aspects of each case rather than just those that were being simulated live.

The use and details of the adaptive learning platform are described in Chapter [10]. Briefly students interacting on the platform make choices about patient assessment and management. The student choices and their input alter the online direction of the case and the feedback the student subsequently receives onliine. Students therefore enter the live simulation setting having committed themselves to specific courses of action. The student and facilitator (in the role of clinical educator) then address the student's clinical reasoning up to a given point, at which time the facilitator guides the reasoning process in transitioning to what the student will do in the live simulation.

The scenarios were about patients with similar conditions to those that the students are likely to see in their upcoming placement. There were no hidden traps or sudden adverse events in the scenarios. Importantly, student performance on the simulation week was confidential and the simulation week was intentionally quarantined from assessment.

Great care was taken to maximize the ability of students to be immersed in the live simulations. It may seem trivial but the author's impression is there is a large difference in the emotional experience, the learning, and the generalizability of the learning when students are truly immersed in the experience rather than 'performing' during the simulated activities. Put another way it is the difference between acting as they would in real life as distinct from 'as if' they were in real life. Techniques employed to promote this authenticity included ensuring that all expectations and ground rules were clearly stated in the pre-simulation briefing; pauses for, and clear delineation of, transitions in and out of the simulation environment; peer or facilitator observers being as unobtrusive as possible; and facilitators modeled expected behaviours and did not transgress the ground rules.

Debriefing throughout T2P generally used a "feedback with good judgement approach" (J. W. Rudolph, Simon, Rivard, Dufresne, & Raemer, 2007). The "pause and discuss" structures (Hogan, Flanagan, & Marshall, 2008) used on Days Two through to Four often included other approaches as were deemed appropriate by the facilitators.

T2P Structure and Rationale

Physiotherapy students at the end of their on-campus semester are considered competent at the individual skills of patient assessment and treatment. Once on a clinical placement, they can appear less able to apply the information they gain from patients to their ongoing reasoning processes particularly while in the midst of the complexities of interacting with a patient. The intentions of the T2P week are to enable students to 'put it all together'. That is, to more effectively gather information in a real life-like situation, to interpret the information they receive and translate that information into meaningful action in real time.

Table 1 demonstrates how the week is structured on each day, and how each day scaffolds the subsequent days. The activities on each day include interaction with the preparatory material on the adaptive learning platform, peer discussion, live simulation, facilitated feedback and debriefing, and follow-up activities performed in the group. Debriefing included discussion with the group of four students. The facilitator often invited the simulated patient into the group discussion where they contributed 'out of role' to provide feedback to the student specifically on how their character responded to the communication strategies used by the student. Generally, to avoid cognitive dissonance of the simulated patient being in and out of role, the input of the simulated patient was not sought if students would be seeing the same simulated patient the following day.

Day One focused on students being able to effectively communicate with the simulated patient and to enact an occasion of service without requiring the usual added cognitive load of clinical reasoning. Days Two through to Four each focused on a specific element of an occasion of service as well as the transitions before and after the element. That is, Day Two focused on history taking, Day Three on physical assessment, and Day Four on treatment. For each day, there were independent activities that the students undertook within their groups following up on that day's simulated patient scenario. These activities included tasks such as recording in writing the patient notes, writing follow-up letters, and administrative tasks for third party insurers. Students also prepared for a follow-up treatment of the simulated patients they had seen that day. The week culminated on Day Five when students were required to put all of the various pieces of the patient engagement together and to perform complete occasions of service as they would be undertaking the following week at the clinical placement site. The following is a more detailed description of the activities on each T2P day.

Day One

On Day One each student worked through the entire assessment and treatment of one simulated patient and also observed a peer with a different simulated patient. The objectives for Day One were for students to understand and experience the flow of a treatment session while communicating with a simulated patient without being burdened by the usual cognitive load of having to make decisions of what to do next

Table 1. Student activities and scenario numbers through the T2P week. The activities performed by students on each day are shown in the grid. Numbers indicate the scenario numbers used on any given day.

Day 1	**Referral Info**	**History**	**Plan Physical**	**Perform Physical**	**Plan Treatment**	**Treat**	**Inter-Professional Activities**	**Plan Follow-Up**	**Second Treatment**
Online prep	1&2	1&2	1&2	1&2	1&2	1&2			
Live simulation	1&2	1&2	1&2	1&2	1&2	1&2			
Independent activities							1&2	1&2	
Day 2									
Online prep	3 &4								
Live simulation		3 &4							1
Online follow-up			3 &4	3 &4	3 &4	3 &4			
Independent activities							3 &4	3 &4	
Day 3									
Online prep	5&6	5&6							
Live simulation				5&6					4
Online follow-up					5&6	5&6			
Independent activities			5&6				5&6	5&6	
Day 4									
Online prep	7&8	7&8	7&8	7&8					
Live simulation						7&8			5
Online follow-up									
Independent activities					7&8		7&8		
Day 5									
Live simulation	9&10	9 &10	9 &10	9&10	9 &10	9 &10			

and how to interpret their findings. To this end, lessons had been constructed on the adaptive learning platform Smartsparrow and these included all aspects of the initial assessment and treatment of the patient in each of the scenarios used on Day One. By working through these lessons prior to the live simulations, students had to use their clinical reasoning and they were guided through all of the decisions they would need to make in the course of seeing that patient. Therefore prior to starting the live simulation, students knew the patient's history, the appropriate physical assessments to perform, the results of the physical assessments, appropriate treatment selection and the effects of those treatments. By having reasoned through all aspects of the scenario prior to the live simulation, students were relieved of much of the cognitive load that would usually have been necessary when interacting with a patient. During the live simulation on Day One, students therefore only needed to 'go through the motions' of what they had already prepared. Going through the motions as a smooth sequence with the added complexity of interacting with the patient was not a trivial task for these novice students.

Having had the above experience of the entire process then reduced the students' cognitive load on the subsequent days enabling them to focus on the learning objectives for those days. Students had approximately one hour in which they undertook the assessment and treatment with a simulated patient and communicated with their simulated clinical educator in a realistic setting. On Day One, each student generally stayed in role for the entire occasion of service and was observed by one other student. The active student was assisted by their facilitator who stayed in the role of clinical educator providing guidance and support as would occur if the student were on clinical placement.

Day Two

The main focus of Day Two was history taking but forty minutes was allocated also for a follow-up occasion of service with one of the simulated patients they had seen on Day One. A student who had seen the simulated patient on the previous day performed the follow-up with the facilitator in the role of clinical educator. This was followed by a debriefing session that also included the other members of the student group.

Each group of students had two new scenarios on Day Two. Students received only the information that they would normally receive prior to seeing a patient on clinical placement such as a referral letter and/or the type of condition the patient was presenting with. One student took the patient's history followed by a debriefing that included the rest of the group. After this initial debriefing, the facilitator had a number of options. For example, the same student or a different student might be asked to repeat all or part of the patient history. Further discussion and practice would then be used to refine the taking and interpreting of the patient's history.

Independent activities then included the students interacting with the adaptive learning platform to work through the patient's physical assessment and treatment. Each group then undertook independent activities similar to Day One including written follow-up activities for each simulated patient and preparation for seeing one of the Day Two simulated patients on Day Three.

Day Three

Day Three of T2P was similar in structure to Day Two except the focus was on the physical assessment. Students engaged in one follow-up session from the previous day and saw two new simulated patients (that is, patients with different clinical scenarios). On Day Three, students worked through the preliminary information, patient history, and planning of the physical assessment using the online adaptive learning platform prior to engaging in the live simulation. The live interaction commenced as would occur during clinical placement, that is, after the student had taken the patient history, the student and their clinical educator would discuss how the student was going to proceed with their physical assessment. A pause, reflect, and re-do approach similar to Day Two was used to refine performance and interpretation of the physical assessment.

Day Four

Day Four of T2P was similar to Days Two and Three with one follow-up simulated patient and two new patients where the focus was on treatment. Prior to the simulation, students were required to have worked through the patient history and physical assessment using the adaptive learning platform; and the live simulation started with a discussion with their clinical educator on how they proposed to proceed to the treatment phase. The pause, reflect, and re-do approach was used in the remainder of the session.

Day Five

Students did not have a follow-up simulated patient to see on Day Five of T2P but each student performed a full assessment and treatment on one simulated patient and observed one other student undertaking the same task on a different simulated patient. Each student would discuss with their clinical educator between sections (history, physical assessment and treatment) as would occur when they were on clinical placement. The debriefing and feedback on Day Five was similar to that undertaken on Day One. Multiple groups of four students were scheduled concurrently, so a global de-brief and summary of the week occurred at the end of Day Five.

Evaluation

Evaluation of the T2P experience was undertaken to understand the effect of the program on student confidence, student perceived impact of the program on their learning, and the effect of the program on student performance while on their subsequent clinical placement.

Students rated their confidence on a five point Likert scale before and after the T2P week in seven areas (establish rapport, explain professional role, conduct effective interview, use appropriate interpersonal skills, identify relevant information, conduct an objective assessment, explain the problem to a patient, discuss management, select appropriate treatment, deliver appropriate treatment, evaluate treatment effectiveness, progress treatment, and interact as a professional). There was a statistically significant increase in confidence from an average of 3.4/5 to 4.0/5.

The self-assessment of student confidence can be difficult because student confidence implies a comparison between the students' perceived abilities and their understanding of an appropriate standard. It is quite possible that a student's perception of an appropriate standard may change with increased understanding gained through an activity such as the T2P week resulting in the student comparing their confidence with a higher bar after the intervention than before the intervention. If that were the case, the increases in confidence found with the current comparisons would under-estimate rather than over-estimate the magnitude of improvement in confidence.

Over 90% of students agreed or strongly agreed that there were benefits to working with peers, feedback from the simulated patients was useful, that simulated learning provided a link between theoretical and practical training, the non-assessability of the T2P week assisted their learning, and that the week better prepared them to assess and manage patients with musculoskeletal conditions.

The aim of the T2P week was to prepare students for their upcoming clinical placement, so the value of the effectiveness of the program was considered to be student performance on their clinical placement. The authors analysed T2P student results from the Assessment of Physiotherapy Practice (APP) scores compared with the previous two cohorts (who had not undertaken T2P) and found a statistically higher overall APP score, with higher scores specifically in the three areas of professional behavior, communication, and evidence-based practice.

The success of the musculoskeletal T2P week has been translated in to a similar T2P experience earlier in Year One of the Master of Physiotherapy graduate-entry program at Griffith University. Students now undertake some limited simulated orthopaedic scenarios in practical sessions in the first semester of the program followed by an orthopaedic T2P week prior to the mid-year orthopaedic in-patient clinical placements.

SOLUTIONS AND RECOMMENDATIONS

In this chapter the authors have discussed the context within which various simulation-based solutions were trialed in order to address issues of access to clinical placements and transition to practice for student physiotherapists at one Australian university. By utilizing an iterative approach to the development of simulation-based learning solutions, we have been able to incorporate the best from a number of strategies into an approach that addresses the specific needs of Griffith Physiotherapy students as well as our clinical partners. The developed strategies may not be suitable or indeed appropriate for every physiotherapy program but the reader might find some guidance in the following recommendations for developing their own strategies for simulation-based learning:

1. Understand the broader context within which the simulation-based learning strategy is to be placed. Be prepared to answer and analyse the answers to the following questions:
    a. How will the strategy be viewed by all stakeholders? How can this view be influenced?
    b. What are the likely benefits and costs of the strategy; and can these be justified in the local context?
    c. What practical aspects of implementing the strategy are required?
2. Be prepared to be open-minded on how the simulation-based learning strategy might be applied. As noted in this chapter, there are many ways in which simulation-based learning can be implemented and no one methodology is likely

to satisfy the learning, teaching and assessment needs of every physiotherapy program.

3. Experiment and evolve your strategies based on the outcomes of each development stage. Simulation-based learning in physiotherapy remains nascent (although maturing) and much can be learned from the evidence. The application of a quality improvement approach to the chosen strategies is a valuable methodology. Be prepared to stop doing some of things that you may have invested in if they are not effective or efficient.
4. Understand exactly what learning outcomes are intended by the inclusion of simulation-based learning in the program of studies, or at various stages of the program. There may be many different ways to achieve such outcomes and simulation-based learning is only one of those ways.

FUTURE RESEARCH DIRECTIONS

The Australian government's financial contribution to the development of simulation-based learning in physiotherapy has been a significant catalyst for the acceptance of simulation-based learning in the profession. It remains to be seen whether the initiatives are sustainable. Wright et al (2016) noted that each Australian university has adapted simulation-based learning in varying ways to fit within the logistical constraints and available funding envelopes. Some of these initiatives directly replaced traditional clinical placement days. Some have utilized simulation-based learning outside of clinical weeks as a way of scaffolding practical learning, for preparing students for placement, or late in the program in order to develop mastery of physiotherapy skills and knowledge for managing complex scenarios. The variations in models lend themselves to be further evaluated so that decision-making regarding the relative value of the various forms of simulation can be better understood. Such evaluations might consider the degree to which psychological fidelity needs to be developed prior to immersion in a simulated-learning environment.

Specific matters that require further investigation regarding utility and cost-effectiveness are those wherein technologies (such as adaptive learning platforms) are integrated in to simulation-based learning and how these might leverage typical methods of simulation-based learning to assist in preparing students for traditional clinical placements. Technologies integrated with simulation-based learning may prove to be highly useful in developing clinical reasoning skills but the measurement and quantification of clinical reasoning remains to be clarified.

The proximity of the simulation-based learning activity to traditional placements, as well as the amount of time devoted to simulation-based learning at various times across a program perhaps also needs further scrutiny. Griffith University has decided to place most of its simulation efforts (specifically T2P) in to the formative teaching and learning in Year 1 of the two year Master of Physiotherapy graduate-entry program. We have made the assumption (based on pedagogical factors as well as more pragmatic budgetary and scheduling factors) that history-taking, physical examination and to some extent treatment skills from the orthopaedic and musculoskeletal areas of practice are transferrable to the other core areas of physiotherapy (neurological and cardiopulmonary) that are addressed in Year 2 of the graduate-entry Master degree program. Further evaluation of matters such as student preparedness for placement, utilising more sensitive measures than those currently available, and their value in improving patient outcomes and increasing occasions of service is important to interrogate. Data regarding the amount of time spent by clinical educators with students who have or have not experienced T2P would assist in understanding the clinical placement outcomes of simulation-based learning.

Given the greater acceptance of simulations in the physiotherapy profession, as the use of simulation-based learning matures, and as virtual reality (VR) and augmented reality (AR) technologies develop, it is expected that the latter too may find a place in the preparation of students for physiotherapy practice. The authors contend that as VR and AR become more accessible and less expensive to universities VR and AR may become an indispensable part of student learning and of professional development and on-site training. As such, it would seem advisable to explore VR and AR as adjuncts to simulation-based learning and to utilise evaluation tools earlier in their take-up, in order to compare the various forms of learning and to develop an admixture of methods that complement each other at different stages of the student lifecycle.

CONCLUSION

This chapter has considered in some detail, the environment in which the preparation of physiotherapy students is taking place in Australia, and the actions taken by the profession in response to significant and on-going pressures in the higher education and clinical placement environs.

In the case of Griffith University we have developed a model of simulation-based learning whereby students experience simulations in limited ways early in their program of learning (to develop history-taking and physical examination skills); and later undertake more comprehensive simulation-based learning that emulates clinical scenarios (in the context of the clinical environment as well as the presenting patient scenario). In the latter, we have integrated a software tool that assists in the development of clinical reasoning. The simulation-based learning model is specifically designed to comply with the Australian and New Zealand practice thresholds and the APC accreditation requirements. The T2P experience aims to prepare students so that they are able not only to learn more during their placements, but also to offer more to the clinical provider at an earlier stage of a clinical placement than they may do otherwise. Simulation-based learning has been found to have a range of benefits and for Griffith University we have found that those benefits are applicable to all of the stakeholders especially the students and the clinical partners.

Griffith University has developed a hybrid model of simulation-based learning that is viable, relatively affordable and contributes to student learning outcomes. These methods and our experience with them will be invaluable for developing the competencies for future teaching and learning required for new areas of learning such as physiotherapist (non-medical) prescribing curricula.

The potential place of technology in simulation-based learning is highly dependent on the specific and desired learning outcomes. We have designed a web-based musculoskeletal clinical reasoning platform that integrates with the students' simulations in the transition to placement week. This hybrid model of simulation and technology-based learning has proven to be very successful.

REFERENCES

Australian Health Practitioner Regulation Agency. (2015). *Physiotherapy practice thresholds in Australia and Aotearoa New Zealand*. Retrieved from https://physiocouncil.com.au/media/1020/physiotherapy-board-physiotherapy-practice-thresholds-in-australia-and-aotearoa-new-zealand-6.pdf

Australian Health Practitioner Regulation Agency. (2017). *Physiotherapy Board of Australia*. Retrieved from http://www.physiotherapyboard.gov.au/About/Statistics.aspx

Australian Physiotherapy Association. (2017). *Physiotherapy in Australia*. Retrieved from http://www.physiotherapy.asn.au/APAWCM/Physio_and_You/physio/APAWCM/Physio_and_You/physio.aspx?hkey=25ad06f0-e004-47e5-b894-e0ede69e0fff

Australian Physiotherapy Council. (2015). *Physiotherapy practice thresholds in Australia and Aotearoa New Zealand.* Retrieved from https://physiocouncil.com.au/media/1020/physiotherapy-board-physiotherapy-practice-thresholds-in-australia-and-aotearoa-new-zealand-6.pdf

Bialocerkowski, A., & Tuttle, N. A. (2013). *The STEPS Project: a Remotely Accessed Simulated Learning Environment to Increase the Viability of Remote Clinic Placements in Physiotherapy and Speech Pathology*. Academic Press.

Blackstock, F. C., Watson, K. M., Morris, N. R., Jones, A., Wright, A., McMeeken, J. M., & Haines, T. P. et al. (2013). Simulation can contribute a part of cardiorespiratory physiotherapy clinical education: Two randomized trials. *Simulation in Healthcare*, *8*(1), 32–42. doi:10.1097/SIH.0b013e318273101a PMID:23250189

Buchanan, J., Jenkins, S., & Scott, L. (2014). *Student clinical education in Australia: a University of Sydney scoping study*. Sydney: The University of Sydney.

Dalton, M., Davidson, M., & Keating, J. L. (2012). The assessment of physiotherapy practice (APP) is a reliable measure of professional competence of physiotherapy students: A reliability study. *Journal of Physiotherapy*, *58*(1), 49–56. doi:10.1016/S1836-9553(12)70072-3 PMID:22341382

Edwards, I., Jones, M., Carr, J., Braunack-Mayer, A., & Jensen, G. M. (2004). Clinical reasoning strategies in physical therapy. *Physical Therapy*, *84*(4), 312. PMID:15049726

Gaba, D. M. (2004). The future vision of simulation in health care. *Quality & Safety in Health Care*, *13*(suppl 1), i2–i10. doi:10.1136/qshc.2004.009878 PMID:15465951

Gann, N., Rogers, C., & Dudley, A. (2002). A comparison of physical therapy students with and without instructions in ultrasound pressure application. *Journal of Allied Health*, *31*(2), 103–105. PMID:12040992

Hassam, M., & Williams, M. (2003). Education via simulation: Teaching safe chest percussion for pre-term infants. *Hong Kong Physiotherapy Journal*, *21*(1), 22–28. doi:10.1016/S1013-7025(09)70036-3

Hila, J., Ellis, E., & Holmes, W. (2002). Feedback withdrawal and changing compliance during manual hyperinflation. *Physiotherapy Research International*, *7*(2), 53–64. doi:10.1002/pri.242 PMID:12109235

Hogan, J., Flanagan, B., & Marshall, S. (2008). What Facilitation Skills Are Required to Assist Students' Learning When Using a Patient Simulator in the 'Pause and Discuss' Mode? *Focus on Health Professional Education: A Multi-Disciplinary Journal*, *10*(2), 36.

Larue, C., Pepin, J., & Allard, É. (2015). Simulation in preparation or substitution for clinical placement: A systematic review of the literature. *Journal of Nursing Education and Practice*, *5*(9), 132. doi:10.5430/jnep.v5n9p132

Mori, B., Carnahan, H., & Herold, J. (2015). Use of simulation learning experiences in physical therapy entry-to-practice curricula: A systematic review. *Physiotherapy Canada. Physiotherapie Canada*, *67*(2), 194–202. doi:10.3138/ptc.2014-40E PMID:25931672

Nestel, D., & Bearman, M. (2014). 0122 The Nhet-sim Program: A National Investment In Faculty Development. *BMJ Simulation and Technology Enhanced Learning*, *1*(Suppl 1), A3–A3. doi:10.1136/bmjstel-2014-000002.6

Ohtake, P. J., Lazarus, M., Schillo, R., & Rosen, M. (2013). Simulation experience enhances physical therapist student confidence in managing a patient in the critical care environment. *Physical Therapy*, *93*(2), 216–228. doi:10.2522/ptj.20110463 PMID:23329555

Rudolph, J. W., Raemer, D. B., & Simon, R. (2014). Establishing a safe container for learning in simulation: The role of the presimulation briefing. *Simulation in Healthcare*, *9*(6), 339–349. doi:10.1097/SIH.0000000000000047 PMID:25188485

Rudolph, J. W., Simon, R., Rivard, P., Dufresne, R. L., & Raemer, D. B. (2007). Debriefing with good judgment: Combining rigorous feedback with genuine inquiry. *Anesthesiology Clinics*, *25*(2), 361–376. doi:10.1016/j.anclin.2007.03.007 PMID:17574196

Sabus, C., Sabata, D., & Antonacci, D. (2011). Use of a virtual environment to facilitate instruction of an interprofessional home assessment. *Journal of Allied Health*, *40*(4), 199–205. PMID:22138875

Stillman, P. L., Burpeau-Di Gregorio, M. Y., Nicholson, G. I., Sabers, D. L., & Stillman, A. E. (1983). Six years of experience using patient instructors to teach interviewing skills. *Academic Medicine*, *58*(12), 941–946. doi:10.1097/00001888-198312000-00004 PMID:6644777

Tuttle, N., Waite, M., & Bialocerkowksi, A. (2015). Increasing external clinical placement capacity and supplementing placement content through a centrally located telemedicine simulated learning environment. *Physiotherapy*, *101*, e1552. doi:10.1016/j.physio.2015.03.1548

Tuttle, N. A., & Bialocerkowski, A. (2014). *Finding a videoconferencing platform for simulated telemedicine is not a trivial pursuit.* Academic Press.

Watson, K., Wright, A., Morris, N., McMeeken, J., Rivett, D., Blackstock, F., & Watson, G. et al. (2012). Can simulation replace part of clinical time? Two parallel randomised controlled trials. *Medical Education*, *46*(7), 657–667. doi:10.1111/j.1365-2923.2012.04295.x PMID:22646319

Wright, A., Moss, P., Watson, K., Rue, S., Jull, G., Mandrusiak, A., & MacIntosh, S. et al. (2015). A profession-wide collaboration to embed role-play simulation into Australian entry-level physiotherapy clinical training. *Physiotherapy*, *101*, e1047. doi:10.1016/j.physio.2015.03.1924

Wright, A., Moss, P., Watson, K., Rue, S., Jull, G., Mandrusiak, A., & Palmer, T. (2016). *Simulation in Physiotherapy Clinical Training*. Academic Press.

Wright, S., Mandrusiak, A., Ramsbotham, N., Hayles, E., & Kelly, K. (2014). The use of simulated learning to enhance cardiorespiratory acute paediatric physiotherapy across Queensland. *Pediatric Critical Care Medicine, 15*(4_suppl), 222.

Chapter 11
Use of E-Portfolios in Health Professions Education

Andrew G. Pearson
Griffith University, Australia

Brooke E. Harris-Reeves
Griffith University, Australia

Lana J. Mitchell
Griffith University, Australia

Jessica J. Vanderlelie
Griffith University, Australia

ABSTRACT

In light of the changing landscape of workforce demand, digital technologies are becoming increasingly important to support students with their studies and professional preparation. As such, tertiary institutions are embedding curriculum approaches focused on the development of employability skills and drawing upon technology in order to prepare students for the real world of work in a manner that is scalable and transferable. Digital technologies such as ePortfolios have become an increasingly utilized platform for reflection, evidencing professional competencies and professional branding. Within this chapter, the authors discuss the benefits and limitations of these platforms from the perspectives of students, staff, professional, and institutional contexts. Case studies are utilzsed to demonstrate ePortfolios in practice across the allied health disciplines and key research questions and solutions for the future are discussed.

DOI: 10.4018/978-1-5225-3850-9.ch011

INTRODUCTION

The use of portfolios as a repository for learning artefacts is not a new phenomenon. Professions such as teacher education (Allan & Cleland, 2012; Lee & Pohio, 2012), construction (Williams, Simmons, Levett-Jones, Sher, & Bowen, 2012) engineering (Faulkner, Aziz, Waye, & Smith, 2013), and the creative arts (Blom & Hitchcock, 2017) have been using portfolios as a means of recording achievements and collating resources for decades. The introduction of the ePortfolio has resulted in an increase in the availability, practicality and assimilation of portfolios, with various forms of technology. The electronic format of the portfolio evolved as a popular alternative to the paper-based approach, due to its functionality and ability to provide instructors the access to evaluate and provide feedback asynchronously. In addition, ePortfolios have the capacity to promote and track student learning, and provide a tool for student reflection as they develop an awareness of what they have learned across a curriculum (Chen & Penny Light, 2010). ePortfolios can be used to document subject, degree and graduate competencies/capabilities as well as provide a space to document and track the development of employability skills with the overarching goal of creating work-ready graduates.

BACKGROUND

A Short History of the Portfolio and ePortfolio

Portfolios have been utilized for career purposes since the early 1800s to showcase achievements in music, fine arts, photography, architecture, and graphic design (Blom & Hitchcock, 2017). Portfolios remain a widely used tool for evidencing professional competencies where selected items of work are compiled to demonstrate the achievements and abilities of the owner.

The use of ePortfolios in education evolved out of print-based student portfolios with significant writing components. Due to the challenges of handling media in the infancy of the internet, ePortfolios emerged as written works in disciplines such as English studies (Connolly, Gould, Hainey, Waugh & Boyle, 2010). Portfolios and ePortfolios have both been used for the owner to analyse and reflect on their work – students collect their work, select examples to showcase, and reflect on what they learned (Yancey, 2001).

With improvements technology, the content in ePortfolios developed to more closely resemble a modern version of an artist's portfolio (Meyer, Abrami, Wade, Aslan & Deault, 2010), containing electronic artefacts such as text, audio, images, video, multimedia, certificates, and digital badges. In addition to the enhanced content options, ePortfolios offer advantages over print portfolios, including the ability to reach vast numbers of people (Rowley, 2008), and the ability to showcase digital tools that are commonly used in the conceptual and creative process (Cleveland & Cleveland, 2004).

Utilization of ePortfolios

Understanding and use of the term 'ePortfolio' varies across discipline areas and institutions. For example - is an ePortfolio defined as a genre, a set of practices, a showcase, a technology, or all four and more? (AAEEBL, 2015). The Australian ePortfolio project reported in 2008 that ePortfolios were being utilized in diverse educational and employment contexts, for varying purposes and target audiences, and implemented across a range of platforms. There was a high level of interest in the use of ePortfolios in higher education, particularly for reflective learning and the capacity to make students' existing and developing skills explicit. Greatest use of ePortfolios was in coursework programs rather than research programs, with a shift beginning to emerge in responsibility for implementation from individual teaching units to a centralised model (Hallam et al., 2008).

A need for open dialogue between government departments, the higher education sector, employers, and ePortfolio stakeholders regarding government policy, technical standards, academic policy, and learning and teaching was identified for effective implementation and use of ePortfolios (Hallam & Creagh, 2010).

There has been an increase in the use of ePortfolios in Australian universities (Hallam, Harper, McAllister, Hauville, & Creagh, 2010; Miller, 2009), though their implementation has varied from a graduate portfolio including as a collection of discrete artefacts, to the documentation of a learning journey (Strampel, Sibson & Main, 2017). Part of the reason for this difference in implementation of ePortfolios has been due to whether their introduction has initiated from the institution, an academic staff member, or an academic developer. Sustained interest, support, and integration of ePortfolios has been most successful where there has been institutional support and ePortfolios have been embedded within Programs (Posey et al., 2015; Siu, 2013; Slade, Murfin, & Readman, 2013). Well-designed pedagogy and purposeful delivery is crucial for ePortfolios to become empowering and regenerative (McAllister & Hauville, 2017). Critical reflection is an iterative process that should be developed throughout a program as core assessment with support to help students learn to write reflectively (O'Connor, Obst, Furlong, & Hansen 2015).

In a pilot study of ePortfolio use by nursing students, many found the technological and logistical challenges of ePortfolio use frustrating, but noted ePortfolios could be useful repositories for documents, reflections and learning experiences. The effectiveness of ePortfolio use in nursing and midwifery education was questioned, particularly, whether ePortfolios have been implemented with misguided and misinformed good intention (Birks, Hartin, Woods, Emmanuel & Hitchins, 2016).

Evidencing and Tracking Competency (Learning Analytics to Ensure Quality)

The process of developing and maintaining an ePortfolio requires students to think critically about their skills, abilities and professional identities. Students who have been through the process of ePortfolio development – through critical reflection on their learning and experience – are more likely to understand their capacity and be able to meet the challenges of graduate recruitment (McAllister & Hauville, 2017).

Where ePortfolios have been embedded across a program of study, they are a valuable tool for the documentation of achievement, professional competencies, and program outcomes across a range of disciplines (Strampel, Sibson & Main, 2017).

Professional Development

The process of creating an ePortfolio is not only valuable for students, it can encourage teachers to reflect on their teaching pedagogy and curriculum, to become more conscious of the theories and assumptions that guide their teaching practice, and engage in collaborative dialogue about teaching (Zeichner & Wray, 2001). Where staff engage in ePortfolio creation and model reflective behaviour, it has resulted in more effective student engagement (Schaub-de Jong, Schönrock-Adema, Dekke, Verkerk, & CohenSchotanus, 2011).

For teachers to successfully implement and embed the use of ePortfolio practices requires the support of an ePortfolio professional learning ecosystem, including professional development and the provision of digital literacy skills. Training is required about a range of issues, including privacy, ownership, security, pedagogy, assessment, and self-reflection (Miller, 2017).

Application of ePortfolios in Health Disciplines

Education in Health Disciplines requires students to develop discipline specific knowledge and skills in addition to key capabilities including self-reflection and professional practice. Assessment of these skills and capabilities occurs through a variety of means including formative and summative subject assessment and clinical placement experiences. ePortfolios have the potential to support students to evidence their skills and capabilities, encourage the documentation of reflection and provide a platform through which to showcase their learnings. For academic staff, the ePortfolio supports the assessment of competencies across the student learning journey with learning activities 'all in one place'. The potential of ePortfolios extends to the support and facilitation of clinical placement and its examination. Providing a platform through which industry networks can assess and contribute to the recorded student learning journey in a manner that occurs in real time and is less labour intensive than traditional paper based methodologies.

Across the Health Disciplines, ePortfolios are emerging as an important platform and the following case studies highlight three separate approaches and platforms for the embedding of ePortfolios.

CASE STUDY 1

The Development of a Platform Starting From Need Rather Than Technology in the Midwifery Discipline

Context

The Griffith University Bachelor of Midwifery (BMid) degree was developed in 2010 to prepare a future-focussed, culturally capable midwifery workforce. Across the program, students are required to complete over 2,000 hours of clinical activity and manual experiences to meet registration requirements. Ongoing industry, professional, student and alumni consultation undertaken by the Midwifery team at Griffith University suggested that the lack of preparedness of the current midwifery workforce was a barrier to the implementation of woman-centered care, hence this was specifically addressed within the curriculum experiences for students.

Rationale

The development of an ePortfolio was considered as part of a broader strategy within the degree program to support preparation for practice through scaffolded professional capability and employability skills training. The Midwifery team investigated a number of commercially available ePortfolio platforms and through the process were unable to find a system that met the diversity of pedagogical requirements. As such, the process of developing a customised ePortfolio solution was undertaken.

The Platform

Utilizing the Smartabase Software system that was originally designed for professional sportspersons, the team developed an online personal learning environment for students termed M@GIE (Midwifery @ Griffith Interactive ePortfolio). M@GIE provides a tool through which students can evidence their learning journey across the degree program. The platform has the built-in capacity for automated feedback from academic staff, tutors and industry professionals, the tracking of clinical hours, the logging of mandatory experiences, and facilitates students and staff to view attainment of the requirements for registration. Additionally, staff can set up performance alerts within the system to encourage students to stay on track with their progress towards professional accreditation requirements.

Currently the platform is being utilized to record and monitor students' clinical performance, attendance and achievement. Elements of teaching have been automated within the system that allow students to practice technical skills in a simulated environment, an activity designed to enhance skills on graduation. There is potential within the system to not only track specific academic fields but to record co-curricular activities and support lifelong learning post-graduation.

Prior to implementation, the Midwifery team developed specialised training and support programs for staff and students regarding system operations and design. Additional high-level training was provided to subject builder and administrators to ensure they have the capacity to build and change components of the system with minimal requirements for technical support.

The Task

One example of the use of M@GIE occurs in a third year Capstone subject. The assessment is based on the industry standard Midwifery Practice Review Program. Students are required to create their portfolio that supplements the logs of competencies and clinical hours also collected within the system. This assessment activity provides students with the opportunity to consolidate learning and demonstrate their readiness for employment. Upon completion of the ePortfolio, students in their final semester have the opportunity to complete a simulated employment interview with industry partners on the panels.

Impact on Students

The Midwifery program at Griffith University, continues to grow in influence and work in partnership with industry to enable students to work at the cutting edge of maternity care. The ePortfolio assessment item was evaluated by a panel of international academics, that acknowledged the clear links to employability and the effectiveness of the item in promoting reflection and application of critical thinking. Formal student evaluation of the assessment identified that while students found the activity time consuming and at times challenging, they recognised how valuable the process was in preparation for employment.

CASE STUDY 2

Programmatic Approach to Embedding PebblePad in the Nutrition and Dietetics Discipline

Context

The dietetic workforce is currently over-supplied in Queensland, a situation that poses a significant challenge for new graduates transitioning to the workforce.

The Bachelor of Nutrition & Dietetics program (BND) at Griffith University is a four-year, undergraduate degree that graduates approximately 60 students each year.

Rationale

To give Griffith graduates an edge in the competitive workforce environment, the Nutrition and Dietetics team developed a tool to actively assist students to translate and articulate their knowledge and skills. The implementation of PebblePad within the Bachelor of Nutrition and Dietetics program occurred as part of the ePortfolios for Dietetic Graduate Employability (eDGE) Project. This was one of several employability initiatives introduced by the Discipline.

The Platform

PebblePad is a personal learning platform and ePortfolio tool. The platform is designed to accommodate a wide variety of learning activities and has the capacity for all assessment to be delivered in some manner through the system. PebblePad has built in capacity for the design interactive workbooks and customisation of existing templates. Students, staff and industry professionals can access components of a student's learning platform and as such can deliver timely feedback to students on their work. Students have complete control over their PebblePad documents and can provide access to individual pages within the system. When deployed across a degree of study the platform facilitates the tracking of learning outcomes, professional competencies and graduate outcomes. PebblePad also contains a personal ePortfolio tool, that provides an opportunity for students to showcase components of their learning journey in a format that is viewable to external audiences.

The Task

Several assessment tasks have been delivered through PebblePad, many of which focused on career planning and the evidencing of graduate employability. In some existing assessment, items were altered to make use of the functionality of PebblePad, while others were introduced for the first time using PebblePad. PebblePad was utilized for the purpose of reflection, with structured reflective tasks, as well as the reflection on learning that occurred throughout a variety of activities, which were also logged through the platform. Work Integrated Learning (WIL) activity logs and class-time activity logs enabled students to collate all related activities and reflect on their learnings from these activities. Students were also required to produce video reflections, which with the assistance of the Pebble Pocket App on smart phones were very easy to create, upload, submit and mark.

Templates were created to encourage students to consider their motivation for enrolment and career goals. PebblePad was also utilized for the purpose of collating placement mandatory documents and evidencing meeting the requirements to embark on WIL placement. Setting of learning goals and logging Continuing Professional Development (CPD) hours is a key requirement of the dietetics profession. Therefore, this key practice has been included in the BND from Year 1 of the degree to motivate students to develop a habit of professional development, encouraging them to select activities that are strongly linked with enhanced employability. The portfolio elements of PebblePad were utilized to allow students to develop their CV from Year 1 of the Program, and to seek out activities to contribute to a strong CV.

Impact on Students

The eDGE Project has been evaluated with the BND students. Their views of the use of PebblePad as a tool for evidencing competency and enhancing employability were evaluated. Students reported that PebblePad encouraged the consolidation of important career planning with the most useful employability feature the collating activities in one place. This functionality facilitated the demonstration of competence and the setting of professional development learning goals across the degree in addition to the capacity to log activities.

CASE 3

Embedding ePortfolios in First Year Health Science

Context

Chemistry of Biological Systems II is a subject offered at Griffith University that enrols 500-600 first year students from a range of health programs including Health Science, Biomedical Science, Exercise Science, Pharmacy, Dental Science, Nutrition and Dietetics, Medical Laboratory Science, Environmental Health, and Public Health. This entry-level science course forms one component of a common Health foundation year. The structure of the foundation year has meant that the embedding of employability skills from first year is uniquely challenging for most programs within the Faculty of Health.

Rationale

As part of a broader university strategy to improve employability outcomes for students Chemistry of Biological Systems II was identified as an ideal candidate to begin specific employability-based education due to the diversity of programs that it supports. To this end, a first year, introductory level employability task was designed that began the process of student ePortfolio development. The assessment item was designed to get first year students thinking about their career path, to start making professional connections, enhance their digital literacy skills.

The Platform

At the time of implementation, the university was without a contractual agreement with any ePortfolio provider. As such students were encouraged to develop their portfolios using publicly available tools. To facilitate flexibility in ePortfolio development, students were given the opportunity to create their ePortfolio on a platform of their choice. To avoid confusion however, four were suggested – the freely available Wix, Weebly and (the now defunct) Re.vu in addition to the licensed platform PebblePad (only available for Nutrition and Dietetics students due to individual licensing). Platforms chosen based on their ease of use, functionality and fact they were freely available online.

The Task

The assessment item was designed as an entry-level activity that required students to develop the basic components of an externally facing ePortfolio that they could continue to develop across the course of their studies. The task comprised of two components – the creation of an ePortfolio and development and linkage of the ePortfolio to a LinkedIn profile.

Within the ePortfolio, students created two tabs – a homepage and an academic skills page. The homepage contained a background image, welcome message, information about themselves and their career path, in addition to a link to their LinkedIn profile. Within the academic skills tab, students wrote a one-paragraph reflection on academic integrity covering why it is important for a future health professional, and their reflections from an online academic integrity module. Digital badges were awarded to students for successful completion of the academic integrity quizzes, and for competent use of a pipette in the laboratory.

For the LinkedIn profile, students were required to include an appropriate photograph, a headline describing their career profile, a career summary, a customised URL, a link to their ePortfolio, their education, employment history, volunteer experience, and skills. To build connections, students were required to join at least four LinkedIn groups. Suggestions for groups included the university careers service, and the Pharmacy Professionals Network. Students also had to make at least 15 LinkedIn connections, and were encouraged to use a personalised message to tailor the introduction.

To support students in building their ePortfolio, the subject convenor created and shared an exemplar, and ran several drop-in tutorials for students to work on their own ePortfolio.

Impact on Students

The quality of work produced was generally excellent, with an average mark of 93% for the combined LinkedIn profile and ePortfolio, which was 10% of the course assessment. Formal evaluation of the assessment task revealed that students found value in the activity despite their reports that it was time consuming. Specifically, students could see the potential for the portfolio to support their employability skills development and as a means through which to showcase their skills. Qualitative comments included *"This is probably one of the best assignments I've had to complete that I know I will use & I bet every other student will as well, so thanks for taking the time to care about our future!"*.

Issues, Controversies Problems

While tertiary institutions in Australia are embracing ePortfolios, it is important to highlight the key considerations and challenges associated with this approach. The issues and controversies of the integration and use of ePortfolios in tertiary settings are recognised to affect students, staff, industry professionals and institutions. Table 1 outlines specific issues and their relevance to different stakeholders and throughout this section the key issues relevant to each stakeholder are discussed.

Students

The use of ePortfolios in student education presents a variety of limitations that may impact on student uptake and utilization of ePortfolios for their learning.

Table 1. Issues and controversies of ePortfolio use for stakeholders

	Students	Staff	Industry Professionals	Institutions
Time Constraints		✓	✓	
Training	✓	✓	✓	✓
IT Support	✓	✓	✓	✓
Increased workload	✓	✓	✓	
Communication of relevance	✓	✓	✓	✓
Curriculum/assessment design		✓		
Digital literacy	✓	✓	✓	
Licensing Cost				✓
Access to technology (devices/websites)	✓		✓	
Student Information Privacy	✓	✓		✓
Professional behaviour	✓	✓	✓	
Access to WiFi	✓			
Policy and Governance		✓		✓
Data and information storage				✓
Professional Accreditation/standards		✓	✓	✓
Assurance of learning		✓		✓
Provision of feedback		✓	✓	

Digital Literacy

Utilizing ePortfolios for learning is ideally suited to today's learners, who often prefer the online and technology-focused environment (Ciocco & Holtzman, 2008). However, it must be acknowledged that not all students feel comfortable in the online environment or with the use of technology. For students, it is important that the chosen ePortfolio tool has a high usability, is intuitive, can conduct file uploads in reasonable timeframes, has labelling/tagging abilities to store and access key resources, and allows for supervisor/marker feedback (Willmarth-Stec & Beery, 2015). Whatever tool is used, adequate training and technological support is required (Willmarth-Stec & Beery, 2015). It is also important that students are shown how to set up their learning environment to enhance organisation and locating of resources for future use (Willmarth-Stec & Beery, 2015). Utilizing tagging functions will assist with this, as well as standard naming conventions (Willmarth-Stec & Beery, 2015). Advancements in portfolio software makes it much more accessible for people without extensive computer programming knowledge, with a more standardised format and less avenue for creativity (Clark, 2009).

Access to Wi-Fi and Internet Networks

Access to Wi-Fi and internet networks is a key limiting factor in the functionality of many ePortfolios if students are required to use these while on placement. Wi-Fi may not be available due to outdoor locations, field trips or patient home visits (Forte, de Souza, da Silva, do Prado, & Rodrigues, 2013). In addition, institutions may also have restrictions on access to external websites that limit the capacity for students to access their portfolio on department computers without internal approval. Some ePortfolio software has navigated this by introducing an app that can be used offline to store work, which is then uploaded when connected to internet Wi-Fi (Pebble Learning Ltd, 2012). However, this does not allow access to current resources within the ePortfolio. This is an issue, for example, when conducting a competency development assessment with a supervisor/ clinical educator on a placement.

Workload/Time Commitments

While ePortfolios are beneficial for the collation of work, the development of a portfolio may be a time-consuming process (Harris, Dolan, & Fairbairn, 2001; Joyce, 2005; Mitchell, 1994). While this is no-doubt made easier with electronic versions rather than paper copies, a great deal of student time may go into these collections. This consideration is a key factor in the recommendation of a scaffolded approach to ePortfolio utilization and the implementation of a consistent platform across an institution, to save students the additional time involved in recreating their portfolio. Academic staff must also be mindful of the associated workload implications of ePortfolio tasks and ensure that clear expectations of what is required for the portfolio are communicated to students. If this is not the case, students have been found to demonstrate increased levels of anxiety, and decreased motivation (Mitchell, 1994).

Relevance

To justify the time commitments associated with portfolio development, it is important that students see the relevance of developing ePortfolio resources to their learning (Harris et al., 2001). This is especially relevant when ePortfolios are not directly assessed (Harris et al., 2001) and may result in a deprioritisation of the task in favour of assessable activities. Additionally, encouragement and support from teaching staff is key to facilitating a greater utilization (Harris et al., 2001).

The benefits of ePortfolio resources on learning and development need to be strongly emphasised to students (Harris et al., 2001); in particular, their potential to allow students to take control of their own learning (Green, Wyllie, & Jackson, 2014;

Joyce, 2005). Reflection is a key element of ePortfolios, however, not all students feel comfortable with this form of writing, as it is much more personal than other academic forms, and requires a greater level of self-awareness and a willingness to explore individual strengths and weaknesses (Harris et al., 2001; Karlowicz, 2000). Using ePortfolios for assessment may result in a student reflecting on what they think they are meant to write, rather than their actual thoughts (Harris et al., 2001). This in turn may limit the value of the reflection to their personal learning.

Privacy (Digital Footprint)

In this digital age, the issue of confidentiality and student privacy has been raised in the context of housing student work online (Joyce, 2005). Once work is shared digitally, a potential exists for this to be copied elsewhere in the online environment. When sharing work with peers, students need to be aware of academic integrity requirements and the potential implications of plagiarism (Turnitin, 2012). Concerns regarding privacy, may limit student openness with their portfolio reflections (Joyce, 2005).

Professional Behaviour

Students need to demonstrate the behaviour that would be expected of them as practicing professionals in their field. As emerging professionals, students require guidance and explicit examples of the kinds of artefacts desirable to collect and present in their ePortfolios (Green et al., 2014). These artefacts need to be beneficial and appropriate for students in the short term as part of their learning and in the long term in their future career (Green et al., 2014). As with the non-online environment, students must maintain patient/client confidentiality, and not include any identifying information within their ePortfolios, in line with their professional standards. This is especially important with the ease of which photographs can be included in ePortfolios. Students need to be reminded of these expectations and how these relate to their ePortfolios (Green et al., 2014).

Staff

Within the broad context of education, there are a myriad of possibilities for the embedding of an ePortfolio in learning and teaching activities. To depict the ePortfolio as merely a tool is to neglect the input required from a staff perspective. Careful consideration and acknowledgement is required regarding the level of staff investment necessary for successful implementation of ePortfolios into the curriculum. Researchers (Hallam & Creagh, 2010) have identified various issues and concerns from a staff perspective including: increased workload; support for training and development of the necessary skills; IT support; and staff compliance.

According to Garrison and Kanuka (2004), increased staff workload is the most significant aspect that requires consideration when integrating ePortfolio technology. Initially, demands on staff time relate to the training required to develop the skills necessary to understand and navigate the technology. This is an essential aspect of successful integration of ePortfolios across the curriculum as a lack of technical skills, understanding and staff buy-in has been identified as a potential barrier to adoption (Peacock, Gordon, Murray, Morss & Dunlop, 2010).

One key approach to obtaining staff buy-in is to acknowledge and highlight how ePortfolio technology aligns with current practice. This can be achieved through identifying existing practice and providing examples of how an ePortfolio can enhance the learning experience. When designing curriculum, it is important that discipline and context specific learning objectives are developed and followed with evaluation of the compatibility of learning activities, assessment and learning outcomes (Aalderink & Veugelers, 2005). This critical approach to curriculum design has been countered by concerns about the increased workload for staff. It is anticipated that effective development and implementation of curriculum, along with support for students will place a strain on teaching staff. An additional workload concern identified by Cheng (2008) relates to assessment, marking and feedback in an online environment. With many educators accustomed to the pen and paper system for marking and providing written feedback, it is perceived by some as a burden to undertake marking directly on a computer screen.

Training, guidance and IT support for staff implementing ePortfolios, is a potential issue influencing the success of ePortfolio based curriculum (Holt et al, 2016). Implementation of new technology often results in staff feeling intimidated and overwhelmed. Appropriate training to ensure staff are adequately skilled is essential given research highlighting student satisfaction is directly related to a teacher's ability and confidence with ePortfolios (Draude and Brace, 1999). Seven factors have been identified as integral staff support approaches (Holt et al, 2016):

1. Communication of ePortfolio relevance;
2. Guidance on how to use ePortfolios;
3. Workshops to support the ePortfolio process;
4. Tutor support;
5. IT help desk support for the teacher;
6. Support for producing media files; and
7. Access to exemplars

The development of integrated and innovative ePortfolio pedagogy takes time to comprehend and support to achieve. The most effective use of ePortfolio practice is realised when students use it to connect their learning journey between subjects and while transitioning through their tertiary studies. The only way this is possible is if there is a shift beyond the 'early-adopters' to take a programmatic and institution-wide approach. Given the 'silo' nature of many faculties and departments within the university setting, staff training and professional development must emphasise a collaborative approach to ePortfolio integration in order to construct a shared direction and achieve a synchronized pedagogical design.

Institutional

Institution-wide ePortfolios can bring about positive, progressive development of practice across the academy. ePortfolios have the potential to streamline the academic planning and development process and provide a vehicle for communication and collaboration between institutions and industry. In order to achieve this, significant time, energy and resources are essential to develop an ongoing institutional ePortfolio. Further, potential issues need to be considered at an institutional level if integration of an ePortfolio is to be successful. Such issues are recognised as being varied and highly challenging including:

1. Support at the policy level for integration of an ePortfolio approach;
2. The provision of resources to support implementation across the institution;
3. Achieving staff and student buy in and understanding of the relevance;
4. Unified curriculum approach across schools and faculties; and
5. Continuing availability for alumni after graduation.

Researchers have recognised the importance of support at policy level as critical to effective ePortfolio implementation and practice (Cosh, 2008; Reese & Levy, 2009). Commitment and support of senior administrators is identified as a major contributing factor leading to successful integration of ePortfolios (Reardon, Lumsden & Meyer, 2005). Research conducted by Hallam et al., (2008) highlights how a strong alignment between strategic, tactical and operational areas within an institution is required for effective ePortfolio practice. For this to occur, clear and precise communication channels are required when integrating an ePortfolio system through institution-wide approach. Communication channels should include a strategic direction, collaborative language, exemplars of good practice and recognition for staff who develop innovative curriculum approaches in the ePortfolio space. Successful integration of any ePortfolio system requires a well-thought-out strategy and a cohesive approach. Technology is a potential factor in how rapidly institutional ePortfolios are adopted and develop. The ongoing support and participation institution-wide of administrators, faculty and IT teams is essential for the organisation of resources and to building an easy to navigate site. Compatibility with existing IT systems are identified as a key determinant to effective institution wide integration (Quinton & Smallbone, 2008). As with any new IT integration, it is imperative to minimise potential technical barriers such as connectivity, navigation between existing learning and teaching platforms, and perceived complexity from both staff and students.

Aside from specific technology issues, Quinton and Smallbone (2008) acknowledged the most significant influence on the success of ePortfolio implementation is the 'people' aspect. The support provided by schools, IT and staff are key to the successful institution wide design and development. Central to the 'people' aspect identified as a pivotal to institution wide ePortfolio success (Quinton and Smallbone, 2008), is the development of a top-down culture. Institutions need to consider the appropriate culture that disseminates a set of core values and assumptions, a unified language, and fundamental educational practices applicable to ePortfolios. With large student cohorts and large numbers of teaching staff, development of a supportive and inclusive culture is crucial to ensure all parties involved understand the purpose of ePortfolios and how they can affect and influence practice. The objective of a cross institutional culture is to support and encourage staff buy-in and student engagement, both of which are key to effective institution-wide integration.

According to researchers (Housego & Parker, 2009; Woodley & Sims, 2011), institution-wide ePortfolios should be integrated into the whole curriculum. The Higher Education Academy (HEA, 2005) acknowledges that effective ePortfolio practices in institutions should include integration with mainstream academic activities and links to program and learning objectives. Staff and curriculum designers are encouraged to introduce ePortfolios in the early stages of a program or degree, providing students with the opportunity to develop and track their own progress as they journey through their studies. Successful implementation is also recognised as one that is understood by students and relevant to each discipline and learning context. Essentially, ePortfolio systems need to be robust, easily accessed and relevant to avoid undesirable levels of adoption. Further, consideration is essential around the access of ePortfolios upon graduation. A system that does not allow students to access their reflections and artefacts for employment purposes upon graduation neglects to take a lifelong learner approach.

Industry Professionals

The use of ePortfolios by industry professionals, or external stakeholders who are involved in students' learning, presents a variety of issues that are similar to those for students and staff as well additional concerns unique to this group.

Digital Literacy

While today's learners are becoming more proficient in the online environment (Ciocco & Holtzman, 2008), this may not be the case for all of the industry professionals who are involved in student education. This must be taken into consideration when implementing the use of ePortfolios for student assessment.

Harris et al, (2001) highlighted the importance of students seeing the relevance of developing ePortfolio resources to their learning to enhance utilization (Harris et al., 2001); however, this is also key in the uptake of new systems for industry professionals. The benefits of ePortfolio resources on learning and development need to be strongly emphasised (Harris et al., 2001); in particular, allowing students to take control of their own learning (Green et al., 2014; Joyce, 2005). In a time-pressured environment, a willingness for change may be limited if not well communicated.

Training and Support

This issue of adequate training and technological support previously identified (Willmarth-Stec & Beery, 2015) is also relevant to industry professionals who are required to access ePortfolio software for student supervision. This is especially true when professionals are assessing student competence and need to interact with the software, rather than just simply view students' work. Initial training in the software is required, and requires dedicated time away from the professional's other work responsibilities, which is often difficult to obtain. For ongoing technological support, it is unlikely that experts in the software are located in the professional's workplace, and therefore they are reliant on telephone support, if available at all. Institutions need to consider the degree of training and support likely required by industry professionals when implementing new software.

Access to External Websites, Online Tools and Software Not Available Within Institution

As with students, industry professionals in some settings may have limited access to external websites and programs due to firewalls within their institutions. If a supervisor / clinical educator on a placement needs to review students' competency assessment forms within an ePortfolio system, it is essential that access is readily available.

Assessment of Students

Issues with consistency of assessment are not unique to online portfolio assessment, however still need to be considered in this context. While institutions and staff must ensure the development of appropriate assessment and marking rubrics, industry professionals should not only be trained in the use of the online tools, but also in the pedagogic underpinning of why ePortfolios are being utilized (Garrett, MacPhee, & Jackson, 2013). Introducing change with the way industry professionals are expected to assess students may result in an unwillingness from the stakeholders, unless the reasons for the change are well justified and communicated clearly. At least initially, ePortfolios may be time consuming to assess (Harris et al., 2001; Joyce, 2005), although once industry professionals become familiar with the new system, workload may decrease. Uptake by each professional may vary, and therefore the quality of assessment, feedback and assistance may vary between supervisors or clinical educators (Harris et al., 2001)

Access to Previous Student Assessment Forms and Feedback

When assessing student competency using ePortfolios, consideration must be made for transparency between placement sites. Institutions should consider the expectations they place on students regarding who they share assessment forms, reflections and learning goals with. While there are benefits of each placement site being able to view previous competency assessment for targeting education to specific needs, this may impact on clinical judgement. While this is not a unique issue to online forms, accessing previous documents may be easier online than in paper format, and expectations regarding this must be clear (Garrett et al., 2013).

SOLUTIONS RECOMMENDATIONS

The following ten points provide a summary of the key best practice strategies for the embedding of ePortfolios in higher education.

1. Pedagogy rather technology should drive the use of ePortfolios.
2. That the introduction of ePortfolio take place early in a degree and scaffolded across all year levels.
3. Wherever possible ePortfolios should be embedded into subject assessment utilizing diverse modalities (peer review, reflection, industry feedback, academic grading).

4. The clear communication to students of the role of the ePortfolios in evidencing the attainment of competencies and visibility within the degree structure and outlines.
5. The provision of structured and scaffolded opportunities to develop reflective capabilities for students (Brandes & Boskic, 2008; Peacock, Gordon, Murray, Morss, & Dunlop 2010).
6. The implementation of a University-wide platform to ensure a consistent student experience for those of undertaking diverse programs of study.
7. The provision for lifetime access for alumni to their ePortfolio.
8. The engagement of Industry professionals in the process of designing assessment and portfolio activities to ensure professional relevance.
9. The provision of comprehensive and inclusive training for students, academic staff and industry partners.
10. Institutions and academics must be cognisant of and develop policy to cover, information privacy, data storage security and student professional behaviour prior to initiating the embedding of ePortfolio solutions.

FUTURE RESEARCH DIRECTIONS

Despite the significant utilization of ePortfolios in higher education, their use in Health Disciplines is still emerging. In this regard, it is important that we collect robust data regarding the student experience of ePortfolio technologies. Greater information regarding the student experience of portfolios, perceptions of workload and relevance during the course of study would assist educators to develop supportive portfolio based activities. However more powerful information will be gained through the exploration of patterns of ePortfolio utilization and perceived professional relevance in continuing practice after graduation. Such data would allow educators to make informed decisions when embedding portfolio based activities and ensure that students are investing time in the creation of a portfolio that has transferability and broad applicability in their emerging and continuing careers.

In addition to the student perspectives, an important piece of work still left to pursue is the exploration of academic staff experiences. Currently there are gaps in our understanding of levels of academic staff digital literacy, and their capacity to embrace ePortfolio technologies to enrich the curriculum. Unpacking the pedagogical benefits of ePortfolios in the context of Health Professions education is fundamental to providing high quality training and support to educators considering the utilization of ePortfolio in their teaching.

Finally, we must consider the resource and training requirements of our clinical educators and industry partners. In many health professions, the transition from paper based student assessment of placement to an ePortfolio solution is not well supported and detailed data regarding the industry professional experience is lacking. Further research in this area will ensure our industry partners are supported in the use of technology such as ePortfolios and as such can articulate the value of this in the changing landscape of the professions. Additionally, the exploration of industry perspective in the relevance of portfolio in the process of graduate recruitment and continuing professional development of the workforce is yet to be explored in the context of the Health Disciplines.

CONCLUSION

ePortfolios offer a powerful tool to capture the student learning journey and evidence the achievement of professional capabilities. Portfolios have been used for over 200 years in the creative disciplines, however their use in the Health disciplines is still considered emerging. The emergence of platforms with greater usability and portability have opened doors to the enrichment of curriculum through the potential offered by ePortfolios. This is particularly evident in the Health Professions through the engagement of industry in the assessment of professional competencies once undertaken through a paper based process that are now more seamlessly delivered through ePortfolio solutions.

For academic staff, ePortfolios afford an unprecedented opportunity to visualise the student learning journey across not only a subject but an entire degree program. The capacity to evidence attainment of University Graduate Attributes / Qualities in addition to professional competencies makes it easier to design curriculum that meets the needs of the student learning journey and ensures key competencies do not 'fall through the gap' due to curriculum drift or staff turnover.

ePortfolios provide an important repository of learning artefacts and reflections of experience that have the capacity to not only evidence performance but enhance the professional maturity and ability of graduates to clearly evidence their skills and achievements. The utilization of externally facing portfolios are becoming more widely recognised across the professions with the existence of such showcase sites a factor that 'sets a graduate apart' in the competitive industrial landscape.

There are several challenges to embedding ePortfolios in the Health professions that require careful consideration by institutions (see Table 1). The privacy and data storage considerations are one of the key issues, with requirements varying dependent upon national laws. In addition to this important policy and procedural consideration, universities also must consider the training and support they provide to staff, students and industry partners. It is not enough to consider that a 21st century academic has the skills to navigate a new technological platform with an eguide to support them and limited 'at elbow' support. What is required is investment in the training in the educational design considerations important when creating ePortfolio assessment and activities. An ePortfolio is more than just a repository for assessment tasks and files; these platforms have the capacity to be transformative to student learning and professional confidence. To achieve this potential, academic staff require support and guidance in pedagogical approaches to ePortfolio embedding that are authentic to their disciplines, industry informed and engaging to the learner.

REFERENCES

Aalderink, W., & Veugelers, M. (2005). ePortfolio practice and opportunities in the knowledge exchange countries (Denmark, Germany, the Netherlands and the United Kingdom). In W. Aalderink & M. Veugelers (Eds.), *Stimulating lifelong learning: The eportfolio in Dutch higher education* (pp. 23–32). Utrecht, The Netherlands: Stichting SURF. Retrieved March 31, 2009 from http://www.surffoundation.nl/download/Stimulating%20Lifelong%20Learning%20-%20ePortfolio.pdf

Allan, C. N., & Cleland, B. (2012). Embedding eportfolios in teacher education: Lessons from a multi-year implementation. In M. Brown, M. Hartwell, & T. Stewart (Eds.), Proceedings of ascilite Wellington 2012: Future challenges, sustainable futures (pp. 197–201). Academic Press.

Authentic Experiential and Evidence Based Learning (AAEEBL). (2015). *Ontology of 'ePortfolio'.* Retrieved from http://www.aaeebl.org/blogpost/1008436/213232/Ontology-ofePortfolio

Birks, M., Hartin, P., Woods, C., Emmanuel, E., & Hitchins, M. (2016). Students' perceptions of the use of eportfolios in nursing and midwifery education. *Nurse Education in Practice, 18*, 46–51. doi:10.1016/j.nepr.2016.03.003 PMID:27235565

Blom, D., & Hitchcock, M. (2017). Perceived Usefulness and Relevance of ePortfolios in the Creative Arts: Investigating Student Views. In ePortfolios in Australian Universities (pp. 155-172). Springer Singapore.

Brandes, G., & Boskic, N. (2008). ePortfolios: From description to analysis. *International Review of Research in Open and Distance Learning, 9*(2), 1–17. doi:10.19173/irrodl.v9i2.502

Chen, H. L., & Penny Light, T. (2010). *Electronic portfolios and student success: effectiveness, efficiency, and learning*. Washington, DC: Association of American Colleges and Universities.

Cheng, G. (2008). Implementation Challenges of the English Language ePortfolio System from Various Stakeholder Perspectives. *Journal of Educational Technology Systems*, *37*(1), 97–118. doi:10.2190/ET.37.1.h

Ciocco, M. D., & Holtzman, D. (2008). Prior Learning Assessment: E-Portfolios and the Millennial Students. *The Journal of Continuing Higher Education*, *56*(3), 69–71. doi:10.1080/07377366.2008.10400165

Clark. (2009). E-portfolios at 2.0-Surveying the Field. *Peer Review: Emerging Trends and Key Debates in Undergraduate Education, 11*(1), 18.

Cleveland, A. O., & Cleveland, M. B. (2004). Coming of age in a digital world: The portfolio grows up. *Theatre Design and Technology*, *40*, 10–17.

Connolly, T., Gould, C., Hainey, T., Waugh, S., & Boyle, B. (2010). An empirical study: The implementation of a virtual learning environment and ePortfolio. *Proceedings of the 7th international conference on networked learning*.

Cosh, J. (2008). *Report on ALSS faculty evaluation of personal development planning (PDP)*. Retrieved from http://www.inspire.anglia.ac.uk/assets/Uploads/Publications/Research/L&T/Evaluation_of_Personal_Development_Planning_in_ALSS_Nov_2007.pdf

Draude, B., & Brace, S. (1999). Assessing the Impact of Technology on Teaching and Learning: Student Perspectives. *Proceedings of the Mid-South Instructional Technology Conference*.

Faulkner, M., Mahfuzul Aziz, S., Waye, V., & Smith, E. (2013). Exploring ways that ePortfolios can support the progressive development of graduate qualities and professional competencies. *Higher Education Research & Development, 32*(6), 871–887. doi:643710.1080/07294360.2013.80

Forte, M., de Souza, W. L., da Silva, R. F., do Prado, A. F., & Rodrigues, J. F. Jr. (2013). A ubiquitous reflective e-portfolio architecture. *International Journal of Medical Informatics*, *82*(11), 1111–1122. doi:10.1016/j.ijmedinf.2013.06.005 PMID:23850148

Garrett, B. M., MacPhee, M., & Jackson, C. (2013). Evaluation of an eportfolio for the assessment of clinical competence in a baccalaureate nursing program. *Nurse Education Today*, *33*(10), 1207–1213. doi:10.1016/j.nedt.2012.06.015 PMID:22789875

Garrison, D. R., & Kanuka, H. (2004). Blended learning: Uncovering its transformative potential in higher education. *The Internet and Higher Education*, *7*(2), 95–105. doi:10.1016/j.iheduc.2004.02.001

Green, J., Wyllie, A., & Jackson, D. (2014). Electronic portfolios in nursing education: A review of the literature. *Nurse Education in Practice*, *14*(1), 4–8. doi:10.1016/j.nepr.2013.08.011 PMID:24090523

Hallam, G., & Creagh, T. (2010). ePortfolio use by university students in Australia: A review of the Australian ePortfolio Project. *Higher Education Research & Development*, *29*(2), 179–193. doi:10.1080/07294360903510582

Hallam, G., Harper, W., McAllister, L., Hauville, K., & Creagh, T. (2010). *Australian ePortfolio project: ePortfolio use by university students in Australian: Informing excellence in policy and practice.* AeP Supplementary report. QUT Department of eLearning.

Hallam, G., Harper, W., McCowan, C., Hauville, K., McAllister, L., Creagh, T., . . . Brooks, C. (2008). ePortfolio use by university students in Australia: Informing excellence in policy and practice. Final project report, August 2008. QUT Department of Teaching and Learning Support Services, Queensland.

Harris, S., Dolan, G., & Fairbairn, G. (2001). Reflecting on the use of student portfolios. *Nurse Education Today*, *21*(4), 278–286. doi:10.1054/nedt.2000.0545 PMID:11339871

Higher Education Academy (HEA). (2005). *Guide for busy academics no.1: Personal development planning*. Retrieved from http://www.heacademy.ac.uk/resources.asp?process5full_record&section5generic&id566

Holt, D., McGuigan, N., Kavanagh, M., Leitch, S., Ngo, L., Salzman, S., & McKay, J. et al. (2016). Academic leaders' perspectives on adopting ePortfolios for developing and assessing professional capabilities in Australian business education. *Australasian Journal of Educational Technology*, *32*(5), 1–18. doi:10.14742/ajet.2666

Housego, S., & Parker, N. (2009). Positioning ePortfolio in an integrated curriculum. *Education + Training*, *51*(5/6), 408–421. doi:10.1108/00400910910987219

Joyce, P. (2005). A framework for portfolio development in postgraduate nursing practice. *Journal of Clinical Nursing, 14*(4), 456–463. doi:10.1111/j.1365-2702.2004.01075.x PMID:15807752

Karlowicz, K. A. (2000). The value of student portfolios to evaluate undergraduate nursing programs. *Nurse Educator, 25*(2), 82–87. doi:10.1097/00006223-200003000-00010 PMID:11052006

Lee, M., & Pohio, L. (2012). An ePortfolio theoretical approach for provisionally registered teachers. In M. Brown, M. Hartwell, & T. Stewart (Eds.), Proceedings of ascilite Wellington 2012: Future challenges, sustainable futures (pp. 550–559). Academic Press.

McAllister, L., & Hauville, K. (2017). Striving for Sustainability: ePortfolio Pedagogy in Australian Higher Education. In ePortfolios in Australian Universities (pp. 13-32). Springer Singapore.

Meyer, E., Abrami, P. C., Wade, C. A., Aslan, O., & Deault, L. (2010). Improving literacy and metacognition with electronic portfolios: Teaching and learning with ePEARL. *Computers & Education, 55*(1), 84–91. doi:10.1016/j.compedu.2009.12.005

Miller, A. (2009). E-portfolios – Managing learner information in the vocational education and training sector. *Learning Communities: International Journal of Learning in Social Contexts,* (2), 16–30.

Miller, A. (2017). Professional Learning Ecosystem Support for ePortfolio Use in Australian Higher Education: An Historical Perspective. In ePortfolios in Australian Universities (pp. 1-11). Springer Singapore.

Mitchell, M. (1994). The views of students and teachers on the use of portfolios as a learning and assessment tool in midwifery education. *Nurse Education Today, 14*(1), 38–43. doi:10.1016/0260-6917(94)90056-6 PMID:8159148

O'Connor, E., Obst, P., Furlong, M., & Hansen, J. (2015). Using the TARL model in psychology: Supporting first and final year students to compose reflections. In *Teaching Reflective Learning in Higher Education* (pp. 77–91). Springer International Publishing. doi:10.1007/978-3-319-09271-3_6

Peacock, S., Gordon, L., Murray, S., Morss, K., & Dunlop, G. (2010). Tutor response to implementing an ePortfolio to support learning and personal development in further and higher education institutions in Scotland. *British Journal of Educational Technology, 41*(5), 827–851. doi:10.1111/j.1467-8535.2009.00986.x

Pebble Learning Ltd. (2012). *Pebble+ Help: Pebble Pocket*. Retrieved from http://www.pebblepad.co.uk/pp3help/helpfile.aspx?t=1&vn=9.0&v=10&tg=3bf540bf-f5a7-4714-a00e-bca93111676b&f=193&v3k=d2a5149c-1595-4e4e-a02a-494a9f52d7c5

Posey, L., Plack, M. M., Snyder, R., Dinneen, P. L., Feuer, M., & Wiss, A. (2015). Developing a pathway for an institution wide eportfolio program. *International Journal of ePortfolio, 5*(1), 75–92.

Quinton, S., & Smallbone, T. (2008). PDP implementation at English universities: What are the issues? *Journal of Further and Higher Education, 32*(2), 99–109. doi:10.1080/03098770701851839

Reardon, R. C., Lumsden, J. A., & Meyer, K. E. (2005). Developing an e-portfolio program: Providing a comprehensive tool for student development, reflection, and integration. *Journal of Student Affairs Research and Practice, 42*(3), 630–642. doi:10.2202/1949-6605.1513

Reese, M., & Levy, R. (2009). Assessing the future: E-portfolio trends, uses, and options in higher education. *Research Bulletin, 4*, 1–12.

Rowley, L. (2008). *How to Market and Sell Your Art, Music, Photographs, and Handmade Crafts Online: Turn Your Hobby Into a Cash Machine*. Atlantic Publishing Company.

Schaub-de Jong, M., Schönrock-Adema, J., Dekker, H., Verkerk, M., & Cohen-Schotanus, J. (2011). Development of a student rating scale to evaluate teachers' competencies for facilitating reflective learning. *Medical Education, 45*(2), 155–165. doi:10.1111/j.1365-2923.2010.03774.x PMID:21208261

Siu, F. K. P. (2013). The incorporation of eportolios into EFL courses: Barriers encountered in the diffusion of technology. *Journal of Interactive Learning Research, 24*(2), 211–231.

Slade, C., Murfin, K., & Readman, K. (2013). Evaluating processes and platforms for potential eportfolio use: The role of the middle agent. *International Journal of ePortfolio, 3*(2), 177–188.

Strampel, K., Sibson, R., & Main, S. (2017). Professional Development to Support the Embedding of ePortfolios in Higher Education Programs. In ePortfolios in Australian Universities (pp. 33-46). Springer Singapore. doi:10.1007/978-981-10-1732-2_3

Turnitin. (2012). *White paper: The Plagiarism Spectrum*. Retrieved from http://go.turnitin.com/paper/plagiarism-spectrum

Williams, A., Simmons, C., Levett-Jones, T., Sher, W., & Bowen, L. (2012). *Facilitating work integrated learning (WIL) through skills-enabled ePortfolios in construction and nursing final report*. Sydney: Office for Learning and Teaching, Department of Industry, Innovation, Science, Research and Tertiary Education. Retrieved from http://www.olt.gov.au/project-facilitating-wil-eportfolios-uon-2009

Willmarth-Stec, M., & Beery, T. (2015). Operationalizing the Student Electronic Portfolio for Doctoral Nursing Education. *Nurse Educator*, *40*(5), 263–265. doi:10.1097/NNE.0000000000000161 PMID:25783814

Woodley, C., & Sims, R. (2011). EPortfolios, professional development and employability: Some student perceptions. *Campus-Wide Information Systems*, *28*(3), 164–174. doi:10.1108/10650741111145698

Yancey, K. B. (2001). Digitized student portfolios. *Electronic portfolios: Emerging practices in student, faculty, and institutional learning*, 15-30.

Zeichner, K., & Wray, S. (2001). The teaching portfolio in US teacher education programs: What we know and what we need to know. *Teaching and Teacher Education*, *17*(5), 613–621. doi:10.1016/S0742-051X(01)00017-8

Chapter 12
Digital Approaches to Embedding Employability

Jessica J. Vanderlelie
Griffith University, Australia

Andrew G. Pearson
Griffith University, Australia

Brooke E. Harris-Reeves
Griffith University, Australia

ABSTRACT

The fourth industrial revolution has seen significant national and international workplace change, with greater emphasis on innovation and digital adaptation. In response, universities across the sector are recognizing the importance of supporting the education of work-ready graduates and the continuing professional development of the existing professional workforce. Digital technologies have the potential to facilitate the development of employability skills such as digital literacy and reflection and foster continuing links to the profession and learning community. This chapter discusses the importance of embedding authentic, digitally enabled employability curriculum across the student and professional lifecycle, and showcases practice in the context of health professional education. A matrix for the selection of technologies that support the development of employability skills is also proposed and discussed.

DOI: 10.4018/978-1-5225-3850-9.ch012

INTRODUCTION

The national and international workplace landscape is in the midst of significant change (Atres, Hooley & Mellors-Bourne, 2017; Taylor, 2015). Technological advances are dramatically shaping the workplace environment, as greater emphasis is placed on innovation and adaptation within the globally connected digital frontier (Davies, Fidler & Gorbis, 2011). Within the next 15 years, up to 40% of Australian jobs have a moderate to high likelihood of disappearing; a statistic that equates to approximately 5.1 million Australian jobs (Johnson, 2015; Taylor, 2015). The reality of this rapidly evolving and economically unstable future is that millennials (individuals born between 1977 and 1997) can expect to have 17 careers across 5 industries over the course of their working lives (Owen, 2016). The impact of technological advances on the workforce is not a new construct, with exponential alterations to labour markets evident since the advent of electricity and the industrial revolution.

Despite the lasting influence of technology on the nature of work, the future industrial landscape will require graduates to adapt more readily to change than ever before and require higher-level competencies in personal reflection and strong understanding of the transferability of their skills. To this end, the quote by Sir Brian Corby, former Chairman of Prudential serves as a call to action to the higher education sector (Taylor & Morison, 1999, p29).

We may not be able to offer long-term employment but we should try to offer long-term employability. (Taylor & Morison, 1999, p29)

It is important to front-end this chapter by explicitly stating that employability is not the same as actual employment. It is a far subtler, multi-layered and essential quality than many universities would concede (Rich, 2015). Employability is the concept which enables graduates to 'hit the ground running' in their first job and is equally valuable as preparation for flexible and productive long-term careers. Employability leads to employment, and the latter back to the former, as graduates change jobs and progress throughout their working lives. So, on that basis, it is vital for universities to provide relevant experiences to all students on both an ethical and a practical level. In response, universities both nationally and internationally are explicitly embedding employability into curriculum to support graduate transitions and workplace success (Atres, Hooley & Mellors-Bourne, 2017; Dibben & Norton, 2017; Blackmore et al., 2016).

A recent report from the Australian Office of Learning and Teaching, identified five (5) key themes for developing student employability that include: development of skills and knowledge; development of self; development of career awareness; capacity to interact with others; and ability to navigate the world (Bennett, Richardson

& MacKinnon, 2016). Across these five themes, institutions provide a variety of curricular and co-curricular activities to encourage students to develop their employability. Digital technologies provide a level of scalability unachievable by other approaches and afford multiple benefits to students including an opportunity to develop digital literacy; profile work widely prior to graduation; and develop a robust record of their achievements and development across a program of study.

This chapter discusses the importance of embedding authentic, digitally–enabled employability curriculum across the student and professional lifecycle and will showcase practice in the varied contexts of health professional education. From this foundation, a matrix for the selection of technologies will be presented that may facilitate institutions and academics to leverage the power of digital technologies in the curriculum.

BACKGROUND

Traditionally, universities have provided career and employability support to students through formalised careers counselling services, in a manner that is separate and discrete from the curriculum (Blackmore et al., 2016; Smith et al., 2009). Students would typically seek out services if they experienced problems with their choice of degree or when beginning their internship or graduate job search. This reactive, service-based model to a career 'problem' provided significant support to a small proportion of students and graduates who were proactive in their approach (Smith et al., 2009).

The role of the university in facilitating students' career development has shifted considerably, with strong interest in graduates' employability driven by data comparing universities on graduate employment outcome rates (Atres, Hooley & Mellors-Bourne, 2017; Folsom & Reardon, 2003), as well as by students' (and their parents') demands for greater return on investment in education (Blackmore et al., 2016; Foskett, 2007; Morley, 2001). This shift has resulted in the need for an explicit definition of employability and a greater exploration of best-practice employability curriculum. For the purpose of this chapter we will define employability as: activities and experiences that support the development of knowledge, professional skills and personal capabilities to enhance a graduate's lifelong professional success.

Developing Employability in Higher Education

The importance of integrating career development authentically within the tertiary curriculum is widely acknowledged (Atres, Hooley & Mellors-Bourne, 2017; Bennett, Richardson & MacKinnon, 2016; Smith et al., 2009; Watts, Sweet, Haines

& McMahon, 2006; Stewart & Knowles, 2001; Lau & Pang, 2000). Taking an integrated approach has established benefits for students and the institution (Atres, Hooley & Mellors-Bourne, 2017; Blackmore et al., 2016; Bimrose, Barnes & Brown, 2005), including:

- Improvement in a student's personal and professional development;
- Increased student confidence;
- Improved satisfaction and retention;
- Greater sense of career direction;
- The formation of strong professional identity and understanding of field;
- Increased ability of students to secure work experience and employment; and
- Improved graduate transitions.

Integration of employability and career development learning is common in the United Kingdom and United States of America (Atres, Hooley & Mellors-Bourne, 2017; Vernick, Reardon & Sampson, 2002) and is becoming more common in Australia (Phillips KPA, 2008). The case for embedding employability into the curriculum has been underscored by the launch of the Higher Education Standards Framework in Australia (TEQSA, 2015) that placed legislative requirements for the support of employability and lifelong learning outcomes to be assessed and assured in curriculum. Additionally there are a number of social and economic factors driving a focus on employability. The realities of a tightening job market and the risk of graduate under-employment (Owen, 2016), has perpetuated pressure to attract quality new students as students and their parents are increasingly considering employment opportunities. This has resulted in competition between higher education providers on graduate employment rates, that carries with it, consequential funding implications (Foskett, 2007; Morley, 2001).

Embedding industry informed, career focused curriculum, through a range of curricular and co-curricular strategies can provide students with opportunities to develop their knowledge, skills, experience and personal attributes, all of which will enhance their employability. However, there is no single strategy or approach to the development and delivery of employability-focused curriculum. Rather the process should be flexible, dynamic and nuanced to specific discipline contexts, the needs of the student cohort and industry requirements (Bennett, Richardson & MacKinnon, 2016; Blackmore et al., 2016; Pegg, Waldock, Hendy-Isaac, Lawton, 2012). As such there are a range of curricular (Table 1) and co-curricular (Table 2) experiences, professional development opportunities and assessment approaches that provide capacity for developing employability.

Table 1. Curricular activities/strategies for building employability skills

Experiences	Assessment Approaches	Professional Development
• Capstone courses • Informational interviews • Guest lectures from industry • Industry placement/WIL • Career development modules • Community engagement • Industry projects • Virtual simulations • Field work and industry visits (national/international) • Research projects • Interprofessional learning	• ePortfolio • Communication skills • Clinical case studies • Reflective journals • Solution-based assessment • Professional practice simulation • Career Development assessment • Peer review • Research reports • Industry market analysis • Authentic assessment • Action Research	• Personal Branding • Professional networking • Selection criteria • Resume development • Interview skills • Professional/personal skills reflection • Entrepreneurial training

Table 2. Co-curricular strategies for building employability skills

Industry Engagement	Professional Development	Experiences
• Networking events • Industry mentoring • Alumni mentoring • Meet the industry events • Work experience • Professional associations	• Seminars and workshops • Professional association events • Student mentoring • Study group facilitation • PASS • Conference attendance	• Orientation activities • International experiences • Volunteer opportunities • Leadership activities • Hackathons • Student representation

EMBEDDING AND EVIDENCING EMPLOYABILITY

Since 1482, when Leonardo da Vinci was credited with the first official resume, professionals have been documenting their skills in an attempt to secure employment (Lempicke, 2011). The resume and Curriculum Vitae (CV) have come a long way from their humble beginnings as letters of reference, to our present day records that border on extinction. The rise of digital records and social media platforms are transforming the way we present our information and the processes through which recruiters now seek to fill vacancies (Gross, 2013).

The affordances of digital platforms enable job seekers to provide a complex and engaging array of information to evidence their employability, outside of the traditional written 2-page skills and experience summary. Recruiters are seeking out those individuals with proven skills in navigating technological environments by assessing an individual's digital presence. Today more than ever before job seekers are required to hone a digital profile and 'market' themselves across multiple media (Lauby, 2011).

The realities of this 'new world of job seeking' means that now, more than ever before, an individual must be able to understand and articulate their 'uniqueness' and the transferability of their skills and capabilities across multiple contexts. The ubiquitous Graduate Attributes statements that pervade tertiary programs of study go some way to supporting students to understand the breadth of the skills they will develop across their university experience (Bridgstock, 2009). However, these statements often do not encompass the more personal capabilities and 'soft skills', and as such students are commonly left to 'unpack' the connections between Graduate Attributes and their experiences both within, and external to the curriculum (Atres, Hooley & Mellors-Bourne, 2017; Bennett, Richardson & MacKinnon, 2016; Oliver, 2013; Bridgstock, 2009).

Technological tools provide a convenient and potentially visible platform upon which students may record, reflect upon and showcase their learning experiences and outputs to the professional marketplace. Each platform provides a range of affordances for the support and assurance of employability learning, as we will discuss.

ePortfolios

In higher education, portfolios have long been utilised to present a collection of work such as assessment submissions, reflections, photographs, academic results, employment history, and professional memberships to evidence professional skills. Technological advances have facilitated the digitization of the portfolio that provides greater opportunities to track student learning across a degree of study and allow students to curate learning artefacts and showcase these in the digital recruitment marketplace. The process of developing an ePortfolio may assist students to reflect on their learning journey, and to recognise and articulate their graduate identity and employability profile (Kinash et al., 2015; Woodley & Sims, 2011). A review of ePortfolios and their use in health professions education is presented in detail in Chapter 11.

As a platform for the curation of learning artefacts evidencing employability experiences across the student learning journey, ePortfolios offer the potential to integrate a number of other technological solutions. Specifically, ePortfolios may form the foundational platform through which students house specific learning outputs such as their digital elevator pitch and other evidence of career development learning; reflect upon their experiences and professional development; and embedded links to social networking profiles such as a LinkedIn. The opportunity to house evidence in one place makes the assurance of learning for institutional employability achievement records easier and also facilitates the award of digital badges and micro-credentials. In this sense the ePortfolio is truly the gold standard repository of employability learning.

One example of an ePortfolio in action exists within the Murdoch University, Bachelor of Nursing degree. The embedding of an ePortfolio across the curriculum in this program allows students to develop their self-directed learning competencies through deep engagement with their learning journey. The development of lifelong learning abilities that promote maintenance of skills, competence, and knowledge are essential requirements for Nursing professional practice, and the ePortfolio facilitates this in a continuing and integrated way by encouraging students to record and evidence their knowledge, skills, and competencies (Dewiyanti & Nilson, 2017).

Social Networking Services

Social networking services such as Facebook, LinkedIn and Twitter are facilitating individuals to develop networks and disseminate their personal and professional brand in new and engaging ways (Tess, 2013; Oliver et al., 2010). Graduates entering the world of work can improve their employability by utilising their existing networking skills to create wider networks through online social networking services (Benson, Morgan & Filippaios, 2014; Rust & Froud, 2011). Each platform differs in its primary purpose, and may be leveraged to develop varying aspects of one's professional brand, with a multifaceted approach recommended to develop a comprehensive digital presence.

Unfortunately, students often underestimate the importance of a professional network and have difficulty engaging in professional dialogue. A number of tertiary institutions are responding to this by supporting students to consider the importance of developing their professional network through LinkedIn. LinkedIn offers today's students unprecedented access to the professional community (Joyce, 2013). Active contribution to the intellectual discussion through engagement in forums, blogs and Twitter, allows students to engage the professional community and develop their reputation prior to graduation. Such engagement can be the key to employment success, with recruiters actively surveying LinkedIn to source talent (Fotrell, 2016).

Griffith University has developed an institution–wide strategy to encourage all final year students to optimize their LinkedIn profile and support its use in job search. To this end, a LinkedIn eModule was developed to provide students with guidance and appropriate resources for the development of their profile including, personal branding, making connections and profile essentials, such as writing a headline and developing a summary. In its initial 12-month phase, a total of 8,930 students and 1226 staff members enrolled into the module (Dobinson & Henly, 2017). A practical extension of this strategy has been the specific embedding of an assessment task in the first year of Health programs from the University, where students utilise the module to develop their LinkedIn portfolio that is then submitted through the ePortfolio and assessed for credit within an introductory Chemistry subject (Pearson, 2017).

Digital Elevator Pitch

The elevator pitch has long been considered one of the most powerful tools for improving student employability (Moran & Jackson, 2012). The traditional elevator pitch was a minute-long summary of an individual's key strengths and capabilities that would be utilized during networking and other face-to-face meetings. Digital technologies have created new frontiers for the standard elevator pitch, with individuals now recording their digital pitch and displaying it on varying outward profiles such as LinkedIn and the ePortfolio (Diaz, 2009).

Deakin University has established a whole of institution strategy to support students to showcase their acquired knowledge, skills and capabilities to prospective employers (Oliver, 2013). The 'Me in a Minute' project at Deakin University (https://blogs.deakin.edu.au/meinaminute/) encourages students to create a digital elevator pitch in the form of a one-minute video. By writing their 'Me in a Minute' script, students must reflect upon their experience, passions, and dreams. Students choose up to three Graduate Learning Outcomes, and include images or videos to evidence their knowledge and capabilities. Videos can then be utilised by students to grow their own professional brand, by including links to their ePortfolio and LinkedIn profile. From the foundation of this work at Deakin, an example has emerged from Griffith University whereby a digital elevator pitch is formulated and assessed as part of a Health Science capstone subject (Vanderlelie, 2017).

Micro-Credentials and Digital Badges

The academic transcript has long been the sole formal recognition of a student's achievements at university. However, the structure and information presented within the transcript means little to an employer and provides no recognition of a student's competency in higher order transferrable skills (Tomlinson, 2007). As universities move to formally support and assess the development of transferrable skills in the curriculum, the emergence of digital badging provides an alternative method to credential engagement, learning, and achievement (Gibson, Ostashewski, Flintoff & Knight, 2015; Mayrath, Clark-Midura & Robinson, 2012).

A digital badge is an authenticated representation of an accomplishment, skill, quality, or interest that can be earned in various learning environments, and contains metadata that provides information such as the badge recipient's name, the badge provider, and what the recipient did to receive the badge (Gibson, Ostashewski, Flintoff & Knight, 2015). The major advantages of the use of digital badges is the ability to track learning in less formal and non-didactic settings, through an approach that incentivizes achievement (Abramovich, Schunn & Higashi, 2013) and that clearly articulates verifiable evidence to a potential employer (Casilli & Hickey, 2016).

Examples of the use of digital badges are wide spread. In the sciences, digital badges recognize practical competencies and digital literacy (Seery et al., 2017; Towns et al., 2015). Within medical education, badges are commonly used to credential entrustable professional activities over the continuum of learning (Mehta et al., 2013). To support institutions to implement badging, a number of providers have emerged, with Open Badges (https://openbadges.org/), Credly (https://credly.com/), and Badgestack (http://badgeos.org/badgestack/) among the most comprehensive.

Work-Integrated Learning

In order to produce work-ready graduates, universities are offering undergraduate students the opportunity to gain real world experience by undertaking work-integrated learning (WIL) as a formal degree requirement. Through WIL, students develop key skills including teamwork, problem solving, communication, information literacy and professionalism (Jackson, 2015). Traditionally WIL experiences are provided in a face-to-face format with students integrated within a workplace environment or through engagement with an industry based project (Jones & Warnock, 2014). These experiences benefit students by reinforcing their learning, increasing self-confidence, and assisting them to establish professional networks (Franks & Oliver, 2012).

The emergence of sophisticated digital technologies has shaped the way we do business across geographic borders and made the virtual workplace a reality. Tertiary providers are leveraging virtual classrooms and digital conferencing, to offer opportunities for students to collaborate on industry specific problems, irrespective of geographical boundaries and reshaping our conceptions of WIL (Patel & Lynch, 2013). A review of emerging technologies for WIL in health professions education is presented in detail in Chapter 13.

The GLOCAL Project (https://glocalclassroom.wordpress.com/about/) is a highly awarded program that supports students to build internationally relevant workplace competencies that include cross cultural communication, negotiation and problem solving. The utilisation of real-time, technology-enabled collaboration software, allows all members of the learning community (academics, practitioners and students) to communicate across four continents, and solve complex industry based problems whilst navigating time, space and cultural difference.

In the Nursing discipline, students studying community-oriented practice were offered a modified problem-based learning unit with either a virtual nursing internship or traditional lectures. The virtual nursing internship students were assigned a community-nursing role in the fictitious town of Killardton. Student outcomes were comparable for both the virtual intern students and the control group. The teaching staff reported that the virtual internships were fun and engaging, and observed that the virtual intern students were more actively involved in class than other students (Ward & Killian, 2011).

Simulation Learning

Simulation learning is used in a variety of health professions education environments to supplement WIL. Simulations replace and amplify real experiences with guided, immersive activities that evoke or replicate substantial aspects of the real world in a fully interactive fashion within the controlled university environment (Bethea, 2014; Lateef, 2010). Simulation learning can improve clinical judgement, develop students' knowledge, skills, and attitudes for clinical situations, whilst protecting patients from unnecessary risks (Harder, 2010; Mayo et al., 2004). Applications of simulation learning in the health professions include skills training (Scalese, Obeso & Issenberg, 2008), competency assessment (Bethea, 2014; Rogers, Jacob & Rashwan et al., 2001), and virtual consults (Naumann, Yang, Thai, Ford & Polly, 2016). The benefits of simulation include that instruction is consistent and reproducible, and can be customised to individual or group needs (Seybert, 2008). Participants respond favourably to simulation learning, reporting increased competence and enthusiasm while learning without fear of patient harm (Steadman, Coates & Huang, et al., 2006).

Emergent technologies have facilitated a range of digital simulations that allow students to attempt complex procedures that are not possible within the realm of standard simulation. At the University of Bradford, final year Pharmacy students used iStan and Müse (CAE Healthcare, http://www.caehealthcare.com/eng/patient-simulators/istan) software to design, develop and run several teaching sessions, drawing upon simulated case studies to demonstrate the effects of an accidental or deliberate drug overdose. The Müse software was used to design suitable simulated experiences that enabled participants to 'experience' the effects of drugs on the patient. Scenarios can then be presented to peers using iStan in a series of small-group teaching sessions. Activities of this nature not only develop theoretical understanding and technical skill, they also support key skills in collaboration and peer review (Bielby-Clarke, 2015).

Within the Medical Laboratory Science discipline, virtual microscopy is being utilized to enhance student learning and readiness to practice. This activity involves the digitization of glass slide specimens in order to create dynamic images that may be manipulated using computer-based technology. Histology classes traditionally taught using light microscopes, glass slides, and PowerPoint presentations of static images, have been replaced with virtual microscopy where specimens are viewed on a computer screen using Aperio's ImageScope technology (Aperio Technologies, http://www.aperio.com) (Nelson, Ziv & Bandali, 2013). Such technology is facilitating a new level of student collaboration, as an entire class has the capacity to view any one of over 2000 available digital slides and compare and contrast several slides simultaneously, by viewing them side by side. Evaluation of the approach identified, that the implementation of virtual microscopy streamlined the learning process and reduced the dependence on traditional glass slide specimens, providing clinical partners and pathologists with meaningful and customised exposure within their clinical environments (Nelson, Ziv & Bandali, 2013).

Simulation learning has also been drawn upon to support the development of interprofessional competencies in the health professions (Cook, Hatala & Brydges, 2011). For health care teams to be effective, team members need to possess emotional intelligence in addition to the pre-requisite technical expertise and knowledge. The Bristol Inquiry in the UK found that to improve patient safety, health professionals need to be educated in communication skills, teamwork, and shared learning across professional boundaries (Department of Health, 2001). Interprofessional learning (IPL) has become a powerful method through which to build professional competency and employability in health professionals (Goldman, 2011).

Digital storytelling has emerged as a contemporary approach to IPL (Frost, Isbel, Kellett & Lawlis, 2017). At the University of Canberra, students enrolled in nursing (undergraduate), nutrition and dietetics, occupational therapy, or physiotherapy (all postgraduate) were presented with a digital patient story through MaskEd. After watching the video, students were asked to identify the roles of different disciplines in the care of the individual portrayed. The results of this innovative approach identified that digital storytelling provided a realistic and engaging learning activity, and supported students to increase their awareness of the importance of working in multidisciplinary teams (Frost, Isbel, Kellett & Lawlis, 2017).

Employability Achievement Records

Co-curricular activities form an important component in the development of a well-rounded employable professional. Indeed, industry is recognizing the benefit of these activities and articulating a preference for talent that have engaged with their communities and participated in experiences outside of the formal curriculum (Roulin & Bangerter, 2013; Callaghan, 2016). Despite the fact that students commonly undertake various activities outside of their university studies, they often struggle to link these experiences to their emerging professional skills and articulate the transferability of these capabilities. A number of institutions across the sector have recognized the importance of co-curricular and extra-curricular experiences in the development of employability skills and have implemented structured programs to encourage and recognize student activity in this space (Clark, 2012; Watson, 2011).

Traditionally employability award programs are not-for-credit, however the award itself is formally recognized by the institution and may appear on a student's exit transcript. Increasingly, universities are working with industry to assist professional partners to understand the meaning of the award and develop programs that encourage students towards activities highly valued by industry partners (Watson, 2011). A key component of each award program is the general requirement for students to reflect upon their experiences and how the skills and capabilities they develop in these experiences contribute towards their emerging professional identity and skills.

Digital technologies are shaping the nature of employability awards, with institutions leveraging the affordances of a number of platforms to provide programs that accurately record activities and reflection in a user-friendly format. Currently, universities are administering their programs through stand-alone websites, ePortfolios and sites within the Learning Management System. More recently an example has emerged from La Trobe University that is managed through an app interface. The La Trobe University Career Ready Advantage program (Brown, 2017) draws upon gamification principles to encourage student engagement with activities to develop key skills required for employability. The foundations of the program were developed through deep industry consultation and as a result students are supported to develop their skills across industry relevant competency themes. The app interface allows students to record their activities and reflections and provides an interactive map of skills and capability development as they progress within the program.

Career Development Learning

For decades, university careers and employment services have been supporting students to develop their employability. These services commonly operate in the co-curricular space and have managed to integrate career development learning into the curriculum to varying degrees in more recent times (Knight & York 2010). Within the Australian higher education context, it remains common for careers services to remain an add-on service. Within the United Kingdom, universities have recognized the importance of career development professionals and their services in supporting graduate employability and have resourced these areas to a greater extent (Dibben and Norton, 2017). Australia and other nations continue to lag in this respect and it is commonplace for careers departments to suffer from the challenges of under-resourcing.

In response to these challenges there is a significant move to embed career development learning activities in the online environment. Online modules are generally provided through the institutions secure servers or within the learning management system. Resume writing, career planning, selection criteria and networking are common examples (McAlpine et al., 2009). Institutions are now building upon these modules by working with academic elements to design tailored career development resources and to support the embedding of these activities within the curriculum. The Griffith University Career Focus module is a recent example of this approach (Vanderlelie & Dobinson, 2017). As part of a whole of faculty approach to embedding employability, academic staff and the Careers and Employment Service developed a collaborative e-module to support first year, first semester students to plan their careers and the curricular and co-curricular experience they will undertake across their degree to improve their employability.

Technology also offers the opportunity for students to gain practical experiences to support their career development. Software such as Big Interview (https://biginterview.com/) and interview stream (https://interviewstream.com/) facilitate students to practice their interview skills by answering common industry specific questions as part of a formalised assessment task. These platforms allow students to record their answers and have their work evaluated by academic staff, industry partners and their peers that provide valuable feedback in this important process of professional development (Anderson, 2014).

Mentoring

Mentoring has long been acknowledged as beneficial to professional development and career success (Goddard & Hughes, 2006). Technology offers new means with which to strengthen university connection with industry and in turn engagement with mentoring. Currently there is an active move to transition existing face-to-face mentoring programs to an online format (Wheeler, 2016; Perren, 2003) This shift not only enables greater participation by industry partners and students, it provides capacity for students to engage in this important professional development opportunity irrespective of geography and with national and international partners.

Digital Technology for Employability Matrix

The following matrix (Table 3) has been developed to capture the strengths of each of the digitally enhanced employability activities discussed above and provide a potential structure from which to assess the relevance of the solution to institutional readiness and processes. Each activity is mapped across the key structural and process considerations that may affect implementation and success.

Table 3. Digital tools for embedding employability matrix

	ePortfolio-Learning Record	ePortfolio - Outward Facing	Employability Achievement Records	LinkedIn	Blogging	Social Media	Digital Badges	Online Career Development Modules	Video Interviewing	Online Mentoring	Virtual WIL	Digital Storytelling	Digital Elevator Pitch
Strengths of the Approach													
Assurance of learning	x						x				x	x	x
Encourages reflection	x		x		x				x	x	x	x	x
Transferrable record of achievement	x	x		x									x
Builds personal and professional brand		x		x	x	x	x			x			
Supports career development skills	x	x	x		x	x		x	x	x			x
Low cost				x	x	x							x
Scalable approach	x	x	x	x	x	x	x	x	x	x			x
Encourages professional engagement			x	x	x	x		x		x	x		
Builds community			x	x	x	x				x	x		
Maintain connection with graduates				x		x							
Encourages co-curricular engagement			x		x	x							

continued on following page

Table 3. Continued

	ePortfolio- Learning Record	ePortfolio - Outward Facing	Employability Achievement Records	LinkedIn	Blogging	Social Media	Digital Badges	Online Career Development Modules	Video Interviewing	Online Mentoring	Virtual WIL	Digital Storytelling	Digital Elevator Pitch
Easily understood by industry		x	x	x	x	x	x	x		x	x		x
Opportunity for peer engagement		x			x				x		x	x	
Facilitates international industry engagement		x		x	x	x			x	x	x		
Preparation for work	x		x	x				x	x		x	x	
Key Considerations/Requirements													
Training and support for students	x	x	x	x	x	x	x		x	x	x	x	x
Training and support for staff	x			x	x	x	x	x	x	x	x	x	
Training and support for industry	x	x	x				x			x	x		
Link to curriculum and assessment	x		x				x	x	x		x	x	x
Platform considerations	x	x	x				x	x	x		x	x	x
Academic/ careers service collaboration	x		x				x		x	x			x

continued on following page

Table 3. Continued

	ePortfolio- Learning Record	ePortfolio - Outward Facing	Employability Achievement Records	LinkedIn	Blogging	Social Media	Digital Badges	Online Career Development Modules	Video Interviewing	Online Mentoring	Virtual WIL	Digital Storytelling	Digital Elevator Pitch
Articulation of value to students		x	x	x	x	x	x	x	x	x			x
Clear presentation of opportunities			x				x	x		x			
Contemporary policy/ procedures				x		x	x				x		
Industry/ alumni engagement		x	x	x		x	x		x	x	x		
Resourcing for careers services			x				x	x	x	x			

ISSUES, CONTROVERSIES, PROBLEMS

While tertiary institutions in Australia are embracing employability, it is important to highlight the key considerations and challenges associated with the implementation of employability focused curriculum. The issues and controversies of designing, developing and implementing curriculum affect a range of stakeholders including students, staff, industry professionals and institutions.

Issues for Students

The key reason students invest time and money into a tertiary qualification is to increase their chance of employment (Yorke, 2006). In the past, a qualification alone was enough to gain employment. Nowadays, while an academic qualification is desirable, it is no longer the only prerequisite to obtain employment (Yorke, 2006). This recent shift has resulted in the need for a curriculum that provides students with opportunities to develop skills outside of their discipline. While there are numerous benefits of employability focused curriculum, the issues and controversies from a student perspective require acknowledgment (Tomlinson, 2008).

Understanding student perceptions and gaining buy-in to employability skill development is one potential barrier to the effectiveness of an employability-based approach. Students often fail to understand the importance and relevance of career planning whilst undertaking tertiary studies (Pegg, Waldock, Hendy-Isaac, Lawton, 2012; Watts, 2006). This is particularly the case in the health professions where students become so focused on obtaining their qualification and entering the profession, that they fail to contemplate a future where employment may not be forthcoming or in which they decide to transition to another profession.

The design and delivery of employability-based curricula can be an integral factor in supporting student engagement. Programs that take a holistic approach to employability skill development through the integration of both curricular and co-curricular opportunities and offer students the opportunity to see employability as central to the experiences offered at university and their professional success, have been found to facilitate deeper engagement (Pegg, Waldock, Hendy-Isaac, Lawton, 2012). Despite evidence to support this approach, educators often focus on discipline specific understandings and fail to support students to make the connections between their curricular and co-curricular experience and their future professional success.

Students are under significant time pressures with assessment deadlines, personal and family commitments and work requirements. In response to these competing pressures, students often opt-out of participation in co-curricular activities. Educators need to assist students to understand the importance of co-curricular experiences and provide meaningful opportunities for students to engage in such activities for professional development purposes, to ensure graduates are equipped with the skills and experiences valued by industry (Bridgstock, 2009).

Finally, students often experience difficulty engaging with the range of employability-based activities offered by an institution. In addition to time pressures, it can be difficult for students to obtain a clear picture of the opportunities provided by an institution. This may be due to siloed organizational structures and convoluted communications methods, that results in the burying of opportunities deep within the layers of an institutional website (Tymon, 2013). Employability award programs offer a means through which to provide a more complete picture of opportunities to students and a framework from which assists students to choose experiences that will develop relevant professional skills (Clark, 2012; Watson, 2011).

Issues for Staff

Academic staff play an important role in preparing graduates for the future of work. Historically the role of academic staff was to teach students the skills and theoretical underpinnings essential to their chosen profession. However, the new world of work has placed an emphasis on a curriculum that prepares students to develop and articulate their theoretical and technical skills in addition to the other employability domains: development of self; development of career awareness; interaction with others and navigation of the world (Bennett, Richardson & MacKinnon, 2016; Pegg, Waldock, Hendy-Isaac, Lawton, 2012). A recent national study across higher education institutions in Australia identified that:

Educators are central to the process of change, but higher education leaders, graduates and students report many educators to be ill equipped for the task. (Bennett, Richardson & MacKinnon, 2016)

The concerns revealed during this study highlight a lack of confidence in academics' knowledge of the contemporary workplace, which is especially true for non-professional programs where staff may have never held a role in industry. The challenges facing academic staff are multifactorial and complex. Indeed, within professional programs significant pressure is placed on the curriculum by external professional accrediting bodies, limiting the capacity of staff to embed experiences that may develop transferrable capabilities. Such overcrowded curricula and the push towards modularised delivery, may in turn limit the scope for creative approaches to discipline nuanced employability curriculum.

It is important to acknowledge that academics across the sector are still grappling with the concept that employability is core academic business. To support academic staff to develop nuanced discipline based employability curriculum requires academic staff to operate in new ways and consider new approaches to assessment that may be foreign to their discipline contexts (Bennett, Richardson & MacKinnon, 2016). There are a number of overlaid technological challenges for staff including a lack of knowledge and personal use of employability-related platforms, such as LinkedIn and Twitter, and reduced confidence in the utilisation of ePortfolio tools and their integration within learning and teaching.

Currently universities offer very little support and training to staff to develop their professional skills in employability curriculum design and technology, meaning that early adopters are often relied heavily upon to carry the burden, rather than encouraging a programmatic approach to embedding employability. Training and support for the development of employability curriculum that leverages the affordances of digital technologies is essential to the successful embedding of employability within the Health professions.

Institutional processes and workload may also contribute to a reluctance to innovate in the design of employability curriculum that leverages technology. The design of authentic employability based curriculum requires strong collaboration between academic staff, career development professionals and industry. In an environment characterized by high academic workloads and under-resourced careers services, such deep collaboration is often difficult to achieve.

Issues for Industry

The engagement of industry in the professional training of students is becoming commonplace across the tertiary sector (Dacre-Pool & Sewell, 2007). Industry currently participate through a variety of mechanisms including membership on advisory boards, participation in industry panel sessions and guest lecturer, mentoring and offering students the opportunity to work on industry projects and within the operations of their professional contexts through WIL. By collaborating with industry, universities ensure the relevance of curriculum to world of work and open students to a range of experiences difficult to provide in a classroom context (Dacre-Pool & Sewell, 2007).

Industry partners experience a number of challenges when engaging with tertiary providers, the largest of which are the time commitments required, and the frustrations that result from difficulties connecting with the varying aspects of an institution (Meredith & Burkle, 2008). The world of industry operates at a vastly different pace and with greater flexibility than the tertiary environment. This reality can make it challenging for industry partners when offering projects for students, when their client's timelines do not fit with a standard academic calendar. Additionally, it can be difficult for industry to navigate the complex organization structure of an institution in order to connect with the 'right person' (Meredith & Burkle, 2008). University websites are designed to offer improved access for students and external individuals to view activities; however, these sites often provide an opaque and disorganized picture of activities and the relevant contacts that can stifle deep engagement.

It is important for universities considering the engagement of industry professionals in the development of curriculum, teaching and supervision of students to also consider the provision of training and support regarding the technological systems in place. As technological solutions are drawn upon to provide a platform for WIL and the external assessment of student work, institutions must deeply consider the impact of these activities upon industry partners and factor in additional time allocations and training accordingly. A more detailed discussion of this issue within the context of ePortfolios is contained within chapters 7 and 11.

Issues for Institutions

As the cost of higher education increases, students, their parents and the government are requiring additional assurance from universities that their teaching approaches and qualifications are industry relevant and leading students on a pathway to professional success (Harvey, 2010). The importance of employability skills development is increasingly acknowledged by the sector and as such it is commonplace for institutions to cite supporting graduate success in statements of strategic intent (Bridgstock, 2009). The implementation of such intent poses a number of challenges for universities.

A focus on developing students' employability skills requires an institution-wide approach that involves a wide range of stakeholders. This appears straightforward on paper, however it involves the deep engagement of staff across the siloed boundaries of academic and professional divisions and a level of resourcing that may be untenable for some providers (Bennett, Richardson & MacKinnon, 2016; Pegg, Waldock, Hendy-Isaac, Lawton, 2012; Knight & York 2010). The integration of industry in the design of curriculum poses an additional challenge, particularly in disciplines that have little natural industry connection (Meredith & Burkle, 2008). As a result, it may be difficult for institutions to gain buy-in from their staff despite a clearly communicated strategic intent.

Technology also adds a layer of complexity to institutional strategic considerations. Whilst it is important for institutions to provide technological solutions to support the embedding of employability, this comes at price beyond the licensing fee, as staff, students and industry partners require training and support in its utilisation. The rapid nature of technological change adds additional complexity, as systems rapidly become out dated and staff opt for unsupported platforms to deliver their innovations. From this standpoint, as is the case with the design of all innovative curriculum, pedagogy should drive the technical solution rather than a retrofitted approach that 'makes do' with the resources at hand, however this may not always be the pervading approach (Watson, 2001).

Finally, the rapid pace of technological advances may mean that institutional policy and procedures lag current practice. The use of social media platforms in the teaching environment is a perfect example. Despite the significant benefits of social media engagement and importance of digital profile development, the vast majority of Australian universities continue to limit connection between staff and students through social networking sites such as Facebook and LinkedIn (New Media Consortium, 2014). In the context of LinkedIn, this policy position may significantly limit a student's capacity to develop their professional network and stifle the opportunity of staff to maintain connection with their students across the course of their professional lives (Tess, 2013). As the value of online professional networks becomes more widely acknowledged and disciplines design assessment activities to support student engagement in professional networking, institutions are being forced to reconsider the boundaries of their social media policy and nuance their approaches.

SOLUTIONS AND RECOMMENDATIONS

Throughout this chapter we have presented a range of digital technologies that support scalable and authentic employability curriculum enhancement. The matrix presented in Table 3 identifies a range of key considerations and requirements that staff and institutions may consider when selecting technology for this purpose. From this work, we can identify eight key recommendations for institutional practice:

1. Development of a statement of clear strategic intent, commitment to resourcing and communication to stakeholders (students, staff, industry) of the employability vision of the institution.
2. Consideration be given to the development of appropriate contemporary policy and procedures to support engagement with technological solutions to build employability.
3. Commitment from institution to pedagogically driven choice of technological solution.
4. Support and leadership for programmatic approaches to embedding employability that leverage technology.
5. Provision of training and support for students, academic staff and industry in the use of technical solutions and development of employability curriculum.
6. Structural support for university staff and students to deeply engage with industry and alumni.

7. Adequate resourcing for career services to facilitate collaboration with academic elements and the development of targeted online resources.
8. Recognition of the workload implications for academic staff.

FUTURE RESEARCH DIRECTIONS

Research regarding the student, academic and industry experience of technological solutions in supporting employability based curriculum and assessment is sparse and often focused in the area of work-integrated learning. As technology rapidly evolves, institutions often move to upgrade systems and approaches, rather than opting for a structured research based framework for implementation and evaluation. As such, small-scale evaluations of the technological platform from a user experience perspective are common and offer little perspectives on the long-term impact of the innovation and technological approach on supporting employability.

As an extension, it is also important to note the complexities of evidencing employability outcomes and the impact of innovations. Timeframes are a major consideration in this respect, as it is realistic for the assessment of any innovation to require upwards of a five-year time period to demonstrate a measurable impact on student and graduate success. At this point it would be remiss not to mention that there remains significant limitations in the metrics used to assess graduate success nationally (Morley, 2001). As institutions continue to embed authentic discipline based employability curricula across programs it will be imperative to evaluate these activities and work towards developing robust graduate success measures that account for the challenges of graduate transitions to the workforce and shifting industrial landscape.

CONCLUSION

Digital technologies have the capacity to support the embedding of employability and the reach of career related experiences to students studying both on and off campus. Each technological solution offers a range of affordances that support its use across multiple contexts. The key for academic staff and institutions developing discipline specific employability experiences for students it to consider the pedagogical requirement before the technological solution. The world of technology is rapidly evolving as new solutions come onto the market every day. By leveraging the power of technology to support our efforts we can help improve the student experience and prepare our graduates to navigate the complexities of the future world of work.

REFERENCES

Abramovich, S., Schunn, C., & Higashi, R. M. (2013). Are badges useful in education?: It depends upon the type of badge and expertise of learner. *Educational Technology Research and Development, 61*(2), 217–232. doi:10.1007/s11423-013-9289-2

Anderson, M. (2014). Evaluating pedagogy for employability: illuminating students' perspectives on an intensive, undergraduate employability module. In *Excavate to Innovate: 'Unearthing' Students' and Tutors' Perceptions of Employability to Energise Work Based Pedagogy*. The University of Northampton. Retrieved from http://nectar.northampton.ac.uk/6788/

Artess, J., Hooley, T., & Mellors-Bourne, R. (2017). *Employability: A Review of the Literature 2012-2016*. York, UK: Higher Education Academy. Retrieved from http://hdl.handle.net/10545/621285

Bennett, D., Richardson, S., & MacKinnon, P. (2016). *Enacting strategies for graduate employability: How universities can best support students to develop generic skill Part A*. Canberra, Australia: Australian Government, Office for Learning and Teaching, Department of Education and Training. Retrieved from http://www.olt.gov.au/project-how-universities-can-best-support-students-develop-generic-skills-enacting-strategies-gradua

Benson, V., Morgan, S., & Filippaios, F. (2014). Social career management: Social media and employability skills gap. *Computers in Human Behavior, 30*, 519–525. doi:10.1016/j.chb.2013.06.015

Bethea, D. P., Castillo, D. C., & Harvison, N. (2014). Use of simulation in occupational therapy education: Way of the future? *The American Journal of Occupational Therapy, 68*(Supplement 2), 32–39. doi:10.5014/ajot.2014.012716 PMID:25397936

Bielby-Clarke, K. (2015). Use of a human patient simulator as a teaching tool by final year pharmacy students. *BMJ Simulation and Technology Enhanced Learning, 1*(Suppl 2), A45. doi:10.1136/bmjstel-2015-000075.110

Bimrose, J., Barnes, S. A., & Brown, J. (2005). *A Systematic Literature Review of Research into Career-related Interventions for Higher Education*. Warwick, UK: Institute for Employment Research, University of Warwick.

Blackmore, P., Bulaitis, Z. H., Jackman, A. H., & Tan, E. (2016). *Employability in higher education: A review of practice and strategies around the world*. London: Pearson.

Blackwell, A., Bowes, L., Harvey, L., Hesketh, A. J., & Knight, P. T. (2001). Transforming work experience in higher education. *British Educational Research Journal, 27*(3), 269–285. doi:10.1080/01411920120048304

Bridgstock, R. (2009). The graduate attributes we've overlooked: Enhancing graduate employability through career management skills. *Higher Education Research & Development, 28*(1), 31–44. doi:10.1080/07294360802444347

Brown, J. (2017). Career Ready Advantage. *National Innovation Case Study Collection*. Retrieved from http://app.iru.edu.au/national-innovation-case-study-collection#browse-by-university/university-details/58be5af15c088326e9f8d3a1/university-case-study-details/5967203e59a41f563590256d/

CAE Healthcare. (n.d.). *iStan and Müse*. Retrieved 20 April, 2017, from http://www.caehealthcare.com/eng/patient-simulators/istan

Callaghan, R. (2016, February 11). Graduate recruitment: Academic results no longer matter as much. *Australian Financial Review*. Retrieved from http://www.afr.com/leadership/careers/graduate-recruitment-academic-results-no-longer-matter-as-much-20160208-gmovnb#ixzz4hgmb6vhf

Casilli, C., & Hickey, D. (2016). Transcending conventional credentialing and assessment paradigms with information-rich digital badges. *The Information Society, 32*(2), 117–129. doi:10.1080/01972243.2016.1130500

Clark, W. (2012). It's about More than Getting a Job. *Adults Learning, 23*(4), 45–47.

Coetzee, M., & Beukes, C. (2010). Employability, emotional intelligence and career preparation support satisfaction among adolescents in the school-to-work transition phase. *Journal of Psychology in Africa, 20*(3), 439–446.

Cole, D., & Tibby, M. (2013). *Defining and developing your approach to employability: A framework for higher education institutions*. Heslington: The Higher Education Academy.

Cook, D. A., Hatala, R., Brydges, R., Zendejas, B., Szostek, J. H., Wang, A. T., & Hamstra, S. J. et al. (2011). Technology-enhanced simulation for health professions education: A systematic review and meta-analysis. *Journal of the American Medical Association, 306*(9), 978–988. doi:10.1001/jama.2011.1234 PMID:21900138

Crebert, G., Bates, M., Bell, B., Patrick, C. J., & Cragnolini, V. (2004). Developing generic skills at university, during work placement and in employment: Graduates' perceptions. *Higher Education Research & Development, 23*(2), 147–165. doi:10.1080/0729436042000206636

Crozier, S. (2001). Career development in the post-secondary curricula. In W. Patton & M. McMahon (Eds.), *Career development programs: Preparation for lifelong career decision making* (pp. 85–93). Melbourne, Australia: ACER Press.

Dacre-Pool, L., & Sewell, P. (2007). The key to employability: Developing a practical model of graduate employability. *Education + Training*, *49*(4), 277–289. doi:10.1108/00400910710754435

Davies, A., Fidler, D., & Gorbis, M. (2011). *Future Work Skills 2020*. Report for the Institute for the Future for Apollo Research Institute.

Deakin University. (2016). *Me in a Minute*. Retrieved 11 April, 2017, from https://blogs.deakin.edu.au/meinaminute/

Department of Health. (2001). *Report of the Public Inquiry into Children's Heart Surgery at the Bristol Royal Infirmary 1984–1995: Learning from Bristol*. London: The Stationery Office.

Dewiyanti, S., & Nilson, C. (2017). Programmatic approach to an ePortfolio in Nursing. *National Innovation Case Study Collection*. Retrieved from https://iru.knack.com/national-innovation-case-study-collection/#browse-by-theme/theme-details/58e5e4d229fe99490ac49677/theme-case-study-details/58e5a223b8ef4658faed35e2/

Diaz, C. S. (2009, July). Teaching the techno-pitch: Taking student innovators beyond the elevator pitch. In *Professional Communication Conference, 2009. IPCC 2009. IEEE International* (pp. 1-7). IEEE. doi:10.1109/IPCC.2009.5208685

Dibben, M., & Norton, S. (2017). *Embedding employability in student programs-it starts with the right language: Reflections from Australia and the UK*. Higher Education Academy. Retrieved 2 May, 2017, from https://www.international.heacademy.ac.uk/node/221

Dobinson, T., & Henly, D. (2017). LinkedIn Employability Strategy and emodule. *National Innovation Case Study Collection*. Retrieved from https://iru.knack.com/national-innovation-case-study-collection/#browse-by-theme/theme-details/58e5e4b57300e05a549c768e/theme-case-study-details/58ed9c298caea04b5143977a/

Duckworth, A., Peterson, C., Matthews, M. D., & Kelly, D. R. (2007). Grit: Perseverance and Passion for Long-Term Goals. *Journal of Personality and Social Psychology*, *92*(6), 1087–1101. doi:10.1037/0022-3514.92.6.1087 PMID:17547490

Folsom, B., & Reardon, R. (2003). College career courses: Design and accountability. *Journal of Career Assessment*, *11*(4), 421–450. doi:10.1177/1069072703255875

Foskett, R. (2007). Collaborative partnership between HE and employers: A study of workforce development. *Journal of Further and Higher Education*, *29*(3), 251–264. doi:10.1080/03098770500166868

Fotrell, Q. (2016, June 16). How recruiters screen you on LinkedIn. *Marketwatch*. Retrieved from http://www.marketwatch.com/story/how-recruiters-screen-you-on-linkedin-2014

Franks, P. C., & Oliver, G. C. (2012). Experiential learning and international collaboration opportunities: Virtual internships. *Library Review*, *61*(4), 272–285. doi:10.1108/00242531211267572

Frost, J., Isbel, S., Kellett, J., & Lawlis, T. (2017). Using digital story telling to assess health students' knowledge of interprofessional roles in the care of the older adult. *BMJ Simulation and Technology Enhanced Learning*, *3*(1), 5–8. doi:10.1136/bmjstel-2016-000136

Gibson, D., Ostashewski, N., Flintoff, K., Grant, S., & Knight, E. (2015). Digital badges in education. *Education and Information Technologies*, *20*(2), 403–410. doi:10.1007/s10639-013-9291-7

Goddard, A., & Hughes, C. (2006). Mentoring and its impact on student employability. *The Higher Education Academy Annual Conference July 2006*.

Goldman, J. (2011). Centre for the Advancement of Interprofessional Education (CAIPE) website: www.caipe.org.uk. *Journal of Interprofessional Care, 25*(5), 386-387.

Gross, D. (2013, July 11) Are Social Media Making the Resume Obsolete? *CNN Tech*. Retrieved from http://edition.cnn.com/2012/07/11/tech/social-media/facebook-jobs-resume/

Harder, B. N. (2010). Use of simulation in teaching and learning in health sciences: A systematic review. *The Journal of Nursing Education*, *49*(1), 23–28. doi:10.3928/01484834-20090828-08 PMID:19731886

Harvey, L. (2010). New realities: The relationships between higher education and employment. *Tertiary Education and Management*, *6*(1), 3–17. doi:10.1080/13583883.2000.9967007

Jackson, D. (2015). Employability skill development in work-integrated learning: Barriers and best practice. *Studies in Higher Education*, *40*(2), 350–367. doi:10.1080/03075079.2013.842221

Johnson, L. (2014). *NMC Horizon Report 2014 Higher Education Edition*. Retrieved from https://www.nmc.org/pdf/2014-nmc-horizon-report-he-EN.pdf

Jones, H. M., & Warnock, L. (2014). *Towards a Competency Framework for Student Work Based Learning*. Higher Education Academy. Retrieved 13 April, 2017, from https://www.heacademy.ac.uk/sites/default/files/resources/towards_a_competency_framework_for_student_work-based_learning.pdf

Joyce, S. P. (2013). Be visible on LinkedIn. *Career Planning and Adult Development Journal*, *29*(3), 88–90.

Kinash, S., Crane, L., Judd, M. M., Mitchell, K., McLean, M., Knight, C., & Schulz, M. et al. (2015). *Supporting graduate employability from generalist disciplines through employer and private institution collaboration*. Sydney: Australian Government Office for Learning and Teaching.

Knight, P. T., & York, M. (2010). Employability and Good Learning in Higher Education. *Teaching in Higher Education*, *8*(1), 3–18. doi:10.1080/1356251032000052294

Lateef, F. (2010). Simulation-based learning: Just like the real thing. *Journal of Emergencies, Trauma and Shock*, *3*(4), 348. doi:10.4103/0974-2700.70743 PMID:21063557

Lau, A., & Pang, M. (2000). Career strategies to strengthen graduate employees' employment position in the Hong Kong labour market. *Education + Training*, *42*(3), 135–149. doi:10.1108/00400910010372689

Lauby, S. (2011). 9 Dynamic Digital Resumes That Stand Out From The Crowd. *Mashable*. Retrieved from http://mashable.com/2011/02/21/dynamic-digital-resumes/#oK_r3LwnIGq7

Lempicke, T. (2011, February 12). History of the Resume. *Business Insider*. Retrieved from https://www.businessinsider.com.au/how-resumes-have-evolved-since-their-first-creation-in-1482-2011-2?r=US&IR=T#the-first-resumes-1

Lowden, K., Hall, S., Elliot, D., & Lewin, J. (2011). *Employers' perceptions of the employability skills of new graduates*. London: Edge Foundation.

Mayo, P. H., Hackney, J. E., Mueck, J. T., Ribaudo, V., & Schneider, R. F. (2004). Achieving house staff competence in emergency airway management: Results of a teaching program using a computerized patient simulator. *Critical Care Medicine*, *32*(12), 2422–2427. doi:10.1097/01.CCM.0000147768.42813.A2 PMID:15599146

Mayrath, M., Clarke-Midura, J., & Robinson, D. (Eds.). (2012). *Technology-Based Assessments for 21st Century Skills: Theoretical and Practical Implications from Modern Research*. Charlotte, NC: Information Age Publishing.

McAlpine, A., Thomson, A., Ridler, G., White, J., & Plaisted, T. (2009). *Designing career development modules into the first year curriculum*. Paper presented at ALTC First Year Experience Curriculum Design Symposium. Retrieved from http://www.fyecd2009.qut.edu.au/resources/FYE_showcaseabstracts_4Feb09_FIN_SJ.pdf

McCorkle, D. E., Alexander, J. F., Reardon, J., & Kling, N. D. (2003, December). Developing self-marketing skills: Are marketing students prepared for the job search? *Journal of Marketing Education*, *25*, 196–207. doi:10.1177/0273475303257517

Mehta, N. B., Hull, A. L., Young, J. B., & Stoller, J. K. (2013). Just imagine: New paradigms for medical education. *Academic Medicine*, *88*(10), 1418–1423. doi:10.1097/ACM.0b013e3182a36a07 PMID:23969368

Meredith, S., & Burkle, M. (2008). Building bridges between university and industry: Theory and practice. *Education + Training*, *50*(3), 199–215. doi:10.1108/00400910810873982

Moran, M., & Jackson, L. (2012). The guide to everlasting employability. 10eightylimited.

Morley, L. (2001). Producing new workers: Quality, equality and employability in higher education. *Quality in Higher Education*, *7*(2), 131–138. doi:10.1080/13538320120060024

Naumann, F., Yang, J. L., Thai, T., Ford, C., & Polly, P. (2016). Virtual patient consultations and the use of an ePortfolio assessment to support student learning of integrated professional skills. *Focus on Health Professional Education: A Multi-Disciplinary Journal, 17*(3), 69.

Nelson, D., Ziv, A., & Bandali, K. S. (2012). Going glass to digital: Virtual microscopy as a simulation-based revolution in pathology and laboratory science. *Journal of Clinical Pathology*, *65*(10), 877–881. doi:10.1136/jclinpath-2012-200665 PMID:22791768

Oliver, B. (2013). Graduate Attributes as a focus for institution-wide curriculum renewal: Innovations and challenges. *Higher Education Research & Development*, *32*(3), 450–463. doi:10.1080/07294360.2012.682052

Oliver, B., von Konsky, B. R., Nikoletatos, P., Wilsinson, H., Ng, J., Quirke, T., & Moore, R. (2010). *Iportfolio, ITunesU, iPhone app: Capturing, tagging and sharing evidence of learning*. Presented at the *Association or Authentic Experiential and Evidence-Based Learning Conference*, Boston, MA.

Owen, J. (2016). *Renewing Australia's Promise Report Card 2016*. Foundation of Young Australians. Retrieved from http://www.fya.org.au

Patel, F., & Lynch, H. (2013). Glocalisation as an alternative to internationalisation in higher education: Embedding positive glocal learning perspectives. *International Journal on Teaching and Learning in Higher Education*, *25*(2), 223–230.

Pegg, A., Waldock, J., Hendy-Isaac, S., & Lawton, R. (2012). *Pedagogy for employability*. Higher Education Academy. Retrieved from: http://oro.open.ac.uk/30792/1/Pedagogy_for_employability_170212_1724.pdf

Pearson, A., & the Centre for Learning Futures. (2017). *ePortfolios to promote employability in Health students*. Retrieved from https://app.griffith.edu.au/explore/entry/3125/view

Perren, L. (2003). The role of e-mentoring in entrepreneurial education and support: A meta- review of academic literature. *Education + Training*, *45*(8), 517–525. doi:10.1108/00400910310508900

Phillips, K. P. A. (2008). *Review of career development services in Australian tertiary institutions*. Canberra, Australia: Department of Education, Employment and Workplace Relations.

Reddan, G. (2008). The benefits of job-search seminars and mock interviews in a work experience course. *Asia Pacific Journal of Cooperative Education*, *9*(2), 113–127.

Rich, J. (2015). *Employability: Degrees of value*. HEPI Occasional Paper 12. Retrieved 20 April, 2017, from www.hepi.ac.uk

Rodger, S., Rodger, J., & Hoffman, S. (2010). Where in the world is interprofessional education? A global environmental scan. *Journal of Interprofessional Care*, *24*(5), 479–491. doi:10.3109/13561821003721329 PMID:20718594

Rogers, P. L., Jacob, H., Rashwan, A. S., & Pinsky, M. R. (2001). Quantifying learning in medical students during a critical care medicine elective: A comparison of three evaluation instruments. *Critical Care Medicine*, *29*(6), 1268–1273. doi:10.1097/00003246-200106000-00039 PMID:11395619

Roulin, N., & Bangerter, A. (2013). Students' use of extra-curricular activities for positional advantage in competitive job markets. *Journal of Education and Work*, *26*(1), 21–47. doi:10.1080/13639080.2011.623122

Rust, C., & Froud, L. (2011). 'Personal literacy': The vital, yet often overlooked, graduate attribute. *Journal of Teaching and Learning for Graduate Employability*, *2*(1), 28–40. doi:10.21153/jtlge2011vol2no1art551

Scalese, R. J., Obeso, V. T., & Issenberg, S. B. (2008). Simulation technology for skills training and competency assessment in medical education. *Journal of General Internal Medicine*, *23*(1), 46–49. doi:10.1007/s11606-007-0283-4 PMID:18095044

Seery, M. K., Agustian, H. Y., Doidge, E. D., Kucharski, M. M., O'Connor, H. M., & Price, A. (2017). Developing laboratory skills by incorporating peer-review and digital badges. *Chemistry Education Research and Practice*, *18*(3), 403–419. doi:10.1039/C7RP00003K

Seybert, A. L., Kobulinsky, L. R., & McKaveney, T. P. (2008). Human Patient Simulation in a Pharmacotherapy Course. *American Journal of Pharmaceutical Education*, *72*(2), 37. doi:10.5688/aj720237 PMID:18483603

Smith, M., Brooks, S., Lichtenberg, A., McIlveen, P., Torjul, P., & Tyler, J. (2009). *Career development learning: Maximising the contribution of work-integrated learning to the student experience*. Final Project Report. University of Wollongong. Careers Central. Academic services Division.

Steadman, R. H., Coates, W. C., Huang, Y. M., Matevosian, R., Larmon, B. R., McCullough, L., & Ariel, D. (2006). Simulation-based training is superior to problem-based learning for the acquisition of critical assessment and management skills. *Critical Care Medicine*, *34*(1), 151–157. doi:10.1097/01.CCM.0000190619.42013.94 PMID:16374169

Stewart, J., & Knowles, V. (2001). Graduate recruitment: Implications for business and management courses in HE. *Journal of European Industrial Training*, *25*(2), 98–108. doi:10.1108/03090590110395771

Taylor, N. (2015) The industrial revolution's next wave. In *CEDA Research Report, Australia's Future Workforce?* Retrieved 17 April, 2017, from http://www.ceda.com.au/research-and-policy/policy-priorities/workforce

Taylor, B. (1999). The Darwinian shake-out in financial services. In Driving strategic change in financial services. Cambridge, UK: Woodhead Publishing Limited. doi:10.1016/B978-1-85573-431-9.50008-6

Tess, P. A. (2013). The Role of Social Media in Higher Education Classes (Real and Virtual)—A Literature Review. *Computers in Human Behavior, 29*, A60–A68.

TEQSA. (n.d.). *Higher Education Standards Framework*. Canberra, Australia: Australian Government. Retrieved from http://www.teqsa.gov.au/teqsa-contextual-overview-hes-framework

University of Queensland. (n.d.). *Three Minute Thesis*. Retrieved 13 April, 2017, from http://threeminutethesis.org/

Tomlinson, M. (2006). 'The degree is not enough': Students' perceptions of the role of higher education credentials for graduate work and employability. *British Journal of Sociology of Education, 29*(1), 49–61. doi:10.1080/01425690701737457

Towns, M., Harwood, C. J., Robertshaw, M. B., Fish, J., & O'Shea, K. (2015). The digital pipetting badge: A method to improve student hands-on laboratory skills. *Journal of Chemical Education, 92*(12), 2038–2044. doi:10.1021/acs.jchemed.5b00464

Tymon, A. (2013). The student perspective on employability. *Studies in Higher Education, 38*(6), 841–856. doi:10.1080/03075079.2011.604408

Vanderlelie, J. (2017). *Development of students professional identity through Me in a Minute presentations*. Retrieved from https://app.secure.griffith.edu.au/explore/entry/3765/view

Vanderlelie, J., & Dobinson, T. (2017). *Enhancing employability within curriculum using the Career Focus Module*. Retrieved from https://app.secure.griffith.edu.au/explore/entry/4625/view

Vernick, S. H., Reardon, R. C., & Sampson, J. P. (2002). *Process and Evaluation of a Career Course: A Replication and Extension (Technical Report 31)*. Tallahassee, FL: Florida State University. Retrieved from http://career.fsu.edu/documents/technical%20reports/Technical%20Report%2031/Technical%20Report%2031.htm

Ward, L. S., & Killian, P. (2011). Virtual Community Internships in the Classroom: Testing an Intervention. *Nurse Educator, 36*(1), 40–44. doi:10.1097/NNE.0b013e3182001e6c PMID:21135684

Watson, D. M. (2001). Pedagogy before technology: Re-thinking the relationship between ICT and teaching. *Education and Information Technologies, 6*(4), 251–266. doi:10.1023/A:1012976702296

Watson, R. (2011). A rationale for the development of an extracurricular employability award at a British university. *Research in Post-Compulsory Education, 16*(3), 371–384. doi:10.1080/13596748.2011.602248

Watts, A. G. (2006). *Career development learning and employability. Learning and Employability Series Two*. York, UK: ESECT and HEA. Retrieved April 12, 2017, from http://www.heacademy.ac.uk/assets/documents/resources/resourcedatabase/id592_career_ development_learning_and_employability.pdf

Watts, A. G., Sweet, R., Haines, C., & McMahon, M. (2006). International symposium on career development and public policy: Synthesis of country papers. *Australian Journal of Career Development, 15*(3), 33–44. doi:10.1177/103841620601500308

Wheeler, A., Austin, S., & Glass, J. (2012). E-mentoring for employability. In Centre for Engineering and Design Education (Ed.), EE2012—Innovation, Practice and Research in Engineering Education (pp. 1–9). Loughborough University.

Williams, B., Boyle, M., Brightwell, R., McCall, M., McMullen, P., Munro, G., & Webb, V. et al. (2013). A cross-sectional study of paramedics' readiness for interprofessional learning and cooperation: Results from five universities. *Nurse Education Today, 33*(11), 1369–1375. doi:10.1016/j.nedt.2012.06.021 PMID:22818954

Woodley, C., & Sims, R. (2011). Eportfolios, professional development and employability: Some student perceptions. *Campus-Wide Information Systems, 28*(3), 164–174. doi:10.1108/10650741111145698

Yorke, M. (2006). Employability in higher education: What it is–what it is not. *Learning and Employability Series, 1*. Higher Education Academy. Retrieved from https://www.heacademy.ac.uk/knowledge-hub/employability-higher-education-what-it-what-it-not

Chapter 13
Implementing Emerging Technologies to Support Work-Integrated Learning in Allied Health Education:
The Journey From Exploration to Adoption

Ganeshan Rao
Griffith University, Australia

Mary-Ann Shuker
Griffith University, Australia

Robert Loudon
Griffith University, Australia

ABSTRACT

The adoption and implementation of new technology to support work-integrated learning (WIL) is often challenging for staff and students. In this chapter, the authors discuss the processes and decisions involved from early piloting to potential institutional adoption of relevant technology (emerging or otherwise) and provide practical tools for the readers' use. The discussion is supported by evidence from allied health programs at a large higher education institution in Australia and identifies issues, controversies, and problems involved in new technology adoption. The importance of clarifying the pedagogical need before looking to technology is reinforced. Guidelines for identifying emerging and/or innovative use of current technologies are described, followed by discussion of considerations for selection of technologies that best align with the educational requirement.

DOI: 10.4018/978-1-5225-3850-9.ch013

INTRODUCTION

Educators today are well aware of the constant evolution of information and communication technologies (ICTs), and how this continually confronts their pedagogical practice. Possible challenges include: re-examination of old practices; pressure from others; evaluating innovative ideas for activities previously not possible; and ever-changing institutional processes to grapple with. The challenges are exciting, but sometimes seem bewildering and even over-whelming, particularly for those who are new to the field.

In this chapter, the place of ICTs in Work Integrated Learning is described, particularly in the context of Allied Health education. This discussion is a map to assist educators and professional support staff in understanding current practices; provide ideas for staying abreast of technological change; and list considerations for effectively selecting, implementing, and further disseminating emerging technologies in their organisation.

It is not a static picture - it is more of a journey to be navigated. The authors contend that this journey should be undertaken with a considered approach which strikes a balance between the speed needed due to the rapid pace of technological change and the caution which is warranted for significant educational investment. Knee-jerk adoption of easily accessible technologies and 'paralysis by analysis' are two extremes to be avoided.

It should be noted that much of the following discussion also applies to the use of ICTs in education more broadly, and to the practice of Work Integrated Learning in other disciplines besides Allied Health. The chapter aims to assist academics in understanding the wider ramifications of technology adoption to minimise risk while maximising innovation.

BACKGROUND

Work Integrated Learning (WIL) is defined by Patrick et al. (2008, p. iv) as "a range of approaches and strategies that integrate theory with the practice of work within a purposefully designed curriculum". WIL provides real world practice on or off campus to improve student employability, understanding of workplace culture, engagement, and retention (Patrick et al., 2008). Similar terms include cooperative education, professional learning, real world learning, and social engagement with the community (Patrick et al., 2008).

Allied Health includes health programs other than medicine and nursing eligible for professional body registration (Campbell, McAllister, & Eley, 2012) who aim to achieve optimal function in their clients (Lowe, Adams, & O'Kane, 2007).

Work Integrated Learning has become integral to Allied Health programs as it is a requirement of many professional accrediting bodies (Exercise and Sports Science Australia, 2016; Nagarajan & McAllister, 2015).

Emerging technologies include both technologies and practices (Veletsianos, 2016) that can significantly change education (Ball & Levy, 2008; Johnson et al., 2016) and which might not be new, except to the context in which they are applied (Veletsianos, 2016). Considerations to implement emerging technologies in WIL in Allied Health are largely characterised by the same tensions that exist between technology and education more generally. The fast and accelerating pace of technological innovation continually challenges the status quo.

Technology is changing fast. "[It] has the shelf life of a banana. By the time you buy it, implement it and train people on it, it's obsolete." (CNBC, 2014). A smartphone today contains more than a million dollars of 1980's technology (Diamandis & Kotler, 2012). Many new technologies offer simple solutions with low learning curves, free entry, and seamless integration via social media accounts like Facebook or Google (Kontaxis, Polychronakis, & Markatos, 2012) making it easy to get started and to mix and match technologies.

Large organisations are unable to change as fast (Fitzgerald, Kruschwitz, Bonnet, & Welch, 2014; Veletsianos, 2016). Security, quality assurance, accessibility, systems integration, adherence to legislation (for example, privacy), sustainability, return on investment, and cost should be considered before a new technology is adopted by the institution (Fitzgerald et al., 2014; Oliveira & Martins, 2011; Zissis & Lekkas, 2012). These could sometimes contribute to the delay in the adoption of a technology. Organisations will monitor their technological profile against developments in the market and actively seek replacement technologies before the predictable end of a technology's life (Smither, Houston, & McIntire, 2016). Gartner created the Hype Cycle to demonstrate the usual path of technology adoption (visibility vs maturity) noting "technologies take years, sometimes decades, to traverse the entire Hype Cycle." (Gartner, 2016). Haldane (2015) notes the virtue of patience as important for growth, but if the institutional technology is too slow to progress, or too confining, academics will seek and adopt technologies to meet their needs on their own (Diaz, 2011).

Academics are motivated by factors such as professional pride, a desire to improve student learning experiences, and to reduce workload (Capelleras, 2005; Davis & Fill, 2007; Newton, 2003). They may be encouraged to adopt a technology by the "carrot" of educational technology's potential as promoted through the media, conferences, literature, and colleagues, or the "stick" of imposed adoption by institutional or Government policies. For example, a policy setting requiring a minimum level of engagement with the learning management system (Griffith University, 2014) is a "stick" approach. Government policy changes can prompt an organisational cultural change and adaptation for staff (Ferns, 2012). For example, the focus on graduate outcomes (Skills Australia, 2010) has been the catalyst for many organisations to adopt ePortfolio technology.

The number of available technology options is a challenge (Diaz, 2011). Technology integration models have been developed to assist academics in choosing technology to meet their pedagogical need (Kimmons & Hall, 2016). Interactive tools have been developed to assist academics in searching for appropriate technologies. For example: the Padagogy Wheel (Carrington, 2015) categorises iPad apps to both Bloom's Cognitive Domains (Krathwohl, 2002) and the SAMR technology adoption model (Puentedura, 2010); University of Minnesota maps technologies to the Gartner Hype Cycle (University of Minnesota, 2017) as an indicator of technology maturation; and University of Arizona maps technologies to teaching practices (ASU Online, 2014). Unfortunately these tools do not develop as fast as the number of new products so academics often encounter new technologies that are not yet curated. The tools listed serve as a starting point, but do not detail all the considerations involved in adopting a new technology, which is the gap this chapter seeks to fill.

These tensions represent a significant challenge to academics and educational institutions wishing to select the most appropriate emerging technology for their need.

TECHNOLOGIES IN WORK INTEGRATED LEARNING

The Pedagogy of Work Integrated Learning

Use of technology in any educational activity should be based on a deliberate and reasoned application of pedagogy (Glover, Hepplestone, Parkin, Rodger, & Irwin, 2016; Sinclair, 2015) and not just because of a vague promise of improved learning (Ehrmann, 2002). This will provide a justification for expenditure of effort and resources, a basis for evaluation, and an awareness of possible negative consequences. Pedagogical thoughtfulness can also lead to innovation as academics seek to solve problems and improve outcomes. Conversely, ignoring pedagogy and acting solely in response to other drivers (such as technological opportunity) can result in no, or even negative, educational benefits. Within an Allied Health context, pedagogy is even more important because of the potential for students to cause harm in real-life situations. Pedagogical requirements include ensuring authentic work activities (placement), providing interprofessional learning, and minimising the potential to do harm.

When designing WIL, ideally supervisors, students and universities will design the learning experiences together (pre-, during and post- placement). WIL therefore provides the opportunity for faculty, students and administrators to form creative partnerships to commit resources towards application of knowledge (Bringle & Hatcher, 1996).

Although a good teacher can excel despite their technological resources (Dron, 2012), technology can enhance teaching practice further. Thomas (2016) notes "When carefully designed and thoughtfully applied, technology can accelerate, amplify, and expand the impact of effective teaching practices".

Despite its promise, technology generally has not transformed learning and teaching (L&T) practice (Jenkins, Browne, Walker, & Hewitt, 2011). Jones (2016) posits that without an understanding of how a technology works, what it does, what it cannot do, it is impossible to think of innovative ways to transform learning with it. Dron (2012) proposes pedagogy is itself a technology, interdependent on other technologies, supporting Ross and Collier's (2016) contention that prior knowledge of technology may influence design in unintentional ways. The danger of choosing technology before considering pedagogy is that innovation is limited by the capabilities of the identified technology.

WIL requires students to recognise their learning experiences in order to improve through effective strategies such as preparation, good supervision and mentoring (Patrick et al., 2008 December). The curriculum should be designed with the pedagogical purpose, to prepare students to meet healthcare needs, understand biopsychosocial health perspectives, develop active learning capabilities, and interprofessional skills (McAllister & Nagarajan, 2016). To maximise their employability, students need to develop skills to work in teams, learn from their peers, reflect on their practice in order to improve, manage time, complex problems and information, develop interpersonal skills, and use technology (Karpati, 2011; McAllister & Nagarajan, 2016). As new work practices and technology are always emerging, it is important for students to develop flexibility and learn how to learn in order to stay abreast of workplace requirements.

Stakeholder assumptions affect the design and development of meaningful learning experiences (Kaider, Henschke, Richardson, & Kelly, 2009) so clear ongoing communication between workplace, student, and university is essential to providing a meaningful experience (Palermo et al., 2016; Winchester-Seeto, Rowe, & Mackaway, 2016).

Allied Health Work Integrated Learning Technologies

Rather than give an exhaustive list of individual technologies, the usage types for Allied Health WIL listed below may assist the categorisation of both existing and new technologies (by the process outlined in the section *Technology adoption process*). The technologies have been categorised by the times that learning potentially occurs

- before, during, and after WIL placement (Nagarajan & McAllister, 2015) as well as how technology can support administration of work integrated learning experiences.

Preparation for WIL

It is important to prepare students for their placement to minimise their fear and increase their effectiveness and safety (Martin & Marsh, 2003; Milkins, Moore, & Spiteri, 2014; Quail, Brundage, Spitalnick, Allen, & Beilby, 2016). Employability skills such as resilience should also be developed throughout the curriculum to improve student productivity on placement (Jackson, 2015; Rook, 2016; Sutherland & Symmons, 2012). Students on health-related WIL placement may have confronting experiences when faced with extremes of health conditions in settings outside of their comfort zone, both social and cultural (Thyer & Simpson, 2016) and technology can help prepare them.

Technologies may be used to provide: pre-placement knowledge (theory delivered via online learning systems), familiarisation (orientation manuals, simulation videos, role play, virtual learning environments such as Second Life, Multimedia Learning Objects, reflection, critical thinking, formative assessment, and scaffolding of skills (adaptive learning).

Simulations are popular in Allied Health WIL as a cost effective method to allow students to apply knowledge to practice, prepare for WIL by familiarising with a workplace and common interactions before arriving, and gain an insight into the roles of other health professionals and work-related interactions in a safe environment (Milkins et al., 2014; Mundkur & Ellickson, 2012). Enhancing simulation with technology allows designing options for students to learn in their own time, repetitively, choosing their own path (adaptive learning) and should they make a decision that results in (virtual) patient harm, they can start again without consequence (Quail et al., 2016).

Many Allied Health accreditation bodies require evidence of interprofessional learning within curricula (Nisbet, O'Keefe, & Henderson, 2016). Simulations can be constructed to provide each profession a significant and balanced role (Boet, Bould, Layat Burn, & Reeves, 2014). Interprofessional simulation using technology reduces the cost and logistical problems inherent in trying to get students and staff from different disciplines together.

Support of Learning While on WIL

It is important for students to feel supported while they are on placement. Keeping in contact and allowing students to share experiences as they are having them can help reduce anxiety. Technology enables this despite students being geographically distributed, using collaboration enablers (online classrooms, blogs, learning circles), skills instruction (video instruction, work manuals), reflection (journals, blogs, reflection tasks), and communication tools (online forums, email, online classrooms).

Due to the Allied Health professional requirement for placement, growth in student numbers and the constant struggle to find enough places, innovative methods of meeting the need supported by technology have developed including paired or group placements (Sealey et al., 2013), overseas placements (Agnew, Pill, & Orrell, 2016; Cameron et al., 2013), virtual WIL (Patrick et al., 2008 December), student led clinics (Hamilton et al., 2015), the jigsaw method of sharing different experiences (Simpson & Thyer, 2016), role-emerging placement in a non-traditional setting with an off-site supervisor (Dancza et al., 2013) and industry based project work on or off campus (Ferns, Russell, & Kay, 2016; James, Demetriades Toftdahl, & Mackey, 2016). These methods increase the requirement for collaborative, communication technologies. Remote, rural, and international placements may introduce more considerations due to lack of access to reliable technology.

The student experience is influenced by the characteristics of the workplace including the supervisor's prior training, the work available at the time, the student's attitude and competence, and the relationship between the student and their assessor (Palermo et al., 2015). Since students' experiences are unique and varied, many universities rely on reflective practice as an assessment supported by technology.

After WIL

Post WIL debriefing, reflection and feedback help students understand the relevance of what they have learned or how best to improve (Constantinou & Kuys, 2013; Palermo et al., 2015). Technology can be used to: debrief, collect evidence of learning/competency (submission tools, supervisor signoffs, certifications), reflect (journals, blogs, reflection tasks), and create linkages to future employment (showcase evidence in portfolios).

Administration of WIL

Technology assists with the huge volume of data collection, status tracking, and workplace relationship management including: placement/industry contact databases, placement allocation/selection tools (for example, SONIA by Planet Software), placement prerequisites databases (agreements, first aid certificates, working with children checks, police checks), monitoring student engagement, support of industry personnel; and supervisor/preceptor training.

Technology can assist supervisors in communication, training, marking and feedback. Areas for improvement include pedagogically sound supervisory methods (McAllister & Nagarajan, 2016). Ferns et al. (2016) have identified strategies to enhance access for industry partners to needed resources in their preferred formats to better enable provision of feedback, designing assessment and delivering authentic experiences reflecting the discipline.

The Need for a Considered Approach

It is important to not introduce new technology for technology's sake as the results can be ineffective, or worse, dangerous (Adams Becker et al., 2017). A new technology can meet a current pedagogical need but may introduce other problems such as student anxiety (Horspool & Lange, 2012) or exposure to privacy, copyright or security risks for students or the university (Hill, 2016; Singer, 2015). Selected technology should take into account the requirements of Allied Health students and the extra challenges posed by WIL placement.

Free technology appears to be the right price, but as (Blue_beetle, 2010) was the first to comment online "If you are not paying for it, you're not the customer; you're the product being sold." highlighting that personal details may be collected and analysed for purposes such as targeted marketing. Another problem with free technology is the lack of control over changes that cause disruption:

- YouTube changed their delivery method mid-academic term causing assessment instructions to be obsolete.
- In January 2017, a Skype change stopped many from attending online meetings (Griffith University, 2017).
- Resumup visual resume service changed from a free service to an annual subscription model then later to a tiered payment system (Severt, 2016). How do academics and students cope when this happens to a mandated application in the middle of a teaching period?

While caution is warranted, it is important to not be so cautious as to never adopt anything new. A pessimistic approach could build an overwhelming list of potential difficulties that may lead to a paralysis stifling all innovation and adoption of new technologies. A thoughtful and reasoned process of selection, implementation, evaluation and review which ensures pedagogical soundness is maintained or improved should be followed.

TECHNOLOGY ADOPTION PROCESS

The authors support the view that technology adoption should be "grounded in the reality that technology alone cannot cultivate education transformation; better pedagogies and more inclusive education models are vital solutions, while digital tools and platforms are enablers and accelerators" (Adams Becker et al., 2017, p. 6).

On the assumption that the pedagogical needs have been identified, in this section the authors discuss the process of an academic identifying, selecting, implementing, monitoring, review and evaluating a new technology. Sometimes the process of adoption may not follow this order, for example, if the institution mandates the use of a new enterprise technology (adopted after an appropriate investigation) then some steps can be omitted.

Identify a Technology/Practice

As new technologies are developed, and as new pedagogical uses for both existing and new technologies are found, there will be new opportunities for ICTs in WIL. The pressure to adopt a new tool can be quite strong, and may arise from various drivers. A new technology may:

- Become mainstream, and popular, outside of education. For example, the general use of mobile devices with smaller screens has led to educational content being redesigned away from large screen formats.
- Become fashionable and lead to educators to think they can "cash in" on its popularity by finding an educational use for it. An example is the 2016 fad for the augmented reality app Pokemon Go.
- Mirror a societal change, and hence become more appropriate than existing technologies or practices. For example, telehealth (Australian Government, 2015) to cope with expanding health needs of baby boomers and Google Translate to support global communications.
- Enable an activity that was hitherto not possible. For example, virtual reality and augmented reality devices have opened up possibilities for a whole new genre of educational experiences.
- Have been widely adopted in an industry or discipline work area, which in turn requires students to become proficient with that technology. For example, electronic medical records.

- Offer cost savings or business efficiencies that are attractive to financial managers. For example, on-premise servers vs. cloud-based servers.
- Replace an ageing technology. For example, an upgrade or replacement of a learning management system.
- Be adopted to fill a pedagogical need across the institution. For example, a portfolio tool supports assessment, reflective practice and presentation of achievement for employment (Hodges, 2011), especially useful for WIL.

It is time consuming to become familiar with what technologies are available and their proven application, so it makes good sense to leverage the efforts and knowledge of others. Contacting the institution's learning and teaching (L&T) unit responsible for technology engaged (or enabled, enhanced) learning is strongly recommended. The L&T unit may well have collated best practices and case scenarios, and may even actively promote certain use cases with full support provided. This unit may include roles such as educational designers, blended learning advisors, or other technology enabled learning team members. Engaging with L&T support staff is a time saving strategy for academics to keep up to date on researched best practices in technology developments.

For an academic proactively seeking to improve teaching practice by adopting an emerging technology, the following strategies can also assist:

- Network with others within the institution or outside including subscribing to online specialist users' forum or groups. For example, find out who is doing what and with what results to achieve the pedagogical outcome being intended within the institution.
- Carry out a regular environmental scan of new trends in educational technology and their uses. For Australia, the annual NMC Horizon Report (Adams Becker et al., 2017) is a valuable resource.
- Follow individual futurists and innovators for creative ideas and trends for example, Bryan Alexander (Alexander, 2017).
- Read educational literature, conference proceedings, and attend demonstrations.
- Utilise tools that map technologies to teaching practice and technology maturation (ASU Online, 2014; Carrington, 2015; University of Minnesota, 2017).
- Visit sites of other adopters.
- Join a relevant professional group/society, community of inquiry, user group or use the networking opportunities provided at conferences.
- Email the authors of articles that mention new technologies in areas of interest.

- Monitor grants awarded for technology adoption.
- Search for existing resources. For example:
    - Search OER Commons – Open Educational Resources (Institute for the Study of Knowledge Management in Education, 2017).
    - Add the keyword *Games* or *Interactives* to topic keywords in a search.
    - If using the Google search engine, search on the topic keywords, then click *Videos* to only view videos (or *Images* to only view images).

Select a Technology

After clearly defining the pedagogical purpose, choose the technology that will best support learning sustainably by careful consideration of the following aspects: students, staff/academics, vendor, workplace, institution, compliance and legislation, cost, pedagogical, and technical considerations discussed below.

Student

Q: How User-Friendly Is the Technology and What Support Is Available to Students?

A new technology is not likely to be adopted or effective if it is hard to use or unreliable. Users will be quickly frustrated if it does not work as expected. The learner interface should be intuitive with up-to-date, easy-to-follow online self-help support resources and preferably a contact help phone line for just-in-time help. The academic may have to create their own step-by-step instructions for students to follow.

Example:

- The online classroom software required 6 steps before students could attend an online class. Realising this to be a potential barrier for students attending online classes, the academic set pre-class activities for students to complete those steps well ahead of the online class time and held a face-to-face session with students bringing their own devices to ensure they were correctly set up before going to their WIL placement.

Q: How Accessible Is It?

Consider if the students will still have the prerequisites for a particular ICT while on placement, for example, smartphone, broadband internet access. Does the tool also provide reasonable accommodations for students with disability (Patrick et al., 2008 December)? If not, using this technology may make the university liable for discrimination claims (for example, in Australia, the *Disability Discrimination Act 1992*).

Examples:

- Students may no longer have access to reliable, high speed internet access on a remote WIL placement which impacts their ability to access online resources or participate in high speed synchronous activities.
- The weekly update video used to keep students feeling connected posted on YouTube in an Australian course is unable to be accessed by students on international placement in China and Borneo because Google software is blocked in those countries.
- If good quality closed captions are not provided, it could breach accessibility regulations.

Q: What Personal Information Will Need to be Provided?

Students should not be forced to expose personal details outside of the academic institution. They should not have to create individual accounts or use single sign-on using their existing internal institutional portal login and not be obliged to provide personal information.

Examples:

- The discussion forum application Piazza requires an account to be created before use. The vendor has been on-selling the personal account details (Hill, 2016). As a consequence, many institutions have ruled out the use of Piazza.
- The results table in a free-to-use software publicly displays a table of student names, student numbers, and their result for activities within that software. This is against information privacy rules in many countries and may incur legal action.

Q How Does the Software Support the Various Needs of the Students in the Course?

Knowing the general characteristics of students can assist the teaching team schedule learning activities and provide appropriate support resources. An instructor should consider technology requirements of all courses the student is likely to be undertaking at the same time to avoid overloading students. Learning to use new technology or switching between technologies could be a cognitive overload.

Examples:

- Students were asked to create a digital story of their placement using software of their choice and submit via YouTube. This created significant angst in students but with encouragement, clear support resources, weekly guidance, and an online forum to discuss issues, all students were successful. Many voiced appreciation for their new skills.
- Not all students have mobile devices, so students were asked to form groups of three in a face-to-face class before engaging in a app based activity, ensuring one member of each group had an internet enabled mobile device.

Q: *How Well Does This Tool Support the Learning Activities Planned?*

Technologies chosen should enhance the educational experience and be relevant to the material being taught including the standards to which a course/program is accredited.

Examples:

- Online classroom software allows communication with students while geographically dispersed. Google Docs software supports collaboration by allowing simultaneous online editing of a document by multiple students in diverse locations.
- The United Kingdom (UK) based Smart Thinking tutoring service sometimes provides advice contrary to the accreditation requirements of Australian Allied Health disciplines potentially adversely impacting student outcomes.

Staff/Academic

Q: *Is the Workflow Involved With the New Technology/Practice Sustainable?*

Consider steps in the workflow including training new staff, setup, use, marking, extracting results, uploading back into the Learning Management System (LMS). Does the new technology/practice offer time savings without impacting student experience and does the proposed benefit outweigh any extra administration time?

Examples:

- Administration time and spreadsheet knowledge required to create accounts and transfer student/group details and assessment results between two systems may be prohibitive, especially as the process has to be repeated for students with extensions.

- One instructor created an online interview assignment in an external tool using a private account. The next offering was convened by a new instructor who was required to repeat the vendor relationship building, assignment resource creation and student account setup in the same technology because the original setup was based on a personal account and unable to be accessed. This required a significant amount of administration time.

Q: Does the Curriculum Allow Time for the Students to Learn the New Tool?

Students need time to become familiar with the new tool before they go on their WIL placement. Consider how much effort is required to develop clear instructions specific to the student's context prior to placement as well as to provide easily accessible support.

Examples:

- Allocate time to implement the training plan for staff and students to become familiar with the new tool, preferably before placement.
- Students asked to submit a digital story have to learn how to use a presentation tool and video recording, editing, and uploading tools.

Q: What Change Management and Training Plans Are in Place?

Training of staff and students may be required before use. Sessional staff often do not get paid for training so may not engage before use. Workplace supervisors may not have time to engage before use, but requiring training before supervision reduces the number of available supervisors in an already tight sphere (Patrick et al., 2008 December). Lack of support for student and workplace supervisors results in poor outcomes.

Examples:

- Soft-launch a new technology with a few early adopters with appropriate support as opposed to a full institutional wide implementation.
- Ensure self-help support resources are in place before asking students or workplace supervisors to engage with a new technology.

Q: Is It Scalable?

What worked for one tutorial may not work for another class or for another discipline. What is cheap for one class may incur prohibitive costs for a school or institution.

Examples:

- Providing feedback on weekly reflections may be achievable for a small cohort but not for a large cohort due to workload implications on the teaching team (or cost of hiring more team members).
- A small class may view/edit a single online document simultaneously (for example, Google Doc), but the file would crash for a large cohort.

Vendor

Q: What Level of Support Is Available or Accessible?

If adopting a technology outside of the organisation, one cannot necessarily rely on the organisation's IT support for help. Is there any support available from the vendor or internally within the institution? What hours is it available? What is the turnaround time from lodging a question to receiving an answer? What self-help resources are available? Are they clear? If vendor support is sparse, and the technology not institutionally supported, the academic must be prepared to personally provide student support or alternate options to achieve the activity.

Examples:

- If considering a United Kingdom (UK) service to be used in Australia, the support service may only be available outside of business hours due to time zone differences, potentially providing no support for students while on placement.
- If the academic is unable to solve problems for an unsupported technology, it can cause anxiety and a significantly greater workload for the academic troubleshooting and implementing workaround solutions.

Q: What Is the Vendor's Track Record?

If the vendor is well established the chances of the continuation of the technology and the business may be higher. If the vendor is new, they may be more responsive to requests for improvement.

Examples:

- The Zaption platform was taken over by another company and shut down mid semester (Zaption, 2016). Two and a half month's notice was given to account holders to migrate their content to the new platform. With the changeover of staff convening a course, the message was not communicated to the right people and the interactive instructional videos disappeared mid semester while students were on WIL, leaving students without instructional information and instructors scrambling to recreate content.

- The School of Pharmacy at Griffith University requested extra functionality in a virtual reality software. The young local business was able to incorporate the changes to meet their needs.

Q: Does the Vendor Provide for Service Level Agreement (SLA)?

A service level agreement is a contract between a vendor and the end user clearly defining the level of service expected from the vendor and what the customer will receive. It should establish the type of service to be provided at what cost and what the vendor will cover in the service including the level of support. The aim is to minimise the risk of the service being unavailable when required and clarify exactly what will be provided.

Examples:

- The SLA for an institution's Learning Management System requires that the technology is readily accessible and reliable when it is needed, for example, during class or while on placement. Maintenance is timetabled when the impact is least and downtime is communicated well in advance.
- When purchasing the School edition of the NearPod classroom technology, a SLA is negotiated to clarify the costs, the service and what the personalised training and support will include.

Workplace

Q: Is the Student Allowed to or Able to Use Technology While at the Workplace?

Workplace rules/policies and firewalls may prevent access or use of ICT. Infrastructure constraints may make some ICTs unavailable, for example, poor or non-existent internet access in rural or overseas locations. Does it require something to be installed on the workplace hardware? Will students have internet access and/or be allowed to use their own mobile devices? Is it for student, workplace supervisor, workplace owner or academic use? There may be different considerations for each.

Examples:

- Government Health and Education workplaces have restricted internet access and firewalls that prevent access to many outside websites and rural/remote workplaces may be disadvantaged due to slow internet speed.
- Some technologies need a small component to be installed before use that some workplace computers might not allow (for example, Webex, Bb Collaborate).

Institution

Q: Does the Institution Support Innovation With Technology?

Large organisations often have cumbersome bureaucracy including lengthy processes and cautious policies, and this tends to stifle innovation and creativity. Policies need to be maintained in a timely fashion to facilitate progress. Does the organisation offer L&T innovation grants that can be used to offset costs of change? Will the IT Support department assist in supporting a technology outside of the enterprise solutions? Does this solution meet organisational policies regarding equity and accessibility?

Examples:

- There is a potential for many different academics to adopt the same technology independently, missing economies of scale or seamless technology integration opportunities.
- Organisational equity policies may require information to be posted within the LMS as not all students have (for example) social media accounts resulting in double the effort for the instructor.

Q: What Are Institutional Technology Adoption Processes and/or Practices?

The institution's L&T unit responsible for technology engaged learning should have tools to guide academics, students, and workplace providers in the interpretation of legislative requirements, including examples of suitable technologies and disseminate these via training and quality assurance reviews.

Examples:

- A new innovation checklist required to be completed as part of a L&T grant process ensures privacy and security have been considered.
- Institutional promotion of, and training in, use cases of the existing and costly technologies, including self-help resources, student guides and support processes, should encourage use and improved experience.

Compliance and Legislation

Q: Would the New Technology/Practice Comply With Legislative/ Regulatory Requirements - Accessibility, Privacy, Information? These Are Usually Reflected in Institutional Policies

It is important not to expose the institution to litigation by breaking the law. Ensure compliance with institutional and national/state policies or legislations. There may be a legal requirement that student information is protected, for example, as per *Information Privacy Act 2009* in Queensland, Australia. It may be possible to seek exemptions to enable a better option to be adopted but this can be a slow process. It is important to follow any internal institutional compliance checklist that may exist to minimise risk. There may also be a requirement to retain student assessment data for a defined period.

Examples:

- Trend Micro studied a number of phone apps and identified 20% leaked information about contacts, location, phone number, and device details (Ferguson, 2014). This practice is against privacy laws.
- Twitter allows students to hone their communications skills and communicate with people from around the world, but if an educational activity is taken out of context, may damage a student's professional image – for example, defending an assigned unpopular position in a debate may incur harassment from the general public. Twitter is also ephemeral. It may be necessary to request students submit a summary of their activity to ensure the information lasts the required amount of time. Alternatively the academic can download relevant tweets regularly for data retention purposes.

Cost

Q: What Would Be the Initial Implementation and Ongoing Support Costs?

Funding implications are key to adoption of technology and support capacity. Costs may include licences, stakeholder time costs, educational design support, opportunity costs (i.e. if this is bought, other items cannot be bought), and ongoing support and maintenance. Where the learning outcome is a generic one, consider collaborating with other departments or other universities to share costs. If a technology is free now, how likely is it to emerge into a fee model later? Will the users be given some form of payment model for use of resources? Is there likely to be a return on investment in terms of enhanced learning experience? What is the difference in price from a single subscription to institution wide?

Examples:

- Consider time and cost of creating closed captions and transcription on video to meet legislation requirements for accessibility. Is this sustainable?

- If small changes are required to an interactive tool developed by an external software company, the changes may take weeks to be made as it is a small job for little revenue. This delay can have significant impact on teaching.

Pedagogical Considerations

Q: What Is the Teaching Style and Intended Learning Outcomes?

Personality and technical confidence/capability of staff can make a huge difference in the success of a technology.

Examples:

- If an academic is not comfortable with new technology, it may be best to stay with institutionally supported tools so they can receive support for every step from development to ongoing use.
- Teaching team members may have different levels of comfort with a proposed technology. It is important to allocate time/resources to up-skill the whole team or select a solution that all are able to use.

Q: How Will User Expectations Be Managed?

Instructors should make their expectations of students clear. A small technological change can have a large impact. Innovations can impact student evaluations negatively. It is best to work with the L&T support professionals and school L&T representatives to minimise the impact of change.

Examples:

- Plan alternate methods of communication/assessment in case a student does not have (access to) the required technology or for instances of technology failure (Murray, 2016).
- Clearly state technology requirements in the course profile (unit outline), in the introductory section of the course site, in the first lecture, and the first emailed announcement. Specific technology needs and support resources should be listed with each assessment. The weekly course emails should explain where students should be up to (including technology skills acquired) with the course materials/assessments and offer support options if they are not. A forum for discussion should be provided for students to seek help and support each other.

Technical Considerations

Q. What Is the Implication of Integration?

If the institution uses a Learning Management System (LMS) then it is important to identify if the selected tool integrates with the LMS and discuss internally the impact of support capacity. Just because a technology can integrate, does not mean the ICT department are willing to, and/or have capacity to, implement the integration.

Examples:

- The new technology may need additional support staff capacity and a change management plan for a wider university implementation.
- Some vendor provided LMS integration packs had wide sweeping permissions allowing access and change rights to far more data than necessary (N. Kays, personal communication, April 13, 2016) creating a security risk for student data.

Q: How Can the Tool/Service Be Monitored for Performance, Issues/ Problems, Potential Upgrades, and Maintenance?

This will inform the forecasting of potential issues and establishing strategies/ solutions to resolve and plan for maintenance schedules. Find out what will be the downtimes, service disruptions, what staff capacity will be needed, and how will these be communicated with clients. The newer the tool, the more there will be unknowns.

Examples:

- An external online testing software was made unavailable for maintenance reasons during the time an online test was scheduled resulting in student anxiety (over and above that created by the assessment) and requiring negotiation of a blanket extension for all students.
- Online classroom software crashed when an online class was scheduled for students on placement the week an assessment was due. The academic recorded the main points and emailed a link to the recording, inviting asynchronous discussion in an online forum instead.

Q: Is the Technology Secure?

Legislation may specify where information may be legally stored. For this reason, it is essential to know what type of data will be submitted, where it will be stored, and how secure it is. A backup copy of student data should be created regularly. Sensitive data requires higher security.

Examples:

- A UK University provided assessment results, student name, and address via a site that could be accessed without logging in, making the data easily extractable by a hacker. This was in violation of the *UK Data Protection Act* (Ghulam, 2016).
- Patient names and WIL placement location should not be identified in reflections in an online blog in order to protect patient confidentiality.

Q: How Sustainable Is It?

Sustainability of tool implementation and hence the service and cost in terms of acquisition, licensing, initial training, ongoing training costs, upgrades, implementation support, and provisions for train the trainers. Another consideration is account creation and permissions management. Is this a single person's responsibility? Maintaining accounts and permissions can increase workload greatly, especially for larger cohorts.

Examples:

- When an externally created interactive module based on a single user account needs updating and the original account owner is no longer available, the resource cannot be maintained.
- When the feedback tool AnswerGarden is used to create a question anonymously without a password, it cannot be edited to block inappropriate answers or clear responses. A new AnswerGarden has to be created and embedded and previous answers copied manually across. If the password is not communicated to the rest of the teaching team, only the original creator can manage the responses. This is a problem if the creator is unavailable when maintenance is required.

To aid comparison between solutions, a table can be used to collect information about how well each technology/practice (columns) meets each requirement (rows). Weighting the requirements based on need will help select the best fit option as shown in Table 1.

After reviewing the questions to inform the selection of a technology, the best result will be obtained if all stakeholders are consulted. An important factor in the final decision is how a proposed technology fits into the wider context of other university systems. A technology roadmap (TRM) should be developed that would "cover a time-based strategic planning process, which helps to line up and communicate needs (why to do) with the corresponding actions (what to do) and the supporting

Table 1. Example of tool comparison

Feature	Tool 1	Tool 2	Tool 3
Q: Is the technology user-friendly?	✓	✓	✓
Q: Is support available to students?	✓	X	✓
Q: Is it accessible?	✓	✓	✓
Q: Does it require personal information to be provided?		✓	✓
Q Does the software support the various needs of the students in the course?	X	X	✓
...			

resources (how to do)" (Bicking & Wimmer, 2011, p. 2). This will enable ease of implementation including support and collaboration from stakeholders and will involve an appropriate change management process.

Implement

Adams Becker et al. (2017) explain that "technology and digital tools have become ubiquitous, but they can be ineffective or dangerous when they are not integrated into the learning process in meaningful ways" (p.7). The users (staff and students) should be able to align the learning outcomes with the use of tools.

Having identified or selected a tool, the following steps will support implementation:

- Develop support resources relevant for staff and students which cover good teaching/learning practice as well as technical how-to guides.
- Consider internet security walls or restrictions on external connections during WIL placements at external locations. If live connections are not possible, the tool needs to be capable of functioning in an offline mode and be able to transfer data once back online. For example, PebblePocket app allows students to collect information offline for later upload to the web based PebblePad application.
- Ensure that the needs of all stakeholders are included in the implementation plan.
- Provide feedback channel (users to vendors and/or users to institutional central support unit).
- Publicly list frequently asked questions and their answers.
- Decide on how to measure success.
- Set up processes to collect statistics for the identified success variables. For an external tool, this may require paying for analytics.

- Comply with copyright regulations.
- Comply with accessibility guidelines (such as World Wide Web Consortium (W3C) enabling use "by people with a diverse range of hearing, movement, sight, and cognitive ability" (W3C, 2016).
- Comply with institutional guidelines and policies relating to use of technology.
- Support a variety of computer equipment including mobile devices.
- Support varying levels of internet connectivity including remote and WiFi.

Monitor Use/Impact

To determine impact, (Johnston & Baker, 2002), argue that it is essential to monitor the implementation efforts and the impact on learning outcomes. The following provides a guide to achieve this:

- Collecting data in a timely manner will enable determination of impact. Some systems may only keep data for a short term so it will be helpful to decide as to what will be collected and how.
- Create feedback channels before, during, and after implementation and adjust software capability and use to meet the needs.
- Observe changing conditions. Conditions that existed when implementation began may change, leading to the need for adjusting delivery. For example, interactive using Adobe Flash would not function due to major browsers stopping Flash support.
- If there are issues emerging or discovered during a trial that may lead to possible reasons to not continue using the technology they should be fully recorded. These will inform decision making for termination of institution-wide implementation.
- Share risk by setting up collaborations across stakeholders within the institution and with other institutions.
- Set up a community of inquiry to share success stories.

Review and Evaluate

As part of evaluation to inform further decision making, Johnston & Baker (2002) present a framework describing the key outcome areas as shown in Table 2.

Adopting methodologies that allow proposed new technologies to be properly evaluated before committing to implementation avoids failed projects and unnecessary expenditure.

Table 2. Key outcome areas

Outcome	Description
Learner Outcomes	• Cognitive domain (skills, abilities and performance). • Affective domain (attitudes, interests, and motivation to learning.
Teacher Outcomes	• Changed pedagogy (improved learning opportunities for students). It will inform changing design and course enhancement. • Improved technology skills (increase in teachers' capability will better expose students to technology based learning).
Technology Integration	An understanding to the type(s) of technology, users (students, teachers and others), learner activities, and cognitive demands required will inform the degree of or ease of integration in L&T.
Dissemination Outcomes	Wider dissemination of lessons learnt from pilots, trials or otherwise will inform other users, institutional level conversations, and decision making. Share with a colleague, share within the discipline, present at a forum.

Expand to an Institutional Technology

The impetus for an institution-wide implementation of a technology may occur from the bottom up or the top down. After a successful pilot, academics share their experience and the use of the technology with colleagues, leading to adoption course by course, until a critical mass is reached and an investigation regarding adoption for the whole institution begins.

Alternatively, the central L&T team may take a proactive approach to identify technology (perhaps following from a successful pilot) and work with the Technology Support team to investigate and adopt the technology. Either way, although the technology adoption process would be similar, an institution-wide approach introduces more factors and stakeholders into the decision making process.

TECHNOLOGY ADOPTION CASES

Case Scenario 1

The authors of this chapter were extensively involved in an institution-wide adoption of a Personal Learning Environment (PLE) / ePortfolio technology. The process went in phases:

Pre-Pilot Phase

The discussions for an institution-wide adoption of an ePortfolio solution took place over some years. An LMS native ePortfolio tool and Google Sites were used by some disciplines but did not allow external reviewers (especially in a WIL situation) to only see what they needed to see.

Phase 1: Pilot

The increasing demand for decisions about such a platform forced two Allied Health Sciences schools to obtain individual licenses for a well-established PLE / ePortfolio platform in their first year courses. At the same time, academics from another discipline conducted the same technology scan and adopted a different PLE technology platform. Their experiences informed further conversations and a subsequent scan for enterprise solutions.

Phase 2: Tool Comparative Evaluation

The central L&T unit initiated a desk-evaluation of this platform, comparing with other platforms that provide a similar service to determine a shortlist of two.

Phase 3: Needs-Case Scenarios

Needs-case scenarios were called for from academic faculty groups. The vendors were invited to demonstrate how their product could meet the needs of each case scenario. Vendors' demonstrations were reviewed and evaluated by attendees at an open invitation forum. Furthermore, very detailed feedback was sought from the authors of the scenarios.

Phase 4: Stakeholder Panel

A panel of stakeholders was formed to make a final informed decision. The panel included Business Owners, Information System Custodian, Data Custodian, Information System Users, and Funding Unit. This phase also included all the considerations outlined above under the section *Select a Technology* and site visits to other institutions who were using the tool. One PLE platform was recommended through a business case to the institutional executive and received strong support and approval, followed by legal and contractual investigations and agreements.

Phase 5: Implementation

The central learning and teaching unit organised an institution-wide open show and tell session during which it launched a call for expressions of interest for early adopters. A PLE Implementation Working Party was formed expanding on the stakeholder panel from Phase 4 to include more representatives from academic disciplines, staff and student support elements. The authors of this chapter were members of this working party.

The implementation, change management, and support framework was jointly crafted involving central and faculty embedded staff and student support elements. The framework included: "train the trainer" workshops by the vendor; demonstration workshops for early adopters; needs scoping conversation with early adopters; specialised workshops to design resources used in the tool; self-help resource and support website; dedicated central support staff as part of L&T systems technical team; and regular conversations with the vendor to improve the tool to meet specific needs.

Case Scenario 2

Chapter 12 of this book by Pearson is an example of a discipline/degree program level implementation. One of the authors of this chapter was involved in the review and use of platforms starting from need rather than technology in the Midwifery discipline. The process began with the formulation of the pedagogical needs by relevant stakeholders, then the identification of relevant technologies that could fulfil those needs. Over a period of six years several platforms were investigated, some selected and implemented.

The use and impact were monitored but as the degree program matured during delivery from year one to year three, and after repeat offerings, clarity emerged based on learner experience and evidence. After each evaluation phase newer platforms were investigated and implemented following the principles outlined in this chapter. The platforms used over this period included ExpoLX Blog/Wiki Tool, Google Sites (with in-house customised user interface) and eventually settled with Smartabase which has been adapted to meet the diversity of pedagogical requirements and the learning journey of a midwifery student through the program.

Case Scenario 3

Chapter 5 of this book by Tuttle is an example of a course level trial of an Adaptive Learning Platform (Smart Sparrow) in an Allied Health Science discipline. As colleagues became aware of this project and its outcomes, and further individual projects using Smart Sparrow were started, the suitability of this tool to meet pedagogical needs was established. This eventually informed and influenced an institutional level investigation and adoption of Smart Sparrow, which followed a similar process to that described in Case Scenario 1 above.

Case Scenario 4

Another example of a small scale to enterprise implementation is the free social networking platform Yammer. A professional staff member started a private network on Yammer from a free account to allow Griffith University staff to share articles of educational interest.

The Social Media Advisor in Griffith's Information Services promoted the use of this private social networking tool in preference to Facebook because the latter contains advertisements and mines user data for marketing purposes. The network grew. Special interest groups were formed. Course based uses for student-student and student-instructor communication were identified.

Eventually an enterprise licence for the product was obtained which provided security for the network beyond a private account. The use of the platform has been promoted more widely especially for course communication and its use continues to grow.

CONCLUSION

Continued change is a certainty in the areas of pedagogical developments and technological advances. The use of ICTs in Allied Health WIL, which already shows much promise, therefore has challenges and opportunities that are both exciting and confronting. In the face of this uncertainty a proactive approach which includes a thoughtful application of pedagogy is recommended. The guidelines and considerations provided within this chapter can be used to inform a careful yet agile process for deciding whether or not to adopt a technology. This process provides a sound pedagogical basis for making a decision, so that intended educational outcomes are achieved, and other undesirable outcomes are avoided.

ACKNOWLEDGMENT

This chapter received no specific grant from any funding agency in the public, commercial, or not-for-profit sectors. Support was received from Griffith University colleagues in the production of the final document.

REFERENCES

W3C. (2016). *Accessibility. Web design and applications.* Retrieved 1 April, 2017, from https://www.w3.org/standards/webdesign/accessibility

Adams Becker, S., Cummins, M., Davis, A., Freeman, A., Hall Giesinger, C., & Ananthanarayanan, V. (2017). *NMC horizon report: 2017 higher education edition.* Austin, TX: The New Media Consortium.

Agnew, D., Pill, S., & Orrell, J. (2016). *Work-integrated learning: Making a contribution to less privileged communities at home and abroad.* Paper presented at the New Zealand Association for Cooperative Education, Takapuna, Auckland, New Zealand.

Alexander, B. (2017). Retrieved 1 April, 2017, from https://bryanalexander.org

ASU Online. (2014). *Third-party tools.* Retrieved 19 February, 2917, from http://teachonline.asu.edu/wp-content/uploads/2014/03/ASU-Online-3rd-Party-Tools.pdf

Australian Government. (2015). *Telehealth.* Retrieved 19 February, 2017, from http://www.health.gov.au/internet/main/publishing.nsf/content/e-health-telehealth

Ball, D. M., & Levy, Y. (2008). Emerging educational technology: Assessing the factors that influence instructors' acceptance in information systems and other classrooms. *Journal of Information Systems Education, 19*, 431–443.

Bicking, M., & Wimmer, M. A. (2011). *Concept to integrate open collaboration in technology roadmapping: Stakeholder involvement in strategic e-government planning.* Paper presented at the 2011 44th Hawaii International Conference on System Sciences.

Blue_beetle. (2010, August 26). Re: User-driven discontent [Blog comment]. Retrieved from http://www.metafilter.com/95152/Userdriven-discontent#32560467

Boet, S., Bould, M. D., Layat Burn, C., & Reeves, S. (2014). Twelve tips for a successful interprofessional team-based high-fidelity simulation education session. *Medical Teacher, 36*(10), 853–857. doi:10.3109/0142159X.2014.923558 PMID:25023765

Bringle, R. G., & Hatcher, J. A. (1996). Implementing service learning in higher education. *The Journal of Higher Education, 67*(2), 221–239. doi:10.1080/00221546.1996.11780257

Cameron, D., Cockburn, L., Nixon, S., Parnes, P., Garcia, L., Leotaud, J., & Williams, T. et al. (2013). Global partnerships for international fieldwork in occupational therapy: Reflection and innovation. *Occupational Therapy International*, *20*(2), 88–96. doi:10.1002/oti.1352 PMID:23661362

Campbell, N., McAllister, L., & Eley, D. (2012). The influence of motivation in recruitment and retention of rural and remote allied health professionals: A literature review. *Rural and Remote Health*, *12*(3), 1900. PMID:22845190

Capelleras, J.-L. (2005). Attitudes of academic staff towards their job and organisation: An empirical assessment. *Tertiary Education and Management*, *11*(2), 147–166. doi:10.1080/13583883.2005.9967144

Carrington, A. (2015). *The padagogy wheel v4.1.* Retrieved 16 February, 2017, from http://designingoutcomes.com/assets/PadWheelV4/PadWheel_Poster_V4.pdf

CNBC. (2014, 7 February). *Technology has the shelf life of a banana: McNealy.* Retrieved from http://video.cnbc.com/gallery/?video=3000242076

Constantinou, M., & Kuys, S. S. (2013). Physiotherapy students find guided journals useful to develop reflective thinking and practice during their first clinical placement: A qualitative study. *Physiotherapy*, *99*(1), 49–55. doi:10.1016/j.physio.2011.12.002 PMID:23219653

Dancza, K., Warren, A., Copley, J., Rodger, S., Moran, M., McKay, E., & Taylor, A. (2013). Learning experiences on role-emerging placements: An exploration from the students' perspective. *Australian Occupational Therapy Journal*, *60*(6), 427–435. doi:10.1111/1440-1630.12079 PMID:24299482

Davis, H. C., & Fill, K. (2007). Embedding blended learning in a university's teaching culture: Experiences and reflections. *British Journal of Educational Technology*, *38*(5), 817–828. doi:10.1111/j.1467-8535.2007.00756.x

Diamandis, P. H., & Kotler, S. (2012). *Abundance: the future is better than you think.* New York, NY: Free Press.

Diaz, V. (2011). Cloud-based technologies: Faculty development, support, and implementation. *Journal of Asynchronous Learning Networks*, *15*(1), 95.

Dron, J. (2012). The pedagogical-technological divide and the elephant in the room. *International Journal on E-Learning*, *11*(1), 23–38.

Ehrmann, S. C. (2002). Improving the outcomes of education: Learning from past mistakes. *EDUCAUSE Review*, *37*, 54–55.

Exercise and Sports Science Australia. (2016). *Course accreditation guide for education providers*. Retrieved April 2, 2016, from https://www.essa.org.au/wp-content/uploads/2016/11/Course-Accreditation-Guide-Oct-2016.pdf

Ferguson, R. (2014, January 2). Snapchat user data exposed in huge data theft [Blog post]. Retrieved from http://countermeasures.trendmicro.eu/snapchat-user-data-exposed-in-huge-data-theft/

Ferns, S. (2012). *Graduate employability: Teaching staff, employer and graduate perceptions*. Paper presented at the Australian Collaborative Education Network National Conference, Geelong, Australia.

Ferns, S., Russell, L., & Kay, J. (2016). Enhancing industry engagement with work-integrated learning: Capacity building for industry partners. *Asia Pacific Journal of Cooperative Education*, *17*(4), 349–375.

Fitzgerald, M., Kruschwitz, N., Bonnet, D., & Welch, M. (2014). Embracing digital technology: A new strategic imperative. *MIT Sloan Management Review*, *55*(2), 1–12.

Gartner. (2016). *Inside Gartner Research: How the art, science and rigor behind our research process and proprietary methodologies help you make the right decisions, every day*. Retrieved from http://www.gartner.com/imagesrv/research/methodologies/inside_gartner_research.pdf

Ghulam, A. (2016, January 16). Is it a security vulnerability if the addresses of university students are exposed? [Blog post]. Retrieved from https://security.stackexchange.com/questions/147222/is-it-a-security-vulnerability-if-the-addresses-of-university-students-are-expos

Glover, I., Hepplestone, S., Parkin, H. J., Rodger, H., & Irwin, B. (2016). Pedagogy first: Realising technology enhanced learning by focusing on teaching practice. *British Journal of Educational Technology*, *47*(5), 993–1002. doi:10.1111/bjet.12425

Griffith University. (2014). *Guidelines for staff engagement with Learning@Griffith*. Retrieved 17 February, 2017, from http://policies.griffith.edu.au/pdf/Staff%20Engagement%20with%20Learning%20at%20Griffith.pdf

Griffith University. (2017). *Skype disruptions on the Griffith network*. Retrieved March 1, 2017, from https://intranet.secure.griffith.edu.au/work/collaboration/self-help/other-collaborative-tools

Haldane, A. G. (2015). Growing, fast and slow. University of East Anglia.

Hill, P. (2016, November 10). Popular discussion platform piazza getting pushback for selling student data. *e-Literate*. Retrieved 27 February, 2016, from http://mfeldstein.com/popular-discussion-platform-piazza-getting-pushback-selling-student-data/

Hodges, D. (2011). The assessment of student learning in cooperative and work-integrated education. In R. K. Coll & K. E. Zegwaard (Eds.), *International Handbook for Cooperative and Work-Integrated Learning: International Perspectives of Theory, Research and Practice* (2nd ed.; pp. 53–62). Lowell, MA: World Association for Cooperative Education.

Horspool, A., & Lange, C. (2012). Applying the scholarship of teaching and learning: Student perceptions, behaviours and success online and face-to-face. *Assessment & Evaluation in Higher Education*, *37*(1), 73–88. doi:10.1080/02602938.2010.496532

Institute for the Study of Knowledge Management in Education. (2017). *OER Commons*. Retrieved from https://www.oercommons.org/

Jackson, D. (2015). Employability skill development in work-integrated learning: Barriers and best practice. *Studies in Higher Education*, *40*(2), 350–367. doi:10.1080/03075079.2013.842221

James, N., Demetriades Toftdahl, S., & Mackey, P. (2016). *Outcomes from Global Scope - a large-scale "virtual micro internship" WIL pilot with NSW State Government*. Paper presented at the WIL 2020: Pushing the boundaries, 2016 Australian Collaborative Education Network National Conference, Sydney, Australia.

Jenkins, M., Browne, T., Walker, R., & Hewitt, R. (2011). The development of technology enhanced learning: Findings from a 2008 survey of UK higher education institutions. *Interactive Learning Environments*, *19*(5), 447–465. doi:10.1080/10494820903484429

Johnson, L., Adams Becker, S., Cummins, M., Estrada, V., Freeman, A., & Hall, C. (2016). *NMC horizon report: 2016 higher education edition*. Austin, TX: The New Media Consortium.

Johnston, J., & Baker, L. T. (2002). *Assessing the impact of technology in teaching and learning: A source book for evaluators*. Ann Arbor, MI: University of Michigan.

Jones, D. (2016, September 11). Which comes first? Pedagogy or technology? [Blog post]. Retrieved from http://djon.es/blog/2016/09/11/which-comes-first-pedagogy-or-technology/

Kaider, F., Henschke, K., Richardson, J., & Kelly, M. P. (2009). *Designing blended spaces to maximise student learning in work integrated learning programs*. Paper presented at the ASCILITE 2009 - The Australasian Society for Computers in Learning in Tertiary Education.

Karpati, A. (2011). *Digital literacy in education*. Moscow, Russia: UNESCO Institute for Information Technologies in Education.

Kontaxis, G., Polychronakis, M., & Markatos, E. P. (2012). Minimizing information disclosure to third parties in social login platforms. *International Journal of Information Security*, *11*(5), 321–332. doi:10.1007/s10207-012-0173-6

Krathwohl, D. R. (2002). A Revision of Bloom's Taxonomy: An Overview. *Theory into Practice*, *41*(4), 212–218. doi:10.1207/s15430421tip4104_2

Lowe, S., Adams, R., & O'Kane, A. (2007). *A framework for the categorization of the Australian health professional workforce - discussion paper*. Retrieved from https://sarrah.org.au/sites/default/files/docs/framework_for_the_categorization_of_the_australian_health_workforce_summary_statement_august_2007.pdf

Martin, A. J., & Marsh, H. W. (2003). Fear of failure: Friend or foe? *Australian Psychologist*, *38*(1), 31–38. doi:10.1080/00050060310001706997

McAllister, L., & Nagarajan, S. V. (2016). Accreditation requirements in allied health education: Strengths, weaknesses and missed opportunities. *Journal of Teaching and Learning for Graduate Employability*, *6*(1), 2–24. doi:10.21153/jtlge2015vol6no1art570

Milkins, L., Moore, C., & Spiteri, J. (2014). *Simulation based education: Professional entry student education and training*. Retrieved from http://www.heti.nsw.gov.au/Global/NSS%20Simulation/SimulationBasedEducation_HETI.pdf

Mundkur, A., & Ellickson, C. (2012). Bringing the real world in: Reflection on building a virtual learning environment. *Journal of Geography in Higher Education*, *36*(3), 369–384. doi:10.1080/03098265.2012.692073

Murray, J. (2016). *Technology in the classroom: What happens when it fails?* Retrieved 15 February, 2017, from http://www.teachhub.com/technology-classroom-what-happens-when-it-fails

Nagarajan, S. V., & McAllister, L. (2015). Integration of practice experiences into the allied health curriculum: Curriculum and pedagogic considerations before, during and after work-integrated learning experiences. *Asia Pacific Journal of Cooperative Education*, *16*(4), 279–290.

Newton, R. (2003). Staff attitudes to the development and delivery of e-learning. *New Library World*, *104*(10), 412–425. doi:10.1108/03074800310504357

Nisbet, G., O'Keefe, M., & Henderson, A. (2016). Twelve tips for structuring student placements to achieve interprofessional learning outcomes. *MedEdPublish*, *5*(3), 23. doi:10.15694/mep.2016.000109

Oliveira, T., & Martins, M. F. (2011). Literature review of information technology adoption models at firm level. *The Electronic Journal Information Systems Evaluation*, *14*(1), 110–121.

Palermo, C., Capra, S., Beck, E. J., Ash, S., Jolly, B., & Truby, H. (2016). Are dietetics educators' attitudes to assessment a barrier to expanding placement opportunities? Results of a Delphi study. *Nutrition & Dietetics: the Journal of the Dietitians Association of Australia*, *73*(3), 254–259. doi:10.1111/1747-0080.12205

Palermo, C., Chung, A., Beck, E. J., Ash, S., Capra, S., Truby, H., & Jolly, B. (2015). Evaluation of assessment in the context of work-based learning: Qualitative perspectives of new graduates. *Nutrition & Dietetics: the Journal of the Dietitians Association of Australia*, *72*(2), 143–149. doi:10.1111/1747-0080.12126

Patrick, C.-j., Peach, D., Pocknee, C., Webb, F., Fletcher, M., & Pretto, G. (2008 December). *The WIL (work integrated learning) report: A national scoping study* [Australian Learning and Teaching Council (ALTC) Final Report]. Brisbane, Australia: Queensland University of Technology.

Puentedura, R. (2010). *SAMR and TPCK: Intro to advanced practice*. Retrieved August 16, 2017, from http://hippasus.com/resources/sweden2010/SAMR_TPCK_IntroToAdvancedPractice.pdf

Quail, M., Brundage, S. B., Spitalnick, J., Allen, P. J., & Beilby, A. J. (2016). Student self-reported communication skills, knowledge and confidence across standardised patient, virtual and traditional clinical learning environments. *BMC Medical Education*, *16*(1), 73. doi:10.1186/s12909-016-0577-5 PMID:26919838

Rook, L. (2016). *Challenges implementing WIL in human resource management*. Paper presented at the WIL 2020: Pushing the boundaries, 2016 Australian Collaborative Education Network National Conference, Sydney, Australia.

Ross, J., & Collier, A. (2016). Complexity, mess, and not-yetness: Teaching online with emerging technologies. In G. Veletsianos (Ed.), *Emergence and innovation in digital learning: foundations and applications* (pp. 17–33). Edmonton, Canada: AU Press. doi:10.15215/aupress/9781771991490.01

Sealey, R., Raymond, J., Groeller, H., Rooney, K., Crabb, M., & Watt, K. (2013). *Current practice of clinical exercise physiology placement supervision in Australia.* 2013 Report.

Severt, N. (2016, October 26). 14 best online resume builders reviewed [Blog post]. Retrieved from https://uptowork.com/blog/best-online-resume-builders

Simpson, P., & Thyer, L. (2016). *Fitting together the pieces: Using the jigsaw classroom to facilitate paramedic WIL.* Paper presented at the WIL 2020: Pushing the boundaries, 2016 Australian Collaborative Education Network National Conference, Sydney, Australia.

Sinclair, N. (2015). How should our pedagogy keep up with rapidly changing technology? *Journal of Initial Teacher Inquiry, 1*, 31–33.

Singer, N. (2015, March 11). Privacy pitfalls as education apps spread haphazardly. *The New York Times.* Retrieved from https://www.nytimes.com/2015/03/12/technology/learning-apps-outstrip-school-oversight-and-student-privacy-is-among-the-risks.html?_r=0

Skills Australia. (2010). *Australian workforce futures: A national workforce development strategy.* Canberra, Australia: Commonwealth of Australia.

Smither, R., Houston, J., & McIntire, S. (2016). *Organization development: Strategies for changing environments.* New York, NY: Routledge.

Sutherland, K., & Symmons, R. (2012). *Development of processes and assessment to facilitate a broad multidisciplinary Work Integrated Learning package.* Paper presented at the Australian Collaborative Education Network National Conference.

Thomas, S. (2016). *Future Ready Learning: Reimagining the Role of Technology in Education. 2016 National Education Technology Plan.* Washington, DC: Office of Educational Technology, US Department of Education.

Thyer, L., & Simpson, M. D. (2016). *Wellness for health students during WIL.* Paper presented at the WIL 2020: Pushing the boundaries, 2016 Australian Collaborative Education Network National Conference, Sydney, Australia.

University of Minnesota. (2017). *Hype cycle for education: Emerging technologies in higher education.* Retrieved 2 February, 2017, from http://hypecycle.umn.edu/

Veletsianos, G. (2016). *Emergence and innovation in digital learning: foundations and applications.* Edmonton, Canada: AU Press. doi:10.15215/aupress/9781771991490.01

Winchester-Seeto, T., Rowe, A., & Mackaway, J. (2016). Sharing the load: Understanding the roles of academics and host supervisors in work-integrated learning. *Asia Pacific Journal of Cooperative Education*, *17*(2), 101–118.

Zaption. (2016, June 30). Zaption joins Workday [Blog post]. Retrieved from http://blog.zaption.com/post/146724427719/zaption-joins-workday

Zissis, D., & Lekkas, D. (2012). Addressing cloud computing security issues. *Future Generation Computer Systems*, *28*(3), 583–592. doi:10.1016/j.future.2010.12.006

KEY TERMS AND DEFINITIONS

Allied Health: Includes health programs other than medicine and nursing eligible for professional body registration.

Compliance: The ability of a technology to be used without breaching governmental legislative or regulatory requirements, and/or institutional policies.

Course: A course is a unit of study within a program receiving a grade upon completion.

Emerging Technology: Technology or practices that are new to the context in which they are applied.

Program: A program is a plan of study, usually made up of courses, leading to an award.

Sustainability: The ability for a technology to continue to be effective without degradation of pedagogical benefit and without significant unexpected resource costs.

Work-Integrated Learning (WIL): Authentic educational activities that are aimed at integrating theory with real-world work practice.

Chapter 14
Digital Technologies for Teaching for Allied Healthcare Students and Future Directions

Roselyn Rose'Meyer
Griffith University, Australia

Indu Singh
Griffith University, Australia

ABSTRACT

Digital technologies are an integral component of the allied healthcare curricula, including dental technology, physiotherapy, pharmacy, nutrition, nursing, and laboratory medicine. Various digital technologies are implemented for the education of allied healthcare students. They have been used for curriculum design, engaging and facilitating the understanding of fundamental concepts in various disciplines, the development of active learning strategies, and designing critical thinking and clinical reasoning education. Online digital atlases and libraries provide flexible resources as study tools for students in the classroom and on industry placement. Adaptive digital learning, communication technologies, and virtual reality for teaching have become an essential component of the allied healthcare education. As students develop skills for their profession, the digital technologies have provided a platform for the documentation of their competencies and progress through industry placement, allowing academic staff to chart their progress and employers to assess the graduate competencies.

DOI: 10.4018/978-1-5225-3850-9.ch014

INTRODUCTION

The purpose of this book is to review the use of digital technologies for the education of students in Allied Health programs including Medical Laboratory Science, Nutrition and Dietetics, Pharmacy, Dental technology and Physiotherapy. It is recognised that there is a rapidly changing work force, where Millennials (individuals born between 1977 and 1997), can expect to have 17 careers across 5 industries over the course of their working lives (Owen, 2016). Not only are universities educating students for their current careers, it is essential that universities endow students with a range of skills that enable them to be employed in their current professions, but flexible and agile enough to adapt to changes within their discipline or enter new or future occupations.

BACKGROUND

All Allied Health students irrespective of the field of study, through meticulous curriculum design, are required to learn concepts relevant to the field, be able to communicate with patients and other Health professionals, use critical analysis or clinical reasoning to devise plans for implementation strategies and, have the skills to test or construct resources. Uniformly across tertiary institutions both nationally and internationally, laboratory teaching hours and access to clinical placements are declining due to the increased pressure of student enrolment numbers. The authors in this discuss innovative ways in which digital technologies have been implemented for curriculum design, for skills development and training and monitoring students during clinical placements. The final chapters discuss the use of digital technologies to document a student's competences and abilities for assessment and employment.

MAIN FOCUS OF THE CHAPTER

Digital Technologies for Curriculum Design

Education is undergoing a significant shift, moving away from teacher led instruction to student centred approaches (Ramsden, 2003). Digital native students have been exposed from an early age to a range of digital technologies and have developed novel learning styles. Students therefore require educational resources other than traditional teaching methods to engage in the learning process (Prensky, 2009), as they expect technology to be integrated into their learning experiences (Berman, Fall, Maloney, & Devine, 2008).

They therefore require educational resources other than traditional teaching methods to engage in the learning process (Prensky, 2009). In this day and age, students expect technology to be integrated into their learning experiences (Berman, Fall, Maloney, & Devine, 2008). However, with the exponential growth of digital technologies and associated resources, we are being inundated with e-learning programs. While e-learning tool designers are producing products that are attractive, they can have limited educational benefit if designed with no specific focus on pedagogy. Pedagogical knowledge amalgamates cognitive, social and developmental theories of learning and how they apply to students in the classroom (Harris, Mishra, & Koehler, 2009). The impact of e-learning tools on student learning is currently evaluated using student attitudes or overall grades without investigating the direct influence of digital technology on learning.

Overall, appropriate education principles for the design of e-learning tools are required so that students are not inundated with too much content, with too many distractions impeding learning due to loss of direction and attention. An understanding as to how students learn and transform information into knowledge is important. Students use distinct processes to learn material, with the auditory system processing narrative information while the visual system processing images (animation). Students learn most effectively when they can see, hear and interact with the e-learning tools. Hence, e-learning tools with animation and narration without too much extraneous information are considered the most superior option for student learning.

Across all the Chapters in this book is the recurrent theme that e-learning tools need to be used as supplementation to lectures and not as a substitute for face to face teaching. Students do not purposefully engage with supplementary teaching materials unless they are reminded and encouraged to do so. E-learning tools and activities need to be developed for specific learning outcomes and as a supplement to the curriculum. The construction of educational activities should be premised on the deliberate and reasoned application of pedagogy (Glover, Hepplestone, Parkin, Rodger, & Irwin, 2016). The main advantages of custom-designed e-learning tools over the functionally limited commercially available tools are that they are designed and developed incorporating the desired educational theories. The content and delivery can be structured and shaped to the particular requirements of a specific curriculum as observed for teaching Pharmacy students (See Chapter 2). The advantage is that the custom-designed e-learning tools can be modified according to learning and teaching needs and educators can easily and economically update the content to encompass evolving course learning objectives, changing practices and new developments in drug discovery and applications. The use of digital technologies and their potential use in Nutrition and Dietetics students is discussed in Chapter 4. As medical evidence emerges for the role of genetics in disease and how nutrition may impact clinical outcomes, curriculum will need to be designed to ensure students appreciate advances in the science of nutritional genomics. Students will need to be able to interrogate and interpret gene databases, review and evaluate data associated with nutrigenetics.

Digital Technologies for the Development of Active Learning

In allied health science education the disciplines lend themselves to the flipped classroom, which encourages students to be more engaged and active in their learning with well constructed learning activities encouraging a better understanding of content and enhancing student performance (Freeman et al., 2014). The combination of digital modules with face-to-face learning activities with peers or staff is required to deliver the desired learning outcomes (Rice & McKendree, 2014). The implementation of technology in a mixed mode approach to teaching supports cognitive learning strategies and provides students with the opportunity to make use of different learning styles to engage with multimedia to maximise and assimilate knowledge.

The digital online resources available include videos, podcasts, databases and scientific articles that are publically available, at a student's disposal and can offer a range of learning experiences. Academics contribute expertise specific to patient cases to create authentic activities to engage students. Digital technologies are used as a supplement for laboratory dissection and prosection session to enhance learning in anatomy (Losco, Grant, Armson, Meyer, & Walker, 2017).

As discussed in Chapter 3 an online digital atlas e-learning resource was successfully implemented at Griffith University for teaching anatomy in the dental program (Bakr, Massey, & Massa, 2016) and digital haematology slides for Medical Laboratory sciences (see Chapter 8). The digital atlas overcomes the barriers of limited cadaver availability, difficulty in observing specimens in large classes and access to rare samples. In anatomy it extends the life expectancy of teaching specimens and provides standardised training for all students. The advantage of a purpose built digital atlas using the University learning platforms is that all students have flexible access to enable self-directed learning activities with the digital repository of images encouraging active learning. Research regarding the learning outcomes of the digital atlases concluded that the teaching of practical skills face to face, needs to be retained rather than be replaced completely by online or digital technologies.

Digital Technologies for Design of Critical Thinking Education

Educational activities for Allied Health students can be structured using digital technologies to create and deliver problem based learning and critical thinking. It requires questions or activities that challenge students' thinking and highlight the most important aspects of the presentation (audiovisual) that relates to common themes. Chapter 7 outlines the use of Pebblepad as a digital platform to connect relevant courses in the Medical Laboratory program across year levels to solve case studies using the different disciplines (ie histology, haematology, clinical biochemistry). In Dental technology education discussed in Chapter 9, learning activities were centred around measurable activities (assessment) that promoted learning and required graduates to move from novice to expert over time, or at least, from knowing to doing (Miller, 1990).

With respect to emerging curriculum design, it was recognised that graduates from Dietetics and Nutrition programs would require training to be able to implement emerging tests and technologies in the treatment of patients, to provide specialised counselling and understand the ethics related to the distribution of relevant information related to health (See Chapter 4). Beyond an understanding of genomics, students must also use critical thinking skills to access, interpret and analyse genetic and peer reviewed scientific publications and understand the hierarchy of evidence for assessing qualitative health research (Daly et al., 2007). Finally, with patient protection of data, graduates need to ensure that digital technologies provide safe sites for data storage of genetic information.

Adaptive Digital Learning for Allied Health Students

Adaptive learning systems may be used to implement/frame/model critical thinking case based problems directly associated with the Allied Health science disciplines. Adaptive learning is a newer digital technology that has been implemented in learning activities for Physiotherapy students (see Chapter 5). Adaptive digital learning allows the development of multi-layered systems such as for Dental students that organise suitable models of student learning styles with advanced pedagogies to create complex learning situations (Baker, 2016) (See Chapter 9). It creates a one-on-one environment to personalise the learning process for students from different abilities, backgrounds, knowledge and behaviours (Crockett, Latham, & Whitton, 2017). Intelligent tutoring systems, which serve as a form of adaptive learning systems, improve the learning and teaching of discipline specific knowledge and manifests as a personal tutoring platform (Stankov, Glavinic, & Rosic, 2011). They are designed to incorporate the learning techniques from artificial intelligence systems to adapt activities and outputs to the individuals who engage with their teaching environments. They are designed to provide competency and knowledge transfer, modelling human behaviours to construct reasoning and problem solve (Khemaja, 2016).

For Physiotherapy students at Griffith University, an adaptive learning module (using SmartSparrow platform), was embedded and implemented to develop case based critical thinking and clinical reasoning skills. The advantage of adaptive learning is that the technology creates an environment that suits the learning processes of individual students and responds to their interactions to provide feedback and support. The technology accounts for students who have various needs and understandings, learn at different rates and distinctive learning styles.

Communication Technologies for Allied Health Programs

Communication skills are an essential component of all of the Allied Health Professions. Graduates must be able to collaborate, talk to patients, or liaise with other Health professionals. There are a significant array of digital technologies used for communication, including social, educational, professional or governance media sites. Social media in particular, engages the millennial student with many utilising Youtube as an online resource for video sharing (Jaffar, 2012). Graduates preferred online media as the primary source of information with students using Facebook, Twitter, LinkedIn and other networking websites (Giordano & Giordano, 2011). Research into the use of social media in education has shown that it promotes cooperation between students and learning from peers (Magro, Sharp, Ryan, & Ryan, 2013) and affords a relaxed learning environment that engages students in learning while accommodating novel learning approaches (Idris & Wang, 2009). Alternatively, other studies found that Facebook was a distraction as a learning tool (Wise, Skues, & Williams, 2011) with a reduced impact on academic performance (Kirschner & Karpinski, 2010). This work demonstrates that social media sites need to be constructed carefully to aid learning.

For teaching purposes digital technologies can facilitate virtual classrooms to provide access for remote or International students to a flexible and interactive learning environment as discussed in Chapter 6. The use of communication technologies enables Inter-professional Learning (IPL) training, where students develop the skills to communicate with clinicians to meet the needs of patients and creates communities of practice (Stephenson et al., 2016). Furthermore as discussed in Chapter 9 communication is required for educational activities such as work integrated learning (WIL), simulation or IPL for training of dentists. Students collaborated with other clinicians and health professionals to create an environment of team based planning. Here students learn teamwork, contribute to peer learning and study evidence based treatment planning strategies (Storrs, Alexander, Sun, Kroon, & Evans, 2015).

Technology allows communication over distances such that students can feel supported while on placement. Although remote, rural and international placements may have problems due to lack of access to reliable technology. Communication technology allows for educators and clinical placement facilitators to discuss student clinical performance and assessment standards and facilitates access to continuing education for practitioners who are placed in rural or remote communities.

Digital Technologies for Skills Development

For some of the Allied Health Professions such as Medical Laboratory Science and Dental Technology, graduates are working with advanced technology in laboratories and dealing with innovative software. For example, the use of fully automated diagnostic equipment in laboratory medicine with remote access communication capacity with multiple information systems across health care industry and the computer assisted designing (CAD) and computer assisted manufacturing (CAM) has transformed how denture products are designed and created in dental laboratories (See Chapter 9). Students are required to be agile and able to adjust to digital changes in order to sustain outputs and productivity in professional practice (Reifeis, Kirkup, Willis, & Browning, 2014). Use of CAD, CAM and 3D printing is now essential components for student education in the Allied Health sciences. For example 3D printing has been used to teach molecular modelling concepts to Pharmacy students at Griffith University (Hall et al., 2017). Hand held computers such as the Rasberry Pi were implemented for educating Medical Laboratory students (See Chapter 7) and provided a low cost alternative for developing computerised laboratories by allowing the digitisation of data from analytical equipment for teaching purposes as well as access to ePortfolios. These devices can be utilised for clinical placement in Industry although data protection would be required. In Chapter 8 the use of digital technologies was discussed with respect to virtual microscopy medical laboratory education. The release of the Aperio digital slide scanners provided the technology to create virtual microscope slides for teaching purposes. The virtual slide presents a large digital image of a section of the blood film to be examined and allows access to an increased number of students with increased flexibility to view slides as required and the slides can be accessed using smartphones at any time. The use of the virtual microscopy has been used for accreditation requirements to determine competencies for national pathology laboratories. An added benefit of virtual slides is that it reduces the biological risks associated with the use of microtomes, and histological stains as well as health and safety concerns associated with patient derived tissues. It also provides access to materials that are ethically difficulty to source for teaching purposes or may be rare.

The virtual slides are designed to complement competency training in the use of microscopes, and do not exempt students from this training as these skills are required in commercial pathology laboratories.

Use of Virtual Reality for Teaching Allied Health Students

The use of virtual reality for teaching in medicine is well established and its use for the education of Allied health students is discussed in Chapter 7. Virtual reality simulators can be used by surgeons to become familiar with a robotic console prior to live surgery (Rajanbabu, Drudi, Lau, Press, & Gotlieb, 2014). Advantages of VR systems include the ability to provide skills assessment and training with no risk to patients and, to create scenarios with increasing levels of difficulty without the resource demands or issues associated with animal based training (Kazemi et al., 2010).

Virtual reality digital technologies have been used to provide preclinical placement training for students in the Medical Laboratory program at Griffith University (See Chapter 7). Virtual reality affords students with laboratory experiences in professional laboratories in readiness for Industry placement. It ensures access to expensive equipment not readily available in teaching laboratories and saves on resources and consumables. Further potential uses for VR technology are identified, including the development of training modules to educate students how to run and trouble shoot apparatus. However, they stressed that 3D resources were used to complement rather than replace the teaching of skills in laboratories and lectures. The advantages of using virtual reality for some disciplines such as teaching anatomical sciences is that it provides a learning tool that is appealing to the millennials without the financial, ethical or manpower restraints of cadaver based classes used in the education of many health related programs. A more recent trend in virtual and augmented reality is haptic simulation which encompasses the sense of touch in simulated practical tasks to enable the training of health practitioners in complex procedures in a risk free environment. Adaptation of the VR technologies has allowed the incorporation of haptic devices, stereographics, adaptive content and assessment into the curriculum. Virtual reality and haptics have been used in medical surgery (Kim, Kim, & Kim, 2017) and restorative dental procedures (Buchanan, 2004).

Use of Digital Technologies for Simulation Training

Simulations are popular in Allied Health sciences as a cost effective way to create an environment where students can apply knowledge to practice and understand the roles of other health professionals prior to entering the workplace. The contribution of digital technologies in simulation based clinical learning is through the use of communication technologies and video recordings. With student centered learning options, they can learn in their own time, make decisions and observe the ramifications of their choices. In simulated learning students can use defined criteria to assess their progress in simulated cases before transition to authentic patient cases in the real world.

Simulated learning environments are an essential part of the Physiotherapy curriculum, and used for training students prior to clinical placements where they are expected to apply their knowledge and skills in a supervised clinical setting. The use of technology in simulated learning provides guided experiences that replicates the real world in an interactive manner and provides the learner with an occasion to refine their skills and make errors in a benevolent and safe setting. Simulation based learning does not replace clinical training but is used as an adjunct in a hybrid model where the activities are built around work integrated learning. Simulation based resources have been created to develop practical learning, prepare students for placement and provide a conduit for students to master skills required to manage complex situations. As the learning activities are designed to facilitate clinical reasoning training prior to placements the authors have indicated that the designers should be prepared to respond to feedback from all stakeholders to modify programs and activities to satisfy learning and teaching requirements. The use of the virtual patient in simulated learning environments has been found to enhance the learning experience but has yet to be evaluated for efficacy and longer-term knowledge retention (Baumann-Birkbeck et al., 2017).

Use of Digital Technologies for Work Integrated Learning

Work integrated learning is mandatory for many of the allied health programs. Technologies can be used for students to prepare for placement and include options for workplace orientation, occupation health and safety and role play. In the area of physiotherapy (see Chapter 10), there are increasing numbers of students being trained requiring clinical placement to meet training needs, however there are insufficient placement sites. Work integrated learning (WIL) students integrate academic and practical knowledge to attain genuine work-based learning in a work based context (Lanning, Wetzel, Baines, & Byrne, 2012). The exchange of students across tertiary institutions and industry globally ensures authentic WIL training opportunities are available through external placements to foster onsite learning and practice (see Chapter 9). Criterion referenced assessment for all procedures is established by national and internationally accrediting bodies and used to compare an individual's performance against criteria for principles and standards (Brown & Knight, 1994). Digital technologies can also be used by students on clinical placements to track their progression as they learn new skills and reflect on their experiences working in the laboratories. The platform also allows staff to review the student experiences and troubleshoot any issues that may arise while students are on placement (see Chapter 7). Digital technologies for WIL can be used for administration including data collection, status tracking, placement prerequisite databases (agreements, health and safety certificates, immunisations, working with children, police checks) and supervisor training.

Digital Technologies for Employment

The focus on graduate outcomes was the driver for many organisations to implement e-portfolio technology (Skills Australia, 2010), with an increase in the use of e-portfolios occurring in the university sector (Hallam & Creagh, 2010). The e-portfolio has been recognised as an important requirement by Allied Health related industries and its use for Allied Health students is discussed in Chapters 7 and 11. A range of e-portfolio platforms are available, including Wiz and Weebly (free), and those that are institutionally licensed and supported such as PebblePad. The software supports students to construct an up to date resume, with modules on self-directed learning, accumulated resources, details related to competency based training skills and critical reflections on what they have learned as they develop over programs (O'Connor, Obst, Furlong, & Hansen, 2015). It allows the accumulation of evidence in tracking competency and ensuring quality of learning outcomes.

Employability is defined as activities and experiences that support the development of knowledge, professional skills and personal capabilities to improve a graduate's lifelong professional success. Strategies for students to identify competences and other evidence to incorporate into their e-portfolios is investigated in Chapter 12. For example, the e-portfolios may document proficiency in new technologies that may be required for use in the workplace. The e-portfolio tool supports assessment, reflective practice and presentation of achievement for employment. After WIL, students can reflect on how to improve, debrief, collect evidence of learning and competency and skills development for their e-portfolio. Adequate training for staff and students in the use of e-portfolios is required (Willmarth-Stec & Berry, 2015), as is internet access, particularly when on clinical placement. It was also recognised that universities should also provide lifetime access to alumni for their e-portfolios.

Consideration of Digital Technologies Options

The choices and use of digital technologies in the education sector is discussed in Chapter 13 and stresses the need to consult with IT specialists prior to implementing new technologies. The proliferation of e-learning tools has made it difficult to determine which products are fit for purpose. As the number of available technology options increases, identifying the most cost effective and efficient programs and platforms becomes more challenging. Educators and e-learning developers need to consider the pros and cons when selecting new technologies, as while it may meet pedagogical requirements, it may cause stress in the students, issues in privacy, copyright or security risks. With the plethora of offerings the Learning and Teaching units should be consulted to identify, relevant educational technologies, identify use across the institution and ease of implementation in the IT infrastructure and use by academic staff and students. As most institutions are enrolling international students through online courses they need to be aware that internet content is blocked in some countries which reduces online course access. To achieve a viable International collaboration a consistent online platform is required. If the technology is outside the organisation then it cannot be supported and may be vulnerable to changes in structure of the platforms or shutdown. Government Health and education workplaces have restricted internet access and firewalls which prevent access to external websites.

The advantages of digital technologies for e-learning for Allied Health students include;

- Students have access to self-directed learning opportunities and activities, access to materials 24 hours on personal hand held devices.
- Digital technologies allow the Nationalisation and Internationalisation of exchanges to facilitate the development of education resources globally, ensuring consistency across disciplines (assuming accreditation requirements are covered) to enable transportability of qualifications.
- Students develop relevant skills sets including critical thinking and clinical reasoning through simulation based training and adaptive learning.
- Investigating the data analytics behind student online engagement provides insight into their e-learning habits.
- The technology can be used to assist industry supervisors and educators in communication, assessment, training, marking and feedback, while students are on industry or clinical placement.

The considerations and possible disadvantages of digital technologies for e-learning for Allied Health students are as follows;

- Currently there is lack of evidence to demonstrate the role of digital technologies for improving student learning, therefore a risk assessment must be considered before investing in and implementing any new digital technology.
- It is important to evaluate the software so that it can be adopted in a timely manner, although the evaluation itself isn't a disadvantage, but the time taken to adequately evaluate to ensure good outcomes need to be considered.
- Costs of software, implementation times and training of staff and students.
- Issues with technology incompatibility of software and hardware.

- Digital technologies make it possible to outsource activities to lower cost economies to save money. The relocation of resources may result in tasks being completed by individuals with minimal training and reduced quality of product may be the outcome.
- Protection of privacy, specifically with public platforms, data storage and professional behaviours is another very important consideration.
- Increased workload with creating and maintaining portfolios could be considered a disadvantage by many educators.
- Consideration needs to be given to the significant gaps in student view and use of the technological resources and their capabilities and the real abilities.
- Inequitable access to software can be a disadvantage for some students who may not have smart phones or similar devices.
- Large digital file sizes increasing download times and causing problems for remote students.
- The requirement for internet access (and a reliable internet connection) can be a barrier to use or disadvantage – to ensure effective use of digital technologies. Connectivity problems associated with internet bandwidth, firewalls at both the university or health provider and remote communities must be considered.
- Cost of production of VR modules of a wide variety of equipment's used in professional laboratories is another limiting barrier.

FUTURE DIRECTIONS

There are numerous digital learning tools / e-learning tools that warrant consideration when designing learning environments for allied health education. It is important that the impact of implementing any e-learning tools be assessed for increased engagement and/or learning. Whereby e-learning tools are evaluated for enhancing or supporting student understanding of content by analysis of performance of assessment tasks that include taxonomic classification of examination answers or through the use of data analytics to determine student engagement. Game-based learning uses video game elements to create web based learning strategies. Developing educational games has been demonstrated to provide learners with a gaming environment including humour, interaction and drama to stimulate and motivate student learning (Su & Cheng, 2015). The game-style learning materials consist of similar elements to video games in that they apply rules, provide rewards, and create scenarios that require students to make meaningful decisions (Coller & Scott, 2009). The development of game based simulation modules will enhance student engagement online and can motivate students to develop basic competencies (Kasemsap, 2017). For the preparation of students for clinical practice further development of resources using adaptive learning, virtual reality or augmented reality technologies is required.

CONCLUSION

In the current educational climate of increased student numbers with declining resources, digital technologies are being developed to enhance student learning and complement traditional teaching tools. As the new generation of students are digital natives, they understand and engage with a variety of media which can be utilised by educational developers to form educational activities such as variety of delivery media and flexible mode of student engagement. The resources including e-learning tools and digital technologies can be used to teach knowledge, develop critical thinking, clinical reasoning skills or laboratory competencies. The underlying theme throughout this book is that educational resources created using the digital technologies must be tailored to relevant and specific tasks and not be expected to replace teaching activities. A criticism of the use of digital technologies is that they do not increase learning, and it is poorly measured in many research papers. The reasons for implementing technology in the classroom are much broader then enhanced learning outcomes. As the millennial student has disengaged with the traditional methods for tertiary teaching, the use of digital technologies are vital in engaging these students and providing a conduit to active learning.

REFERENCES

Baker, R. S. (2016). Stupid tutoring systems, intelligent humans. *International Journal of Artificial Intelligence in Education*, *26*(2), 600–614. doi:10.1007/s40593-016-0105-0

Bakr, M. M., Massey, W. L., & Massa, H. M. (2016). Digital Cadavers: Online 2D Learning Resources Enhance Student Learning in Practical Head and Neck Anatomy within Dental Programs. *Education Research International*, *10*. doi:10.1155/2016/8506251

Baumann-Birkbeck, L., Florentina, F., Karatas, O., Sun, J., Tang, T., Thaung, V., & Anoopkumar-Dukie, S. et al. (2017). (in press). Appraising the role of the virtual patient for therapeutics health education. *Currents in Pharmacy Teaching and Learning*. doi:10.1016/j.cptl.2017.05.012

Berman, N., Fall, L., Maloney, C., & Devine, D. (2008). Computer-assisted instruction in clinical education: A roadmap to increasing CAI implementation. *Advances in Health Sciences Education: Theory and Practice*, *13*(3), 373–383. doi:10.1007/s10459-006-9041-3 PMID:17089076

Brown, S., & Knight, P. (1994). *Assessing learning in higher education*. London: Kogan Page.

Buchanan, J. A. (2004). Experience with virtual reality-based technology in teaching restorative dental procedures. *Journal of Dental Education*, *68*, 1258–1265. PMID:15576814

Coller, B. D., & Scott, M. J. (2009). Effectiveness of using a video game to teach a course in mechanical engineering. *Computers & Education*, *53*(3), 900–912. doi:10.1016/j.compedu.2009.05.012

Crockett, K., Latham, A., & Whitton, N. (2017). On predicting learning styles in conversational intelligent tutoring systems using fuzzy decision trees. *International Journal of Human-Computer Studies*, *97*, 98–115. doi:10.1016/j.ijhcs.2016.08.005

Daly, J., Willis, K., Small, R., Green, J., Welch, N., Kealy, M., & Hughes, E. (2007). A hierarchy of evidence for assessing qualitative health research. *Journal of Clinical Epidemiology*, *60*(1), 43–49. doi:10.1016/j.jclinepi.2006.03.014 PMID:17161753

Freeman, S., Eddy, S. L., McDonough, M., Smith, M. K., Okoroafor, N., Jordt, H., & Wenderoth, M. P. (2014). Active learning increases student performance in science, engineering, and mathematics. *Proceedings of the National Academy of Sciences of the United States of America*, *111*(23), 8410–8415. doi:10.1073/pnas.1319030111 PMID:24821756

Giordano, C., & Giordano, C. (2011). Health Professions Students' Use of Social Media. *Journal of Allied Health*, *40*(2), 78–81. PMID:21695367

Glover, I., Hepplestone, S., Parkin, H. J., Rodger, H., & Irwin, B. (2016). Pedagogy first: Realising technology enhanced learning by focusing on teaching practice. *British Journal of Educational Technology*, *47*(5), 993–1002. doi:10.1111/bjet.12425

Hall, S., Grant, G., Arora, D., Karaksha, A., McFarland, A., Lohning, A., & Anoopkumar-Dukie, S. (2017). A pilot study assessing the value of 3D printed molecular modelling tools for pharmacy student education. *Currents in Pharmacy Teaching and Learning*, *9*(4), 723–728. doi:10.1016/j.cptl.2017.03.029

Hallam, G., & Creagh, T. (2010). ePortfolio use by university students in Australia: A review of the Australian ePortfolio Project. *Higher Education Research & Development*, *29*(2), 179–193. doi:10.1080/07294360903510582

Harris, J., Mishra, P., & Koehler, M. (2009). Teachers' technological pedagogical content knowledge and learning activity types: Curriculum-based technology integration reframed. *Journal of Research on Technology in Education*, *41*(4), 393–416. doi:10.1080/15391523.2009.10782536

Idris, Y., & Wang, Q. (2009). Affordances of Facebook for learning. *International Journal of Continuing Engineering Education and Lifelong Learning*, *19*(2/3), 247–255. doi:10.1504/IJCEELL.2009.025031

Jaffar, A. A. (2012). YouTube: An emerging tool in anatomy education. *Anatomical Sciences Education*, *5*(3), 158–164. doi:10.1002/ase.1268 PMID:22383096

Kasemsap, K. (2017). *Mastering educational computer games, educational video games, and serious games in the digital age*. IGI Global. doi:10.4018/978-1-5225-1034-5.ch003

Kazemi, H., Rappel, J. K., Poston, T., Lim, B. H., Burdet, E., & Teo, C. L. (2010). Assessing suturing techniques using a virtual reality surgical simulator. *Microsurgery*, *30*(6), 479–486. doi:10.1002/micr.20766 PMID:20201052

Khemaja, M. (2016). Using a knapsack model to optimize continuous building of a hybrid intelligent tutoring system: Application to information technology professionals. *International Journal of Human Capital and Information Technology Professionals*, *7*(2), 1–18. doi:10.4018/IJHCITP.2016040101

Kim, Y., Kim, H., & Kim, Y. O. (2017). Virtual reality and augmented reality in plastic surgery: A review. *Archives of Plastic Surgery*, *44*(3), 179–187. doi:10.5999/aps.2017.44.3.179 PMID:28573091

Kirschner, P. A., & Karpinski, A. C. (2010). Facebook® and academic performance. *Computers in Human Behavior*, *26*(6), 1237–1245. doi:10.1016/j.chb.2010.03.024

Lanning, S. K., Wetzel, A. P., Baines, M., & Byrne, B. E. (2012). Evaluation of a revised curriculum: A four year qualitative study of student perceptions. *Journal of Dental Education*, *76*(10), 1323–1333. PMID:23066131

Losco, C. D., Grant, W. D., Armson, A., Meyer, A. J., & Walker, B. F. (2017). Effective methods of teaching and learning in anatomy as a basic science: A BEME systematic review: BEME guide no. 44. *Medical Teacher*, *39*(3), 234–243. doi:10.1080/0142159X.2016.1271944 PMID:28129720

Magro, M., Sharp, J., Ryan, K., & Ryan, S. (2013). Investigating Ways to Use Facebook at the University Level: A Delphi Study. *Proceedings of the Informing Science and Information Technology Education Conference.*

Miller, G. E. (1990). The assessment of clinical skills/competence/performance. *Journal of Academic Medicine*, *65*(9), S63–S67. doi:10.1097/00001888-199009000-00045 PMID:2400509

O'Connor, E., Obst, P., Furlong, M., & Hansen, J. (2015). Using the TARL model in psychology: Supporting first and final year students to compose reflections. In *Teaching Reflective Learning in Higher Education* (pp. 77–91). Springer International Publishing. doi:10.1007/978-3-319-09271-3_6

Owen, J. (2016). *Renewing Australia's promise Report Card*. Foundation of Australians. Retrieved from http://www.fya.org.au/report/renewing-australias-promise-report-card-2016/

Prensky, M. (2009). H. Sapiens digital: From immigrants and digitalnatives to digital wisdom. *Innovate: Journal of Online Education*, *5*(3), 1–9.

Rajanbabu, A., Drudi, L., Lau, S., Press, J. Z., & Gotlieb, W. H. (2014). Virtual reality surgical simulators: A prerequisite for robotic surgery. *Indian Journal of Surgical Oncology*, *5*(2), 125–127. doi:10.1007/s13193-014-0314-7 PMID:25114465

Ramsden, P. (2003). *Learning to teach in higher education; approaches to learning* (2nd ed.). London: Routledge.

Reifeis, P. E., Kirkup, M. L., Willis, L. H., & Browning, W. D. (2014). Introducing CAD/CAM into a predoctoral dental curriculum: A case study. *Journal of Dental Education*, *78*(10), 1432–1441. PMID:25281677

Rice, S., & McKendree, J. (2014). e-learning. In T. Swantick (Ed.), Understanding medical education (pp. 161-173). Oxford, UK: Wiley and Sons.

Skills Australia. (2010). *Australian workforce futures: A national workforce development strategy.* Retrieved from https://docs.education.gov.au/system/files/doc/other/wwf_strategy-2010.pdf

Stankov, S., Glavinic, V., & Rosic, M. (2011). *Intelligent tutoring systems in e-learning environments: Design, implementation and evaluation.* IGI Global. doi:10.4018/978-1-61692-008-1

Stephenson, C. R., Wang, A. T., Szostek, J. H., Bonnes, S. L., Ratelle, J. T., Mahapatra, S., & Wittich, C. M. et al. (2016). Flipping the Continuing Medical Education Classroom: Validating a Measure of Attendees' Perceptions. *The Journal of Continuing Education in the Health Professions*, *36*(4), 256–262. doi:10.1097/CEH.0000000000000113 PMID:28350306

Storrs, M. J., Alexander, H. G. I., Sun, J., Kroon, J., & Evans, J. L. (2015). Measuring teams-based interprofessional education outcomes in clinical dentistry: Psychometric evaluation of a new scale at an Australian dental school. *Journal of Dental Education*, *79*(3), 249–258. PMID:25729018

Su, C. H., & Cheng, C. H. (2015). A mobile gamification learning system for improving the learning motivation and achievements. *Journal of Computer Assisted Learning*, *31*(3), 268–286. doi:10.1111/jcal.12088

Willmarth-Stec, M., & Beery, T. (2015). Operationalizing the Student Electronic Portfolio for Doctoral Nursing Education. *Nurse Educator*, *40*(5), 263–265. doi:10.1097/NNE.0000000000000161 PMID:25783814

Wise, I., Skues, J., & Williams, B. (2011). *Facebook in Higher Education Promotes Social but not Academic Engagement.* Paper presented at the Annual Australasian Society of Computers in Learning in Tertiary Education (ASCILITE), Hobart, Australia.

Compilation of References

AACP. (2011). *American Association of Colleges of Pharmacy, Commission to Implement Change in Pharmaceutical Education "What is the Mission of Pharmaceutical Education?"*. Retrieved from www.aacp.org/resources/historicaldocuments/BackgroundPaper1.pdf

Aalderink, W., & Veugelers, M. (2005). ePortfolio practice and opportunities in the knowledge exchange countries (Denmark, Germany, the Netherlands and the United Kingdom). In W. Aalderink & M. Veugelers (Eds.), *Stimulating lifelong learning: The eportfolio in Dutch higher education* (pp. 23–32). Utrecht, The Netherlands: Stichting SURF. Retrieved March 31, 2009 from http://www.surffoundation.nl/download/Stimulating%20Lifelong%20Learning%20-%20ePortfolio.pdf

Abid, B., Hentati, N., Chevallier, J.-M., Ghorbel, A., Delmas, V., & Douard, R. (2010). Traditional versus three-dimensional teaching of peritoneal embryogenesis: A comparative prospective study. *Surgical and Radiologic Anatomy*, *32*(7), 647–652. doi:10.1007/s00276-010-0653-1 PMID:20352215

Abramovich, S., Schunn, C., & Higashi, R. M. (2013). Are badges useful in education?: It depends upon the type of badge and expertise of learner. *Educational Technology Research and Development*, *61*(2), 217–232. doi:10.1007/s11423-013-9289-2

Adams Becker, S., Cummins, M., Davis, A., Freeman, A., Hall Giesinger, C., & Ananthanarayanan, V. (2017). *NMC horizon report: 2017 higher education edition*. Austin, TX: The New Media Consortium.

Adams, A. M. (2004). Pedagogical underpinnings of computer-based learning. *Journal of Advanced Nursing*, *46*(1), 5–12. doi:10.1111/j.1365-2648.2003.02960.x PMID:15030437

Agnew, D., Pill, S., & Orrell, J. (2016). *Work-integrated learning: Making a contribution to less privileged communities at home and abroad*. Paper presented at the New Zealand Association for Cooperative Education, Takapuna, Auckland, New Zealand.

Ahlgren, J., Nordgren, A., Perrudin, M., Ronteltap, A., Savigny, J., van Trijp, H., & Gorman, U. et al. (2013). Consumers on the Internet: Ethical and legal aspects of commercialization of personalized nutrition. *Genes & Nutrition*, *8*(4), 349–355. doi:10.1007/s12263-013-0331-0 PMID:23471853

Ahmad, I. (2010). Risk management in clinical practice. Part 5. Ethical considerations for dental enhancement procedures. *British Dental Journal*, *209*(5), 207–214. doi:10.1038/sj.bdj.2010.769 PMID:20829856

Ahmed, K., Rowland, S., Patel, V., Khan, R. S., Ashrafian, H., Davies, D. C., & Paraskeva, P. A. et al. (2010). Is the structure of anatomy curriculum adequate for safe medical practice? *The Surgeon*, *8*(6), 318–324. doi:10.1016/j.surge.2010.06.005 PMID:20950770

Aken, B. L., Ayling, S., Barrell, D., Clarke, L., Curwen, V., Fairley, S., & Searle, S. M. et al. (2016). The Ensembl gene annotation system. *Database (Oxford)*, *2016*, baw093. doi:10.1093/database/baw093 PMID:27337980

Aklillu, E., Carrillo, J. A., Makonnen, E., Hellman, K., Pitarque, M., Bertilsson, L., & Ingelman-Sundberg, M. (2003). Genetic polymorphism of CYP1A2 in Ethiopians affecting induction and expression: Characterization of novel haplotypes with single-nucleotide polymorphisms in intron 1. *Molecular Pharmacology*, *64*(3), 659–669. doi:10.1124/mol.64.3.659 PMID:12920202

Alexander, B. (2017). Retrieved 1 April, 2017, from https://bryanalexander.org

Ali, M., Vlaskamp, J. H. A., Eddin, N. N., Falconer, B., & Oram, C. (2013). *Technical development and socioeconomic implications of the Raspberry Pi as a learning tool in developing countries*. Paper presented at the Computer Science and Electronic Engineering Conference (CEEC), 2013 5th. doi:10.1109/CEEC.2013.6659454

Ali, K., Tredwin, C., Kay, E. J., Slade, A., & Pooler, J. (2014). Preparedness of dental graduates for foundation training: A qualitative study. *British Dental Journal*, *217*(3), 145–149. doi:10.1038/sj.bdj.2014.648 PMID:25104700

Allan, C. N., & Cleland, B. (2012). Embedding eportfolios in teacher education: Lessons from a multi-year implementation. In M. Brown, M. Hartwell, & T. Stewart (Eds.), Proceedings of ascilite Wellington 2012: Future challenges, sustainable futures (pp. 197–201). Academic Press.

Anderson, M. (2014). Evaluating pedagogy for employability: illuminating students' perspectives on an intensive, undergraduate employability module. In *Excavate to Innovate: 'Unearthing' Students' and Tutors' Perceptions of Employability to Energise Work Based Pedagogy*. The University of Northampton. Retrieved from http://nectar.northampton.ac.uk/6788/

Anderson, L. W., & Krathwohl, D. R. (Eds.). (2001). *A taxonomy for teaching, learning and assessing: A revision of Bloom's taxonomy of educational objectives*. New York: Longman.

Anderson, L. W., Krathwohl, D. R., & Bloom, B. S. (2001). *A taxonomy for learning, teaching, and assessing: a revision of Bloom's taxonomy of educational objectives*. Longman.

Antonenko, P., Toy, S., & Niederhauser, D. (2004). *Modular Object-Oriented Dynamic Learning Environment: What Open Source Has to Offer*. Association for Educational Communications and Technology.

Arena, G., Kruger, E., Holley, D., Millar, S., & Tennant, M. (2007). Western Australian dental graduates' perceptions of preparedness to practice: A five-year follow-up. *Journal of Dental Education*, *71*(9), 1217–1222. PMID:17761629

Armellini, A., & Padilla Rodriguez, B. C. (2016). Are Massive Open Online Courses (MOOCs) pedagogically innovative? *Journal of Interactive Online Learning*, *14*(1), 17–28.

Artess, J., Hooley, T., & Mellors-Bourne, R. (2017). *Employability: A Review of the Literature 2012-2016*. York, UK: Higher Education Academy. Retrieved from http://hdl.handle.net/10545/621285

ASU Online. (2014). *Third-party tools*. Retrieved 19 February, 2917, from http://teachonline.asu.edu/wp-content/uploads/2014/03/ASU-Online-3rd-Party-Tools.pdf

Attardi, S. M., & Rogers, K. A. (2015). Design and implementation of an online systemic human anatomy course with laboratory. *Anatomical Sciences Education*, *8*(1), 53–62. doi:10.1002/ase.1465 PMID:24920278

Australian Government. (2015). *Telehealth*. Retrieved 19 February, 2017, from http://www.health.gov.au/internet/main/publishing.nsf/content/e-health-telehealth

Australian Health Practitioner Regulation Agency. (2015). *Physiotherapy practice thresholds in Australia and Aotearoa New Zealand*. Retrieved from https://physiocouncil.com.au/media/1020/physiotherapy-board-physiotherapy-practice-thresholds-in-australia-and-aotearoa-new-zealand-6.pdf

Australian Health Practitioner Regulation Agency. (2017). *Physiotherapy Board of Australia*. Retrieved from http://www.physiotherapyboard.gov.au/About/Statistics.aspx

Australian Physiotherapy Association. (2017). *Physiotherapy in Australia*. Retrieved from http://www.physiotherapy.asn.au/APAWCM/Physio_and_You/physio/APAWCM/Physio_and_You/physio.aspx?hkey=25ad06f0-e004-47e5-b894-e0ede69e0fff

Australian Physiotherapy Council. (2015). *Physiotherapy practice thresholds in Australia and Aotearoa New Zealand*. Retrieved from https://physiocouncil.com.au/media/1020/physiotherapy-board-physiotherapy-practice-thresholds-in-australia-and-aotearoa-new-zealand-6.pdf

Authentic Experiential and Evidence Based Learning (AAEEBL). (2015). *Ontology of 'ePortfolio'*. Retrieved from http://www.aaeebl.org/blogpost/1008436/213232/Ontology-ofePortfolio

Avery, D. (2012). The globalization of the dental laboratory industry. *Journal of Esthetic and Restorative Dentistry*, *24*(2), 79–82. doi:10.1111/j.1708-8240.2012.00507.x PMID:22524712

Azer, S. A., & Azer, S. (2016). 3D Anatomy Models and Impact on Learning: A Review of the Quality of the Literature. *Health Profession Education*, *2*(2), 80–98. doi:10.1016/j.hpe.2016.05.002

Babu, P. V., Liu, D., & Gilbert, E. R. (2013). Recent advances in understanding the anti-diabetic actions of dietary flavonoids. *The Journal of Nutritional Biochemistry*, *24*(11), 1777–1789. doi:10.1016/j.jnutbio.2013.06.003 PMID:24029069

Badyal, D., Bala, S., & Kathuria, P. (2010). Student evaluation of teaching and assessment methods in pharmacology. *Indian Journal of Pharmacology*, *42*(2), 87. doi:10.4103/0253-7613.64502 PMID:20711372

Bagley, C. H., Gillott, E., & Gunasekera, A. (2011). Undergraduate Anatomy Teaching: Are we Failing a Generation of Future Surgeons? *The Bulletin of the Royal College of Surgeons of England*, *93*(1), 26–28. doi:10.1308/147363511X545456

Baker, R. S. (2016). Stupid tutoring systems, intelligent humans. *International Journal of Artificial Intelligence in Education*, *26*(2), 600–614. doi:10.1007/s40593-016-0105-0

Bakr, M. M., Massey, W. L., & Alexander, H. (2013). Evaluation of Simodont® Haptic 3D Virtual Reality Dental Training Simulator. *International Journal of Dental Clinics*, *5*(4).

Bakr, M. M., Massey, W. L., & Alexander, H. (2014). Students' Evaluation of a 3DVR Haptic Device (Simodont®). Does Early Exposure to Haptic Feedback During Preclinical Dental Education Enhance the Development of Psychomotor Skills? *International Journal of Dental Clinics*, *6*(2), 1–7.

Bakr, M. M., Massey, W. L., & Alexander, H. (2015). Can Virtual Simulators Replace Traditional Preclinical Teaching Methods: A Students' Perspective? *International Journal of Dentistry and Oral Health*, *2*(1). doi:10.16966/2378-7090.149

Bakr, M. M., Massey, W. L., & Massa, H. M. (2016a). Digital Cadavers: Online 2D Learning Resources Enhance Student Learning in Practical Head and Neck Anatomy within Dental Programs. *Education Research International*, *10*. doi:10.1155/2016/8506251

Bakr, M. M., Massey, W. L., & Massa, H. M. (2016b). Flipping a Dental Anatomy Course: A Retrospective Study Over Four Years. *Education Research International*, *9*. doi:10.1155/2016/7097398

Ball, D. M., & Levy, Y. (2008). Emerging educational technology: Assessing the factors that influence instructors' acceptance in information systems and other classrooms. *Journal of Information Systems Education*, *19*, 431–443.

Barajas, M., & Owen, M. (2000). Implementing Virtual Learning Environments: Looking for Holistic Approach. *Journal of Educational Technology & Society*, *3*(3), 39–53.

Bareither, M. L., Arbel, V., Growe, M., Muszczynski, E., Rudd, A., & Marone, J. R. (2013). Clay modeling versus written modules as effective interventions in understanding human anatomy. *Anatomical Sciences Education*, *6*(3), 170–176. doi:10.1002/ase.1321 PMID:23027681

Barker, M. (2011). *The GIHE Good Practice Guide to Internationalising the Curriculum*. Retrieved from https://www.griffith.edu.au/__data/assets/pdf_file/0006/345291/Internationalising-the-Curriculum.pdf

Barnett, R., & Coate, K. (2005). *Engaging the curriculum in higher education*. McGraw-Hill Education.

Baumann-Birkbeck, L., Florentina, F., Karatas, O., Sun, J., Tang, T., Thaung, V., & Anoopkumar-Dukie, S. et al. (2017). (in press). Appraising the role of the virtual patient for therapeutics health education. *Currents in Pharmacy Teaching and Learning*. doi:10.1016/j.cptl.2017.05.012

Beetham, H., & Sharpe, R. (2013). *Rethinking Pedagogy for a Digital Age: Designing for 21st Century Learning*. Routledge.

Benjamin, L. T. (1988). A history of teaching machines. *The American Psychologist*, *43*(9), 703–712. doi:10.1037/0003-066X.43.9.703

Bennett, B. (2006). Certification from the American Board of Pathology: Getting it and keeping it. *Human Pathology*, *37*(8), 978–981. doi:10.1016/j.humpath.2006.02.023 PMID:16867858

Bennett, D., Richardson, S., & MacKinnon, P. (2016). *Enacting strategies for graduate employability: How universities can best support students to develop generic skill Part A*. Canberra, Australia: Australian Government, Office for Learning and Teaching, Department of Education and Training. Retrieved from http://www.olt.gov.au/project-how-universities-can-best-support-students-develop-generic-skills-enacting-strategies-gradua

Benson, V., Morgan, S., & Filippaios, F. (2014). Social career management: Social media and employability skills gap. *Computers in Human Behavior*, *30*, 519–525. doi:10.1016/j.chb.2013.06.015

Bergmann, J., & Sams, A. (2013). Flip your students' learning. *Educational Leadership*, *70*(6), 16–20.

Berman, N., Fall, L., Maloney, C., & Levine, D. (2008). Computer-assisted instruction in clinical education: A roadmap to increasing CAI implementation. *Advances in Health Sciences Education: Theory and Practice*, *13*(3), 373–383. doi:10.1007/s10459-006-9041-3 PMID:17089076

Berry, J., Nesbit, M., Saberi, S., & Petridis, H. (2014). Communication methods & production techniques in fixed prosthodontics fabrication: A UK based survey. Part 2: Production techniques. *British Dental Journal*, *217*(6), E13. doi:10.1038/sj.bdj.2014.644 PMID:25257017

Berry, J., Nesbit, M., Saeri, S., & Petridis, H. (2014). Communication methods and production techniques in fixed prosthesis fabrication: A UK based survey. Part 1: Communication methods. *British Dental Journal*, *217*(6 (E12)). doi:10.1038/sj.bdj.2014.643

Bethea, D. P., Castillo, D. C., & Harvison, N. (2014). Use of simulation in occupational therapy education: Way of the future? *The American Journal of Occupational Therapy*, *68*(Supplement 2), 32–39. doi:10.5014/ajot.2014.012716 PMID:25397936

Bialocerkowski, A., & Tuttle, N. A. (2013). *The STEPS Project: a Remotely Accessed Simulated Learning Environment to Increase the Viability of Remote Clinic Placements in Physiotherapy and Speech Pathology*. Academic Press.

Bicking, M., & Wimmer, M. A. (2011). *Concept to integrate open collaboration in technology roadmapping: Stakeholder involvement in strategic e-government planning*. Paper presented at the 2011 44th Hawaii International Conference on System Sciences.

Bielby-Clarke, K. (2015). Use of a human patient simulator as a teaching tool by final year pharmacy students. *BMJ Simulation and Technology Enhanced Learning*, *1*(Suppl 2), A45. doi:10.1136/bmjstel-2015-000075.110

Biggs, J. (2003). Setting the stage for effective teaching. In Teaching for quality learning at university: What the student does (2nd ed.; pp. 56-73). Buckingham, UK: SRHE and Open University Press.

Biggs, J., & Tang, C. (2007a). Designing Intended Learning Outcomes. In Teaching for Quality Learning at University (3rd ed.). Open University Press (McGraw-Hill Education).

Biggs, J., & Tang, C. (2007b). Teaching according to how students learn. In Teaching for quality learning at university (4th ed.; pp. 15-30). Berkshire, UK: Open University Press (McGraw-Hill Education).

Biggs, J., & Tang, C. (2010). *Applying constructive alignment to outcomes-based teaching and learning*. Paper presented at the Training material for "quality teaching for learning in higher education" workshop for master trainers, Ministry of Higher Education, Kuala Lumpur, Malaysia.

Billett, S. (Ed.). (2010). *Learning Through Practice*. Dordrecht, The Netherlands: Springer. doi:10.1007/978-90-481-3939-2

Bimrose, J., Barnes, S. A., & Brown, J. (2005). *A Systematic Literature Review of Research into Career-related Interventions for Higher Education*. Warwick, UK: Institute for Employment Research, University of Warwick.

Birks, M., Hartin, P., Woods, C., Emmanuel, E., & Hitchins, M. (2016). Students' perceptions of the use of eportfolios in nursing and midwifery education. *Nurse Education in Practice*, *18*, 46–51. doi:10.1016/j.nepr.2016.03.003 PMID:27235565

Blackmore, P., Bulaitis, Z. H., Jackman, A. H., & Tan, E. (2016). *Employability in higher education: A review of practice and strategies around the world*. London: Pearson.

Blackstock, F. C., Watson, K. M., Morris, N. R., Jones, A., Wright, A., McMeeken, J. M., & Haines, T. P. et al. (2013). Simulation can contribute a part of cardiorespiratory physiotherapy clinical education: Two randomized trials. *Simulation in Healthcare*, *8*(1), 32–42. doi:10.1097/SIH.0b013e318273101a PMID:23250189

Blackwell, A., Bowes, L., Harvey, L., Hesketh, A. J., & Knight, P. T. (2001). Transforming work experience in higher education. *British Educational Research Journal*, *27*(3), 269–285. doi:10.1080/01411920120048304

Blau, N. (2016). Genetics of Phenylketonuria: Then and Now. *Human Mutation*, *37*(6), 508–515. doi:10.1002/humu.22980 PMID:26919687

Blom, D., & Hitchcock, M. (2017). Perceived Usefulness and Relevance of ePortfolios in the Creative Arts: Investigating Student Views. In ePortfolios in Australian Universities (pp. 155-172). Springer Singapore.

Blom, D., Rowley, J., Bennett, D., Hitchcock, M., & Dunbar-Hall, P. (2013). Two-way impact: Institutional e-learning policy/educator practices in creative arts through ePortfolio creation. *Proceedings of the 12th European conference on e-learning.*

Blue_beetle. (2010, August 26). Re: User-driven discontent [Blog comment]. Retrieved from http://www.metafilter.com/95152/Userdriven-discontent#32560467

Boet, S., Bould, M. D., Layat Burn, C., & Reeves, S. (2014). Twelve tips for a successful interprofessional team-based high-fidelity simulation education session. *Medical Teacher, 36*(10), 853–857. doi:10.3109/0142159X.2014.923558 PMID:25023765

Boyer, E. L. (1991). Highlights of the Carnegie Report: The Scholarship of Teaching from "Scholarship Reconsidered: Priorities of the Professoriate". *College Teaching, 39*(1), 11–13. do i:10.1080/87567555.1991.10532213

Bradford, P., Porciello, M., Balkon, N., & Backus, D. (2007). The Blackboard learning system: The be all and end all in educational instruction? *Journal of Educational Technology Systems, 35*(3), 301–314. doi:10.2190/X137-X73L-5261-5656

Bradley, D., Noonan, P., Nugent, H., & Scales, B. (2008). *Review of higher education: Final report.* Retrieved from http://www.voced.edu.au/content/ngv%3A32134

Brandes, G., & Boskic, N. (2008). ePortfolios: From description to analysis. *International Review of Research in Open and Distance Learning, 9*(2), 1–17. doi:10.19173/irrodl.v9i2.502

Brand, H. S., Kamell, H., Kharbanda, A. K., & Dozic, A. (2013). Students' Perceptions of Materials and Techniques Used at European Dental Schools in the Education of Fixed Prosthodontics. *Journal of Dental Education, 77*(9), 1140–1146. PMID:24002851

Bridges, S., Chang, J. W. W. W., Chu, C. H., & Gardener, K. (2014). Blended learning in situated contexts: 3-year evaluation of an online peer review project. *European Journal of Dental Education, 18*(3), 170–179. doi:10.1111/eje.12082 PMID:24460682

Bridgstock, R. (2009). The graduate attributes we've overlooked: Enhancing graduate employability through career management skills. *Higher Education Research & Development, 28*(1), 31–44. doi:10.1080/07294360802444347

Bringle, R. G., & Hatcher, J. A. (1996). Implementing service learning in higher education. *The Journal of Higher Education, 67*(2), 221–239. doi:10.1080/00221546.1996.11780257

Brinson, J. R. (2015). Learning outcome achievement in non-traditional (virtual and remote) versus traditional (hands-on) laboratories: A review of the empirical research. *Computers & Education, 87*, 218–237. doi:10.1016/j.compedu.2015.07.003

Brooks-Young, S. (2008). Got moodle? The free, open source program enjoys great appeal among K-12 teachers, as it allows them to get the upper hand on course management and assessment. *T.H.E. Journal, 35*(4), 28.

Brown, J. (2017). Career Ready Advantage. *National Innovation Case Study Collection.* Retrieved from http://app.iru.edu.au/national-innovation-case-study-collection#browse-by-university/university-details/58be5af15c088326e9f8d3a1/university-case-study-details/5967203e59a41f563590256d/

Brown, S., & Knight, P. (1994). *Assessing learning in higher education.* London: Kogan Page.

Brueggeman, M. S., Swinehart, C., Yue, M. J., Conway-Klaassen, J. M., & Wiesner, S. M. (2012). Implementing virtual microscopy improves outcomes in a hematology morphology course. *Clinical Laboratory Science, 25,* 149. PMID:22953514

Bucat, R. (2004). Pedagogical content knowledge as a way forward: Applied research in chemistry education. *Chemistry Education Research and Practice, 5*(3), 215–228. doi:10.1039/B4RP90025A

Buchanan, G., Ma, M., & Rea, P. M. (2014). A multimedia package for patient understanding and rehabilitation of non-contact anterior cruciate ligament injuries. *International Journal of Medical Imaging, 2*(3), 44–53. doi:10.11648/j.ijmi.20140203.11

Buchanan, J. A. (2004). Experience with Virtual Reality-Based Technology in Teaching Restorative Dental Procedures. *Journal of Dental Education, 68*(12). PMID:15576814

Buchanan, J. A. (2004). Experience with virtual reality-based technology in teaching restorative dental procedures. *Journal of Dental Education, 68,* 1258–1265. PMID:15576814

Buchanan, J. A. (2004). Use of simulation technology in dental education. *Journal of Dental Education, 68*(12), 1258–1265. PMID:15576814

Buchanan, J., Jenkins, S., & Scott, L. (2014). *Student clinical education in Australia: a University of Sydney scoping study.* Sydney: The University of Sydney.

Buckridge, M., Krause, K.-L., & Alexander, H. (2010). *Scholarship of Learning and Teaching.* Retrieved from http://www.griffith.edu.au/__data/assets/pdf_file/0010/119467/SOLT-GPG.pdf

Bukowski, E. L. (2002). Assessment outcomes: Computerised instruction in a human gross anatomy course. *Journal of Allied Health, 31*(3), 153–158. PMID:12227266

Bullock, A., & deJong, P. G. (2014). Technology-enhanced learning. In T. Swanwick (Ed.), *Understanding medical education: Evidence, theory and practice* (2nd ed.; pp. 149–160). Oxford, UK: John Wiley & Sons.

Burke, W. (2004). Clinical validity and clinical utility of genetic tests. Curr Protoc Hum Genet, 9. doi:10.1002/0471142905.hg0915s42

Burthem, J., Brereton, M., Ardern, J., Hickman, L., Seal, L., Serrant, A., & De la Salle, B. et al. (2005). The use of digital 'virtual slides' in the quality assessment of haematological morphology: Results of a pilot exercise involving UK NEQAS (H) participants. *British Journal of Haematology, 130*(2), 293–296. doi:10.1111/j.1365-2141.2005.05597.x PMID:16029459

Cadorin, L., Bagnasco, A., Rocco, G., & Sasso, L. (2014). An integrative review of the characteristics of meaningful learning in healthcare professionals to enlighten educational practices in health care. *Nursing Open*, *1*(1), 3–14. doi:10.1002/nop2.3 PMID:27708790

CAE Healthcare. (n.d.). *iStan and Müse*. Retrieved 20 April, 2017, from http://www.caehealthcare.com/eng/patient-simulators/istan

Callaghan, R. (2016, February 11). Graduate recruitment: Academic results no longer matter as much. *Australian Financial Review*. Retrieved from http://www.afr.com/leadership/careers/graduate-recruitment-academic-results-no-longer-matter-as-much-20160208-gmovnb#ixzz4hgmb6vhf

Cameron, D., Cockburn, L., Nixon, S., Parnes, P., Garcia, L., Leotaud, J., & Williams, T. et al. (2013). Global partnerships for international fieldwork in occupational therapy: Reflection and innovation. *Occupational Therapy International*, *20*(2), 88–96. doi:10.1002/oti.1352 PMID:23661362

Campbell, M., Herrington, A., & Verenikina, I. (2009). Journeying from college to work: The changing identity of early-career policep. *The Journal of Cooperative Education and Internships*, *43*(1), 55–64.

Campbell, N., McAllister, L., & Eley, D. (2012). The influence of motivation in recruitment and retention of rural and remote allied health professionals: A literature review. *Rural and Remote Health*, *12*(3), 1900. PMID:22845190

Camp, K. M., & Trujillo, E. (2014). Position of the Academy of Nutrition and Dietetics: Nutritional genomics. *Journal of the Academy of Nutrition and Dietetics*, *114*(2), 299–312. doi:10.1016/j.jand.2013.12.001 PMID:24439821

Candler, C., Ihnat, M., & Huang, G. (2007). Pharmacology education in undergraduate and graduate medical education in the United States. *Clinical Pharmacology and Therapeutics*, *82*(2), 134–137. doi:10.1038/sj.clpt.6100266 PMID:17632538

Cant, R. P., & Cooper, S. J. (2010). Simulation-based learning in nurse education: Systematic review. *Journal of Advanced Nursing*, *66*(1), 3–15. doi:10.1111/j.1365-2648.2009.05240.x PMID:20423432

Capelleras, J.-L. (2005). Attitudes of academic staff towards their job and organisation: An empirical assessment. *Tertiary Education and Management*, *11*(2), 147–166. doi:10.1080/13583883.2005.9967144

Carbonaro, M., King, S., Taylor, E., Satzinger, F., Snart, F., & Drummond, J. (2008). Integration of E-Learning Technologies in an Interprofessional Health Science Course. *Medical Teacher*, *30*(1), 25–33. doi:10.1080/01421590701753450 PMID:18278648

Carr, A. B., & Brown, D. T. (2011). Work authorizations for removable partial dentures. In A. B. Carr & D. T. Brown (Eds.), *McCracken's removable partial prosthodontics* (12th ed.; pp. 284–288). St. Louis, MO: Mosby. doi:10.1016/B978-0-323-06990-8.00019-1

Carrington, A. (2015). *The padagogy wheel v4.1*. Retrieved 16 February, 2017, from http://designingoutcomes.com/assets/PadWheelV4/PadWheel_Poster_V4.pdf

Carroll, C., Booth, A., Papaioannou, D., Sutton, A., & Wong, R. (2009). UK health-care professionals' experience of on-line learning techniques: A systematic review of qualitative data. *The Journal of Continuing Education in the Health Professions*, *29*(4), 235–241. doi:10.1002/chp.20041 PMID:19998474

Casilli, C., & Hickey, D. (2016). Transcending conventional credentialing and assessment paradigms with information-rich digital badges. *The Information Society*, *32*(2), 117–129. doi:10.1080/01972243.2016.1130500

Chan, C. C., Tsui, M. S., Chan, M. Y. C., & Hong, J. H. (2002a). Applying the Structure of the Observed Learning Outcomes (SOLO) Taxonomy on Student's Learning Outcomes: An empirical study. *Assessment & Evaluation in Higher Education*, *27*(6), 511–527. doi:10.1080/0260293022000020282

Chaoyi, M., Liwei, Z., Li, Y., Min, Z., & Haiyang, Y. (2012). Current status, crisis and trends in Chinese dental technicians. *International Dental Journal*, *62*(2), 79–83. doi:10.1111/j.1875-595X.2011.00093.x PMID:22420476

Charsky, D., & Ressler, W. (2011). "Games are made for fun": Lessons on the effects of concept maps in the classroom use of computer games. *Computers & Education*, *56*(3), 604–615. doi:10.1016/j.compedu.2010.10.001

Cheng, G. (2008). Implementation Challenges of the English Language ePortfolio System from Various Stakeholder Perspectives. *Journal of Educational Technology Systems*, *37*(1), 97–118. doi:10.2190/ET.37.1.h

Chen, H. L., & Penny Light, T. (2010). *Electronic portfolios and student success: effectiveness, efficiency, and learning*. Washington, DC: Association of American Colleges and Universities.

Chen, J., Lieffers, J., Bauman, A., Hanning, R., & Allman-Farinelli, M. (2017). The use of smartphone health apps and other mobile health (mHealth) technologies in dietetic practice: A three country study. *Journal of Human Nutrition and Dietetics*, *30*(4), 439–452. doi:10.1111/jhn.12446 PMID:28116773

Chen, P.-S. D., Lambert, A. D., & Guidry, K. R. (2010). Engaging online learners: The impact of Web-based learning technology on college student engagement. *Computers & Education*, *54*(4), 1222–1232. doi:10.1016/j.compedu.2009.11.008

Chickering, A. W., & Ehrmann, S. (1986). *Implementing the seven prinicples: Technology as a lever.* American Association of Higher Education. Retrieved from https://case.edu/ucite/media/caseedu/ucite/documents/seven_principles.pdf

Chickering, A. W., & Gamson, Z. F. (1997). Seven prinicples of good practice in undergraduate education. *AAHE Bulletin*, 3–7. Retrieved from https://eric.ed.gov/?id=ED282491

Ciocco, M. D., & Holtzman, D. (2008). Prior Learning Assessment: E-Portfolios and the Millennial Students. *The Journal of Continuing Higher Education*, *56*(3), 69–71. doi:10.1080/07377366.2008.10400165

Clark. (2009). E-portfolios at 2.0-Surveying the Field. *Peer Review: Emerging Trends and Key Debates in Undergraduate Education, 11*(1), 18.

Clark, W. (2012). It's about More than Getting a Job. *Adults Learning*, *23*(4), 45–47.

Cleveland, A. O., & Cleveland, M. B. (2004). Coming of age in a digital world: The portfolio grows up. *Theatre Design and Technology*, *40*, 10–17.

CNBC. (2014, 7 February). *Technology has the shelf life of a banana: McNealy*. Retrieved from http://video.cnbc.com/gallery/?video=3000242076

Codd, A. M., & Choudhury, B. (2011). Virtual reality anatomy: Is it comparable with traditional methods in the teaching of human forearm musculoskeletal anatomy? *Anatomical Sciences Education*, *4*(3), 119–125. doi:10.1002/ase.214 PMID:21480538

Coetzee, M., & Beukes, C. (2010). Employability, emotional intelligence and career preparation support satisfaction among adolescents in the school-to-work transition phase. *Journal of Psychology in Africa*, *20*(3), 439–446.

Cole, D., & Tibby, M. (2013). *Defining and developing your approach to employability: A framework for higher education institutions*. Heslington: The Higher Education Academy.

Cole, M. (2009). Using Wiki technology to support student engagement: Lessons from the trenches. *Computers & Education*, *52*(1), 141–146. doi:10.1016/j.compedu.2008.07.003

Coller, B. D., & Scott, M. J. (2009). Effectiveness of using a video game to teach a course in mechanical engineering. *Computers & Education*, *53*(3), 900–912. doi:10.1016/j.compedu.2009.05.012

Colson, N. J., Naug, H. L., Nikbakht, E., Zhang, P., & McCormack, J. (2017). The impact of MTHFR 677 C/T genotypes on folate status markers: A meta-analysis of folic acid intervention studies. *European Journal of Nutrition*, *56*(1), 247–260. doi:10.1007/s00394-015-1076-x PMID:26497154

Connolly, T., Gould, C., Hainey, T., Waugh, S., & Boyle, B. (2010). An empirical study: The implementation of a virtual learning environment and ePortfolio. *Proceedings of the 7th international conference on networked learning.*

Constantinou, M., & Kuys, S. S. (2013). Physiotherapy students find guided journals useful to develop reflective thinking and practice during their first clinical placement: A qualitative study. *Physiotherapy*, *99*(1), 49–55. doi:10.1016/j.physio.2011.12.002 PMID:23219653

Cook, D. A., Hatala, R., Brydges, R., Zendejas, B., Szostek, J. H., Wang, A. T., & Hamstra, S. J. et al. (2011). Technology-enhanced simulation for health professions education: A systematic review and meta-analysis. *Journal of the American Medical Association, 306*(9), 978–988. doi:10.1001/jama.2011.1234 PMID:21900138

Cooper, G. (1998). *Research into Cognitive Load Theory and Instructional Design at UNSW.* Retrieved from New South Wales, Australia: http://dwb4.unl.edu/Diss/Cooper/UNSW.htm

Cooper, L., Orrell, J., & Bowden, M. (2010). *Work-integrated Learning: A guide to effective practice.* New York: Taylor and Francis.

Cordier, R., McAuliffe, T., Wilson, N. J., Totino, R., Dender, A., Smith, C., & Stephens, M. (2016). The appropriateness and feasibility of an online e-Portfolio for assessment of undergraduate allied health students. *Australian Occupational Therapy Journal, 63*(3), 154–163. doi:10.1111/1440-1630.12226 PMID:26449172

Corella, D., Coltell, O., Sorli, J. V., Estruch, R., Quiles, L., Martinez-Gonzalez, M. A., & Ordovas, J. M. et al. (2016). Polymorphism of the Transcription Factor 7-Like 2 Gene (TCF7L2) Interacts with Obesity on Type-2 Diabetes in the PREDIMED Study Emphasizing the Heterogeneity of Genetic Variants in Type-2 Diabetes Risk Prediction: Time for Obesity-Specific Genetic Risk Scores. *Nutrients, 8*(12), 793. doi:10.3390/nu8120793 PMID:27929407

Cornelis, M. C., El-Sohemy, A., Kabagambe, E. K., & Campos, H. (2006). Coffee, CYP1A2 genotype, and risk of myocardial infarction. *Journal of the American Medical Association, 295*(10), 1135–1141. doi:10.1001/jama.295.10.1135 PMID:16522833

Cornelis, M. C., Qi, L., Kraft, P., & Hu, F. B. (2009). TCF7L2, dietary carbohydrate, and risk of type 2 diabetes in US women. *The American Journal of Clinical Nutrition, 89*(4), 1256–1262. doi:10.3945/ajcn.2008.27058 PMID:19211816

Cosh, J. (2008). *Report on ALSS faculty evaluation of personal development planning (PDP).* Retrieved from http://www.inspire.anglia.ac.uk/assets/Uploads/Publications/Research/L&T/Evaluation_of_Personal_Development_Planning_in_ALSS_Nov_2007.pdf

Covolo, L., Rubinelli, S., Ceretti, E., & Gelatti, U. (2015). Internet-Based Direct-to-Consumer Genetic Testing: A Systematic Review. *Journal of Medical Internet Research, 17*(12), e279. doi:10.2196/jmir.4378 PMID:26677835

Crebert, G., Bates, M., Bell, B., Patrick, C. J., & Cragnolini, V. (2004). Developing generic skills at university, during work placement and in employment: Graduates' perceptions. *Higher Education Research & Development, 23*(2), 147–165. doi:10.1080/0729436042000206636

Crockett, K., Latham, A., & Whitton, N. (2017). On predicting learning styles in conversational intelligent tutoring systems using fuzzy decision trees. *International Journal of Human-Computer Studies, 97*, 98–115. doi:10.1016/j.ijhcs.2016.08.005

Crompton, H. (2014). A diachronic overview of technology contributing to mobile learning: A shift towards student-centred pedagogies. *Increasing Access, 7.*

Crosslin, M. (2016). From Instructivism to Connectivism: Theoretical Underpinnings of MOOCs. *Current Issues in Emerging eLearning, 3*(1), 6.

Crozier, S. (2001). Career development in the post-secondary curricula. In W. Patton & M. McMahon (Eds.), *Career development programs: Preparation for lifelong career decision making* (pp. 85–93). Melbourne, Australia: ACER Press.

Dacre-Pool, L., & Sewell, P. (2007). The key to employability: Developing a practical model of graduate employability. *Education + Training, 49*(4), 277–289. doi:10.1108/00400910710754435

Dahlman, I., Linder, K., Arvidsson Nordstrom, E., Andersson, I., Liden, J., Verdich, C., & Arner, P. et al. (2005). Changes in adipose tissue gene expression with energy-restricted diets in obese women. *The American Journal of Clinical Nutrition, 81*(6), 1275–1285. PMID:15941876

Dalgarno, B., & Lee, M. J. (2010). What are the learning affordances of 3-D virtual environments? *British Journal of Educational Technology, 41*(1), 10–32. doi:10.1111/j.1467-8535.2009.01038.x

Dalton, M., Davidson, M., & Keating, J. L. (2012). The assessment of physiotherapy practice (APP) is a reliable measure of professional competence of physiotherapy students: A reliability study. *Journal of Physiotherapy, 58*(1), 49–56. doi:10.1016/S1836-9553(12)70072-3 PMID:22341382

Daly, J., Willis, K., Small, R., Green, J., Welch, N., Kealy, M., & Hughes, E. (2007). A hierarchy of evidence for assessing qualitative health research. *Journal of Clinical Epidemiology, 60*(1), 43–49. doi:10.1016/j.jclinepi.2006.03.014 PMID:17161753

Dancza, K., Warren, A., Copley, J., Rodger, S., Moran, M., McKay, E., & Taylor, A. (2013). Learning experiences on role-emerging placements: An exploration from the students' perspective. *Australian Occupational Therapy Journal, 60*(6), 427–435. doi:10.1111/1440-1630.12079 PMID:24299482

Davies, A., Fidler, D., & Gorbis, M. (2011). *Future Work Skills 2020*. Report for the Institute for the Future for Apollo Research Institute.

Davis, H. C., & Fill, K. (2007). Embedding blended learning in a university's teaching culture: Experiences and reflections. *British Journal of Educational Technology, 38*(5), 817–828. doi:10.1111/j.1467-8535.2007.00756.x

Davis, M. C., Can, D. D., Pindrik, J., Rocque, B. G., & Johnston, J. M. (2016). Virtual interactive presence in global surgical education: International collaboration through augmented reality. *World Neurosurgery, 86*, 103–111. doi:10.1016/j.wneu.2015.08.053 PMID:26342783

Day-Black, C., & Merrill, E. B. (2015). Using Mobile Devices in Nursing Education. *The ABNF Journal, 26*(4), 78–84. PMID:26665501

de Jong, T., Linn, M. C., & Zacharia, Z. C. (2013). Physical and virtual laboratories in science and engineering education. *Science, 340*(6130), 305–308. doi:10.1126/science.1230579 PMID:23599479

De Waard, I., Abajian, S., Gallagher, M. S., Hogue, R., Keskin, N., Koutropoulos, A., & Rodriguez, O. C. (2011). Using mLearning and MOOCs to understand chaos, emergence, and complexity in education. *The International Review of Research in Open and Distributed Learning*, *12*(7), 94–115. doi:10.19173/irrodl.v12i7.1046

Deakin University. (2016). *Me in a Minute*. Retrieved 11 April, 2017, from https://blogs.deakin.edu.au/meinaminute/

Dee, F. R. (2009). Virtual microscopy in pathology education. *Human Pathology*, *40*(8), 1112–1121. doi:10.1016/j.humpath.2009.04.010 PMID:19540551

Del Mar, C., Doust, J., & Glasziou, P. (2006). *Clinical Thinking: evidence, communication and decision-making*. Malden, MA: BMJ/Blackwell. doi:10.1002/9780470750568

Department of Health. (2001). *Report of the Public Inquiry into Children's Heart Surgery at the Bristol Royal Infirmary 1984–1995: Learning from Bristol*. London: The Stationery Office.

Dewhurst, D. G., & Norris, T. A. M. (2003). Helping teachers to embed e-learning materials into undergraduate pharmacology courses. *Bioscience Education*, *1*(1), 1–16. doi:10.3108/beej.2003.01010006

Dewiyanti, S., & Nilson, C. (2017). Programmatic approach to an ePortfolio in Nursing. *National Innovation Case Study Collection*. Retrieved from https://iru.knack.com/national-innovation-case-study-collection/#browse-by-theme/theme-details/58e5e4d229fe99490ac49677/theme-case-study-details/58e5a223b8ef4658faed35e2/

Diamandis, P. H., & Kotler, S. (2012). *Abundance: the future is better than you think*. New York, NY: Free Press.

Diaz, C. S. (2009, July). Teaching the techno-pitch: Taking student innovators beyond the elevator pitch. In *Professional Communication Conference, 2009. IPCC 2009. IEEE International* (pp. 1-7). IEEE. doi:10.1109/IPCC.2009.5208685

Diaz-Perez, J. A., Raju, S., & Echeverri, J. H. (2014). Evaluation of a teaching strategy based on integration of clinical subjects, virtual autopsy, pathology museum, and digital microscopy for medical students. *Journal of Pathology Informatics*, *5*(1), 25. doi:10.4103/2153-3539.137729 PMID:25191624

Diaz, V. (2011). Cloud-based technologies: Faculty development, support, and implementation. *Journal of Asynchronous Learning Networks*, *15*(1), 95.

Dibben, M., & Norton, S. (2017). *Embedding employability in student programs- it starts with the right language: Reflections from Australia and the UK*. Higher Education Academy. Retrieved 2 May, 2017, from https://www.international.heacademy.ac.uk/node/221

Dickey, R. M., Srikishen, N., Lipshultz, L. I., Spiess, P. E., Carrion, R. E., & Hakky, T. S. (2016). Augmented reality assisted surgery: A urologic training tool. *Asian Journal of Andrology*, *18*(5), 732. doi:10.4103/1008-682X.166436 PMID:26620455

Dixon, P. C., Loh, J. J., Michaud-Paquette, Y., & Pearsall, D. J. (2017). biomechZoo: An open-source toolbox for the processing, analysis, and visualization of biomechanical movement data. *Computer Methods and Programs in Biomedicine*, *140*, 1–10. doi:10.1016/j.cmpb.2016.11.007 PMID:28254065

Djordjevic, N., Ghotbi, R., Jankovic, S., & Aklillu, E. (2010). Induction of CYP1A2 by heavy coffee consumption is associated with the CYP1A2 -163C>A polymorphism. *European Journal of Clinical Pharmacology*, *66*(7), 697–703. doi:10.1007/s00228-010-0823-4 PMID:20390257

Dobinson, T., & Henly, D. (2017). LinkedIn Employability Strategy and emodule. *National Innovation Case Study Collection.* Retrieved from https://iru.knack.com/national-innovation-case-study-collection/#browse-by-theme/theme-details/58e5e4b57300e05a549c768e/theme-case-study-details/58ed9c298caea04b5143977a/

Donaldson, M. E., Gadbury-Amyot, C. C., Khajotia, S. S., Natterstad, A., Norton, N., Zubiaurre, L. A., & Turner, S. P. (2007). Dental education in a flat world: Advocating for increased global collaboration and standardization. *Journal of Dental Education*, *72*(4), 408–421. PMID:18381847

Donnelly, L., Patten, D., White, P., & Finn, G. (2009). Virtual human dissector as a learning tool for studying cross-sectional anatomy. *Medical Teacher*, *31*(6), 553–555. doi:10.1080/01421590802512953 PMID:19288305

Doody, C., & McAteer, M. (2002). Clinical reasoning of expert and novice physiotherapists in an outpatient orthopaedic setting. *Physiotherapy*, *88*(5), 258–268. doi:10.1016/S0031-9406(05)61417-4

Doolittle, P. E. (2002). *Multimedia Learning: Empirical Results and Practical Applications*. Paper presented at the Irish Educational Technology Users' Conference, Carlow, Ireland.

Drake, R. L., McBride, J. M., Lachman, N., & Pawlina, W. (2009). Medical education in the anatomical sciences: The winds of change continue to blow. *Anatomical Sciences Education*, *2*(6), 253–259. doi:10.1002/ase.117 PMID:19890982

Draude, B., & Brace, S. (1999). Assessing the Impact of Technology on Teaching and Learning: Student Perspectives. *Proceedings of the Mid-South Instructional Technology Conference.*

Dron, J. (2012). The pedagogical-technological divide and the elephant in the room. *International Journal on E-Learning*, *11*(1), 23–38.

Duckworth, A., Peterson, C., Matthews, M. D., & Kelly, D. R. (2007). Grit: Perseverance and Passion for Long-Term Goals. *Journal of Personality and Social Psychology*, *92*(6), 1087–1101. doi:10.1037/0022-3514.92.6.1087 PMID:17547490

Dunne, J. R., & McDonald, C. L. (2010). Pulse!!: A model for research and development of virtual-reality learning in military medical education and training. *Military Medicine*, *175*(7Suppl), 25–27. doi:10.7205/MILMED-D-10-00158 PMID:23634475

Edwards, I., Jones, M., Carr, J., Braunack-Mayer, A., & Jensen, G. M. (2004). Clinical reasoning strategies in physical therapy. *Physical Therapy*, *84*(4), 312. PMID:15049726

Ehrmann, S. C. (2002). Improving the outcomes of education: Learning from past mistakes. *EDUCAUSE Review*, *37*, 54–55.

Erickson, S. R., Chang, A., Johnson, C. E., & Gruppen, L. D. (2003). Lecture Versus Web Tutorial for Pharmacy Students' Learning of MDI Technique. *The Annals of Pharmacotherapy*, *37*(4), 500–505. doi:10.1345/aph.1C374 PMID:12659603

Estevez, M. E., Lindgren, K. A., & Bergethon, P. R. (2010). A Novel Three-Dimensional Tool for Teaching Human Neuroanatomy. *Anatomical Sciences Education*, *3*(6), 309–317. doi:10.1002/ase.186 PMID:20939033

Euzent, P., Martin, T., Moskal, P., & Moskal, P. (2011). Assessing student performance and perceptions in lecture capture vs. face-to-face course delivery. *Journal of Information Technology Education*, *10*, 295–307.

Evans, J. L., Henderson, A. J., & Johnson, N. W. (2010). The future of education and training in dental technology: Designing a dental curriculum that facilitates teamwork across the oral health professions. *British Dental Journal*, *208*(5), 227–230. doi:10.1038/sj.bdj.2010.208 PMID:20228758

Evans, J. L., Henderson, A. J., & Johnson, N. W. (2012). Interprofessional learning enhances knowledge of roles but is less able to shift attitudes: A case study from dental education. *European Journal of Dental Education*, *16*(4), 239–245. doi:10.1111/j.1600-0579.2012.00749.x PMID:23050506

Evans, J. L., Henderson, A., Haugen, H., Myhrer, T., Nordin-Ivanow, K., Maryan, C., & Johnson, N. W. et al. (2015). The value of interprofessional education: A comparative study of dental technology students' perceptions across four countries. *British Dental Journal*, *218*(8), 481–487. doi:10.1038/sj.bdj.2015.296 PMID:25908364

Exercise and Sports Science Australia. (2016). *Course accreditation guide for education providers*. Retrieved April 2, 2016, from https://www.essa.org.au/wp-content/uploads/2016/11/Course-Accreditation-Guide-Oct-2016.pdf

Fallaize, R., Macready, A. L., Butler, L. T., Ellis, J. A., & Lovegrove, J. A. (2013). An insight into the public acceptance of nutrigenomic-based personalised nutrition. *Nutrition Research Reviews*, *26*(1), 39–48. doi:10.1017/S0954422413000024 PMID:23561449

Faulkner, M., Mahfuzul Aziz, S., Waye, V., & Smith, E. (2013). Exploring ways that ePortfolios can support the progressive development of graduate qualities and professional competencies. *Higher Education Research & Development*, *32*(6), 871–887. doi:643710.1080/07294360.2013.80

Fenech, M., El-Sohemy, A., Cahill, L., Ferguson, L. R., French, T. A., Tai, E. S., & Head, R. et al. (2011). Nutrigenetics and nutrigenomics: Viewpoints on the current status and applications in nutrition research and practice. *Journal of Nutrigenetics and Nutrigenomics*, *4*(2), 69–89. doi:10.1159/000327772 PMID:21625170

Ferguson, R. (2014, January 2). Snapchat user data exposed in huge data theft [Blog post]. Retrieved from http://countermeasures.trendmicro.eu/snapchat-user-data-exposed-in-huge-data-theft/

Ferguson, L. R., De Caterina, R., Gorman, U., Allayee, H., Kohlmeier, M., Prasad, C., & Martinez, J. A. et al. (2016). Guide and Position of the International Society of Nutrigenetics/Nutrigenomics on Personalised Nutrition: Part 1 - Fields of Precision Nutrition. *Journal of Nutrigenetics and Nutrigenomics*, *9*(1), 12–27. doi:10.1159/000445350 PMID:27169401

Fernandez, M., Nimmo, A., & Behar-Horenstein, L. (2016). Digital denture fabrication in pre- and postdoctoral education: A Survey of U.S. dental schools. *Journal of Prosthodontics*, *25*(1), 83–90. doi:10.1111/jopr.12287 PMID:26098406

Ferns, S. (2012). *Graduate employability: Teaching staff, employer and graduate perceptions.* Paper presented at the Australian Collaborative Education Network National Conference, Geelong, Australia.

Ferns, S., Russell, L., & Kay, J. (2016). Enhancing industry engagement with work-integrated learning: Capacity building for industry partners. *Asia Pacific Journal of Cooperative Education*, *17*(4), 349–375.

Fitzgerald, M., Kruschwitz, N., Bonnet, D., & Welch, M. (2014). Embracing digital technology: A new strategic imperative. *MIT Sloan Management Review*, *55*(2), 1–12.

Fletcher, J. D. (1990). *Effectiveness and Cost of Interactive Video Disk Instruction in Defense Training and Education.* Academic Press.

Foley, N. M., Maher, B. M., & Corrigan, M. A. (2014). Social Media and Tomorrow's Medical Students—How Do They Fit? *Journal of Surgical Education*, *71*(3), 385–390. doi:10.1016/j.jsurg.2013.10.008 PMID:24797855

Folsom, B., & Reardon, R. (2003). College career courses: Design and accountability. *Journal of Career Assessment*, *11*(4), 421–450. doi:10.1177/1069072703255875

Food4me. (n.d.). *An integrated analysis of opportunities and challenges for personalised nutrition.* Retrieved from www.food4me.org

Forte, M., de Souza, W. L., da Silva, R. F., do Prado, A. F., & Rodrigues, J. F. Jr. (2013). A ubiquitous reflective e-portfolio architecture. *International Journal of Medical Informatics*, *82*(11), 1111–1122. doi:10.1016/j.ijmedinf.2013.06.005 PMID:23850148

Foskett, R. (2007). Collaborative partnership between HE and employers: A study of workforce development. *Journal of Further and Higher Education*, *29*(3), 251–264. doi:10.1080/03098770500166868

Fossum, M., Fruhling, A., Moe, C. E., & Thompson, C. B. (2016). Crossing Borders: An Online Interdisciplinary Course in Health Informatics for Students From Two Countries. *Computers, Informatics, Nursing*. doi:10.1097/cin.0000000000000323 PMID:28002116

Fotrell, Q. (2016, June 16). How recruiters screen you on LinkedIn. *Marketwatch*. Retrieved from http://www.marketwatch.com/story/how-recruiters-screen-you-on-linkedin-2014

Francis, B., Mauriello, S. M., Phillips, C., Englebardt, S., & Grayden, S. K. (2000). Assessment of Online Continuing Dental Education in North Carolina. *The Journal of Continuing Education in the Health Professions*, *20*(2), 76–84.

Franklin, T., & Van Harmelen, M. (2007). *Web 2.0 for content for learning and teaching in higher education*. Retrieved from http://www.jisc.ac.uk/media/documents/programmes/digital_repositories/web2-content-learning-and-teaching.pdf

Franks, P. C., & Oliver, G. C. (2012). Experiential learning and international collaboration opportunities: Virtual internships. *Library Review*, *61*(4), 272–285. doi:10.1108/00242531211267572

Franzone, J. M., Kennedy, B. C., Merritt, H., Casey, J. T., Austin, M. C., & Daskivich, T. J. (2015). Progressive independence in clinical training: Perspectives of a national, multispecialty panel of residents and fellows. *Journal of Graduate Medical Education*, *7*(4), 700–704. doi:10.4300/JGME-07-04-51 PMID:26692998

Freeman, S., Eddy, S. L., McDonough, M., Smith, M. K., Okoroafor, N., Jordt, H., & Wenderoth, M. P. (2014). Active learning increases student performance in science, engineering, and mathematics. *Proceedings of the National Academy of Sciences of the United States of America*, *111*(23), 8410–8415. doi:10.1073/pnas.1319030111 PMID:24821756

Friedman, T. L. (2006). *The world is flat: a brief history of the twenty first century*. New York: Farrar, Straus & Giroux.

Fritz, D., Hu, A., Wilson, T., Ladak, H., Haase, P., & Fung, K. (2011). Long-term retention of a 3-dimensional educational computer model of the larynx: A follow-up study. *Archives of Otolaryngology--Head & Neck Surgery*, *137*(6), 598–603. doi:10.1001/archoto.2011.76 PMID:21690512

Frosst, P., Blom, H. J., Milos, R., Goyette, P., Sheppard, C. A., Matthews, R. G., & Rozen, R. et al. (1995). A candidate genetic risk factor for vascular disease: A common mutation in methylenetetrahydrofolate reductase. *Nature Genetics*, *10*(1), 111–113. doi:10.1038/ng0595-111 PMID:7647779

Frost, J., Isbel, S., Kellett, J., & Lawlis, T. (2017). Using digital story telling to assess health students' knowledge of interprofessional roles in the care of the older adult. *BMJ Simulation and Technology Enhanced Learning*, *3*(1), 5–8. doi:10.1136/bmjstel-2016-000136

Gaba, D. M. (2004). The future vision of simulation in health care. *Quality & Safety in Health Care*, *13*(suppl 1), i2–i10. doi:10.1136/qshc.2004.009878 PMID:15465951

Gabril, M. Y., & Yousef, G. M. (2010). Informatics for practicing anatomical pathologists: Marking a new era in pathology practice. *Modern Pathology*, *23*(3), 349–358. doi:10.1038/modpathol.2009.190 PMID:20081805

Gann, N., Rogers, C., & Dudley, A. (2002). A comparison of physical therapy students with and without instructions in ultrasound pressure application. *Journal of Allied Health*, *31*(2), 103–105. PMID:12040992

Garg, A. X., Norman, G. R., Eva, K. W., Spero, L., & Sharan, S. (2002). Is There Any Real Virtue of Virtual Reality?: The Minor Role of Multiple Orientations in Learning Anatomy from Computers. *Academic Medicine*, *77*(10Supplement), S97–S99. doi:10.1097/00001888-200210001-00030 PMID:12377717

Garrett, B. M., MacPhee, M., & Jackson, C. (2013). Evaluation of an eportfolio for the assessment of clinical competence in a baccalaureate nursing program. *Nurse Education Today*, *33*(10), 1207–1213. doi:10.1016/j.nedt.2012.06.015 PMID:22789875

Garrison, D. R., & Kanuka, H. (2004). Blended learning: Uncovering its transformative potential in higher education. *The Internet and Higher Education*, *7*(2), 95–105. doi:10.1016/j.iheduc.2004.02.001

Gartner. (2016). *Inside Gartner Research: How the art, science and rigor behind our research process and proprietary methodologies help you make the right decisions, every day*. Retrieved from http://www.gartner.com/imagesrv/research/methodologies/inside_gartner_research.pdf

Genetic Alliance, & the New England Public Health Genetics Education Collaborative. (2010). *Understanding Genetics: A New England Guide for Patients and Health Professionals*. Retrieved from https://www.ncbi.nlm.nih.gov/books/NBK132187/

Gervasini, G., Ghotbi, R., Aklillu, E., San Jose, C., Cabanillas, A., Kishikawa, J., & Carrillo, J. A. et al. (2013). Haplotypes in the 5′-untranslated region of the CYP1A2 gene are inversely associated with lung cancer risk but do not correlate with caffeine metabolism. *Environmental and Molecular Mutagenesis*, *54*(2), 124–132. doi:10.1002/em.21747 PMID:23138776

Ghotbi, R., Christensen, M., Roh, H. K., Ingelman-Sundberg, M., Aklillu, E., & Bertilsson, L. (2007). Comparisons of CYP1A2 genetic polymorphisms, enzyme activity and the genotype-phenotype relationship in Swedes and Koreans. *European Journal of Clinical Pharmacology*, *63*(6), 537–546. doi:10.1007/s00228-007-0288-2 PMID:17370067

Ghulam, A. (2016, January 16). Is it a security vulnerability if the addresses of university students are exposed? [Blog post]. Retrieved from https://security.stackexchange.com/questions/147222/is-it-a-security-vulnerability-if-the-addresses-of-university-students-are-expos

Gibbs, G., & Coffey, M. (2004). The Impact Of Training Of University Teachers on their Teaching Skills, their Approach to Teaching and the Approach to Learning of their Students. *Active Learning in Higher Education*, *5*(1), 87–100. doi:10.1177/1469787404040463

Gibson, D., Ostashewski, N., Flintoff, K., Grant, S., & Knight, E. (2015). Digital badges in education. *Education and Information Technologies*, *20*(2), 403–410. doi:10.1007/s10639-013-9291-7

Gilbert, J. K., & Treagust, D. F. (2009). *Towards a coherent model for macro, submicro and symbolic representations in chemical education. In Multiple representations in chemical education* (pp. 333–350). Springer.

Giordano, C., & Giordano, C. (2011). Health Professions Students' Use of Social Media. *Journal of Allied Health*, *40*(2), 78–81. PMID:21695367

Glittenberg, C., & Binder, S. (2006). Using 3D computer simulations to enhance ophthalmic training. *Ophthalmic & Physiological Optics*, *26*(1), 40–49. doi:10.1111/j.1475-1313.2005.00358.x PMID:16390481

Glover, I., Hepplestone, S., Parkin, H. J., Rodger, H., & Irwin, B. (2016). Pedagogy first: Realising technology enhanced learning by focusing on teaching practice. *British Journal of Educational Technology*, *47*(5), 993–1002. doi:10.1111/bjet.12425

Goddard, A., & Hughes, C. (2006). Mentoring and its impact on student employability. *The Higher Education Academy Annual Conference July 2006.*

Goldman, J. (2011). Centre for the Advancement of Interprofessional Education (CAIPE) website: www.caipe.org.uk. *Journal of Interprofessional Care, 25*(5), 386-387.

Goldstein, R. E. (1998). *Esthetics in Dentistry* (2nd ed.). Ontario, Canada: D C Decker.

Gorman, U., Mathers, J. C., Grimaldi, K. A., Ahlgren, J., & Nordstrom, K. (2013). Do we know enough? A scientific and ethical analysis of the basis for genetic-based personalized nutrition. *Genes & Nutrition*, *8*(4), 373–381. doi:10.1007/s12263-013-0338-6 PMID:23471854

Graham, C. R. (2006). Blended learning systems. The handbook of blended learning, 3-21.

Grauerholz, L., & Zipp, J. F. (2008). How to do the Scholarship of Teaching and Learning. *Teaching Sociology*, *36*(1), 87–94. doi:10.1177/0092055X0803600111

Green, J., Wyllie, A., & Jackson, D. (2014). Electronic portfolios in nursing education: A review of the literature. *Nurse Education in Practice*, *14*(1), 4–8. doi:10.1016/j.nepr.2013.08.011 PMID:24090523

Green, M., Lea, J. H., & McNair, C. L. (2014). Reality check: Augmented reality for school libraries. *Teacher Librarian*, *41*(5), 28.

Green, R. A., & Whitburn, L. Y. (2016). Impact of introduction of blended learning in gross anatomy on student outcomes. *Anatomical Sciences Education*, *9*(5), 422–430. doi:10.1002/ase.1602 PMID:26929149

Griffith University. (2014). *Guidelines for staff engagement with Learning@Griffith.* Retrieved 17 February, 2017, from http://policies.griffith.edu.au/pdf/Staff%20Engagement%20with%20 Learning%20at%20Griffith.pdf

Griffith University. (2017). *Skype disruptions on the Griffith network.* Retrieved March 1, 2017, from https://intranet.secure.griffith.edu.au/work/collaboration/self-help/other-collaborative-tools

Grigg, P., & Stephens, C. D. (1998). Computer-assisted learning in dentistry a view from the UK. *Journal of Dentistry*, *26*(5-6), 387–395. doi:10.1016/S0300-5712(98)00012-8 PMID:9699427

Groenewald, T. (2004). Toward a Definition for Cooperative Education. In R. K. Coll & C. Eames (Eds.), International Handbook for Cooperative Education: An International Perspective of the Theory, Research, and Practice of Work-Integrated Learning (pp. 17-25). Boston: World Association for Cooperative Education.

Gross, D. (2013, July 11) Are Social Media Making the Resume Obsolete? *CNN Tech*. Retrieved from http://edition.cnn.com/2012/07/11/tech/social-media/facebook-jobs-resume/

Grunwald, T., & Charisse, C.-M. (2006). Guidelines for Cognitively Efficient Multimedia Learning Tools: Educational Strategies, Cognitive Load, and Interface Design. *Academic Medicine*, *81*(3), 213–223. doi:10.1097/00001888-200603000-00003 PMID:16501261

Gupta, Y., Morgan, M., Singh, A., & Ellis, H. (2008). Junior doctors' knowledge of applied clinical anatomy. *Clinical Anatomy (New York, N.Y.)*, *21*(4), 334–338. doi:10.1002/ca.20628 PMID:18428998

Haggis, T. (2006). Pedagogies for diversity: Retaining critical challenge amidst fears of 'dumbing down'. *Studies in Higher Education*, *31*(5), 521–535. doi:10.1080/03075070600922709

Hahne, A. J., Keating, J. L., & Wilson, S. C. (2004). Do within-session changes in pain intensity and range of motion predict between-session changes in patients with low back pain? *The Australian Journal of Physiotherapy*, *50*(1), 17–23. doi:10.1016/S0004-9514(14)60244-0 PMID:14987188

Haldane, A. G. (2015). Growing, fast and slow. University of East Anglia.

Hallam, G., Harper, W., McAllister, L., Hauville, K., & Creagh, T. (2010). *Australian ePortfolio project: ePortfolio use by university students in Australian: Informing excellence in policy and practice.* AeP Supplementary report. QUT Department of eLearning.

Hallam, G., Harper, W., McCowan, C., Hauville, K., McAllister, L., Creagh, T., . . . Brooks, C. (2008). ePortfolio use by university students in Australia: Informing excellence in policy and practice. Final project report, August 2008. QUT Department of Teaching and Learning Support Services, Queensland.

Hallam, G., & Creagh, T. (2010). ePortfolio use by university students in Australia: A review of the Australian ePortfolio Project. *Higher Education Research & Development*, *29*(2), 179–193. doi:10.1080/07294360903510582

Halliday, A. C., Devonshire, I. M., Greenfield, S. A., & Dommett, E. J. (2010). Teaching medical students basic neurotransmitter pharmacology using primary research resources. *Advances in Physiology Education*, *34*(4), 205–212. doi:10.1152/advan.00005.2010 PMID:21098388

Hall, S., Grant, G., Arora, D., Karaksha, A., McFarland, A., Lohning, A., & Anoopkumar-Dukie, S. (2017). A pilot study assessing the value of 3D printed molecular modelling tools for pharmacy student education. *Currents in Pharmacy Teaching and Learning*, *9*(4), 723–728. doi:10.1016/j.cptl.2017.03.029

Hamat, A., Embi, M. A., & Abu Hassan, H. (2012). The Use of Social Networking Sites among Malaysian University Students. *International Education Studies*, *5*(3), 56–66. doi:10.5539/ies.v5n3p56

Hamilton, P. W., Wang, Y., & McCullough, S. J. (2012). Virtual microscopy and digital pathology in training and education. *APMIS*, *120*(4), 305–315. doi:10.1111/j.1600-0463.2011.02869.x PMID:22429213

Hamosh, A., Scott, A. F., Amberger, J. S., Bocchini, C. A., & McKusick, V. A. (2005). Online Mendelian Inheritance in Man (OMIM), a knowledgebase of human genes and genetic disorders. *Nucleic Acids Research*, *33*(Database issue), D514–D517. doi:10.1093/nar/gki033 PMID:15608251

Hampton, B. S., & Sung, V. W. (2010). Improving medical student knowledge of female pelvic floor dysfunction and anatomy: A randomized trial. *American Journal of Obstetrics and Gynecology*, *202*(6), 601.e601–601.e608. doi:10.1016/j.ajog.2009.08.038 PMID:20430356

Hansen, M. M. (2008). Versatile, Immersive, Creative and Dynamic Virtual 3-D Healthcare Learning Environments: A Review of the Literature. *Journal of Medical Internet Research*, *10*(3), e26. doi:10.2196/jmir.1051 PMID:18762473

Harder, B. N. (2010). Use of simulation in teaching and learning in health sciences: A systematic review. *The Journal of Nursing Education*, *49*(1), 23–28. doi:10.3928/01484834-20090828-08 PMID:19731886

Harorli, O., & Harorli, H. E. (2014). Evaluation of internet search trends of some common oral problems, 2004 to 2014. *Community Dental Health*, *31*, 188–192. PMID:25300156

Harris, J., Mishra, P., & Koehler, M. (2009). Teachers' technological pedagogical content knowledge and learning activity types: Curriculum-based technology integration reframed. *Journal of Research on Technology in Education*, *41*(4), 393–416. doi:10.1080/15391523.2009.10782536

Harris, S., Dolan, G., & Fairbairn, G. (2001). Reflecting on the use of student portfolios. *Nurse Education Today*, *21*(4), 278–286. doi:10.1054/nedt.2000.0545 PMID:11339871

Hartley, J., & Cameron, A. (1967). Some observations on the effeciency of lecturing. *Educational Review*, *20*(1), 30–37. doi:10.1080/0013191670200103

Harvey, L. (2010). New realities: The relationships between higher education and employment. *Tertiary Education and Management*, *6*(1), 3–17. doi:10.1080/13583883.2000.9967007

Hassam, M., & Williams, M. (2003). Education via simulation: Teaching safe chest percussion for pre-term infants. *Hong Kong Physiotherapy Journal*, *21*(1), 22–28. doi:10.1016/S1013-7025(09)70036-3

Hays, R., Veitch, J., & Lam, A. (2005). Teaching clinical pathology by flexible delivery in rural sites. *The Australian Journal of Rural Health*, *13*(4), 232–235. doi:10.1111/j.1440-1584.2005.00707.x PMID:16048465

HEFCE. (2010). *The higher education workforce framework*. Retrieved from Horgan, J. (2003). Lecturing for learning. In H. Fry, S. Ketteridge, & S. Marshall (Eds.), *A Handbook for Teaching and Learning in Higher Education* (2nd ed.; pp. 75–90). London: Kogan Page.

Heidger, P. M., Dee, F., Consoer, D., Leaven, T., Duncan, J., & Kreiter, C. (2002). Integrated approach to teaching and testing in histology with real and virtual imaging. *The Anatomical Record*, *269*(2), 107–112. doi:10.1002/ar.10078 PMID:12001217

Henderson-King, D., & Henderson-King, E. (2005). Acceptance of cosmetic surgery: Scale development and validation. *Body Image*, *2*(2), 137–149. doi:10.1016/j.bodyim.2005.03.003 PMID:18089182

Henry, M., Pooley, J. A., & Omari, M. (2014). *Student motivations for studying online: A qualitative study*. Academic Press.

Hew, K. F., & Cheung, W. S. (2014). Students' and instructors' use of massive open online courses (MOOCs): Motivations and challenges. *Educational Research Review*, *12*, 45–58. doi:10.1016/j.edurev.2014.05.001

Hickey, S. E., Curry, C. J., & Toriello, H. V. (2013). ACMG Practice Guideline: Lack of evidence for MTHFR polymorphism testing. *Genetics in Medicine*, *15*(2), 153–156. doi:10.1038/gim.2012.165 PMID:23288205

Higher Education Academy (HEA). (2005). *Guide for busy academics no.1: Personal development planning*. Retrieved from http://www.heacademy.ac.uk/resources.asp?process5full_record&section5generic&id566

Hila, J., Ellis, E., & Holmes, W. (2002). Feedback withdrawal and changing compliance during manual hyperinflation. *Physiotherapy Research International*, *7*(2), 53–64. doi:10.1002/pri.242 PMID:12109235

Hilbelink, A. J. (2007). *The effectiveness and user perception of 3-dimensional digital human anatomy in an online undergraduate anatomy laboratory*. University of South Florida, Scholar Commons.

Hill, P. (2016, November 10). Popular discussion platform piazza getting pushback for selling student data. *e-Literate*. Retrieved 27 February, 2016, from http://mfeldstein.com/popular-discussion-platform-piazza-getting-pushback-selling-student-data/

Hodges, D. (2011). The assessment of student learning in cooperative and work-integrated education. In R. K. Coll & K. E. Zegwaard (Eds.), *International Handbook for Cooperative and Work-Integrated Learning: International Perspectives of Theory, Research and Practice* (2nd ed.; pp. 53–62). Lowell, MA: World Association for Cooperative Education.

Hoffman, H., & Vu, D. (1997). Virtual reality: Teaching tool of the twenty-first century? *Academic Medicine*, *72*(12), 1076–1081. doi:10.1097/00001888-199712000-00018 PMID:9435714

Hogan, J., Flanagan, B., & Marshall, S. (2008). What Facilitation Skills Are Required to Assist Students' Learning When Using a Patient Simulator in the 'Pause and Discuss' Mode? *Focus on Health Professional Education: A Multi-Disciplinary Journal, 10*(2), 36.

Høivik, H. (2016). *Introduction to the IN:Code Project 2016-2017.* Paper presented at the International Joint Course Development (IN:Code) Oslo and Akershus University of Applied Sciences, Norway.

Hoivik, H., Cong, J. B., Haihuang, F., & Xiaochun, W. (2015). Teaching and learning in the digital age. In H. Holvik (Ed.), *Experiential approaches to learning design in Norway and China* (pp. s107–s128). Capital Normal University Press.

Holdsworth, A., Watty, K., & Davies, M. (2009). *Developing capstone experiences.* Melbourne Centre for Study of Higher Education, University of Melbourne.

Holland, L., & Bosch, B. (2006). Medical students' perceptions of pathology and the effect of the second-year pathology course. *Human Pathology, 37*(1), 1–8. doi:10.1016/j.humpath.2005.10.004 PMID:16360409

Hollands, G. J., French, D. P., Griffin, S. J., Prevost, A. T., Sutton, S., King, S., & Marteau, T. M. (2016). The impact of communicating genetic risks of disease on risk-reducing health behaviour: Systematic review with meta-analysis. *BMJ (Clinical Research Ed.), 352*, i1102. doi:10.1136/bmj.i1102 PMID:26979548

Holt, D., McGuigan, N., Kavanagh, M., Leitch, S., Ngo, L., Salzman, S., & McKay, J. et al. (2016). Academic leaders' perspectives on adopting ePortfolios for developing and assessing professional capabilities in Australian business education. *Australasian Journal of Educational Technology, 32*(5), 1–18. doi:10.14742/ajet.2666

Hopkins, R., Regehr, G., & Wilson, T. D. (2011). Exploring the Changing Learning Environment of the Gross Anatomy Lab. *Academic Medicine, 86*(7), 883–888. doi:10.1097/ACM.0b013e31821de30f PMID:21617516

Horigan, G., McNulty, H., Ward, M., Strain, J. J., Purvis, J., & Scott, J. M. (2010). Riboflavin lowers blood pressure in cardiovascular disease patients homozygous for the 677C-->T polymorphism in MTHFR. *Journal of Hypertension, 28*(3), 478–486. doi:10.1097/HJH.0b013e328334c126 PMID:19952781

Horne, J., Madill, J., & O'Connor, C. (2016). Exploring Knowledge and Attitudes of Personal Nutrigenomics Testing among Dietetic Students and its Value as a Component of Dietetic Education and Practice. *The Canadian Journal of Clinical Nutrition, 4*(1), 50–62. doi:10.14206/canad.j.clin.nutr.2016.01.07

Horspool, A., & Lange, C. (2010). Applying the scholarship of teaching and learning: Student perceptions, behaviours and success online and face-to-face. *Assessment & Evaluation in Higher Education, 37*(1), 73–88. doi:10.1080/02602938.2010.496532

Housego, S., & Parker, N. (2009). Positioning ePortfolio in an integrated curriculum. *Education + Training*, *51*(5/6), 408–421. doi:10.1108/00400910910987219

Hoyek, N., Collet, C., Di Rienzo, F., De Almeida, M., & Guillot, A. (2014). Effectiveness of three-dimensional digital animation in teaching human anatomy in an authentic classroom context. *Anatomical Sciences Education*, *7*(6), 430–437. doi:10.1002/ase.1446 PMID:24678034

Hu, A., Wilson, T., Ladak, H., Haase, P., & Fung, K. (2009). Three-dimensional educational computer model of the larynx: Voicing a new direction. *Archives of Otolaryngology--Head & Neck Surgery*, *135*(7), 677–681. doi:10.1001/archoto.2009.68 PMID:19620589

Hughes, I. (2003). Teaching Pharmacology in 2010 - New Knowledge, New Tools, New Attitudes. *Nihon yakurigaku zasshi. Folia pharmacologica Japonica, 122*(5), 411 - 418.

Hughes, I. (2002). Computer-Based Learning - an Aid to Successful Teaching of Pharmacology? *Naunyn-Schmiedeberg's Archives of Pharmacology*, *366*(1), 77–82. doi:10.1007/s00210-002-0552-z PMID:12107637

Idris, Y., & Wang, Q. (2009). Affordances of Facebook for Learning. *International Journal of Continuing Engineering Education and Lifelong Learning*, *19*(2/3), 247–255. doi:10.1504/IJCEELL.2009.025031

Imai, K., Kricka, L. J., & Fortina, P. (2011). Concordance study of 3 direct-to-consumer genetic-testing services. *Clinical Chemistry*, *57*(3), 518–521. doi:10.1373/clinchem.2010.158220 PMID:21159896

Institute for the Study of Knowledge Management in Education. (2017). *OER Commons*. Retrieved from https://www.oercommons.org/

Ioannou, N. K., Ioannidis, G. S., Papadopoulos, G. D., & Tapeinos, A. E. (2014). *A novel educational platform, based on the Raspberry-Pi: Optimised to assist the teaching and learning of younger students*. Paper presented at the Interactive Collaborative Learning (ICL), 2014 International Conference on.

Jackson, D. (2015). Employability skill development in work-integrated learning: Barriers and best practice. *Studies in Higher Education*, *40*(2), 350–367. doi:10.1080/03075079.2013.842221

Jacob, R. R., Allen, P. M., Ahrendt, L. J., & Brownson, R. C. (2017). Learning About and Using Research Evidence Among Public Health Practitioners. *Am J Prev Med, 52*(3S3), S304-S308. doi: 10.1016/j.amepre.2016.10.010

Jaffar, A. A. (2012). YouTube: An emerging tool in anatomy education. *Anatomical Sciences Education*, *5*(3), 158–164. doi:10.1002/ase.1268 PMID:22383096

Jaffar, A. A. (2014). Exploring the use of a facebook page in anatomy education. *Anatomical Sciences Education*, *7*(3), 199–208. doi:10.1002/ase.1404 PMID:24022984

Jamali, S. S., Shiratuddin, M. F., Wong, K. W., & Oskam, C. L. (2015). Utilising Mobile-Augmented Reality for Learning Human Anatomy. *Procedia: Social and Behavioral Sciences*, *197*, 659–668. doi:10.1016/j.sbspro.2015.07.054

James, N., Demetriades Toftdahl, S., & Mackey, P. (2016). *Outcomes from Global Scope - a large-scale "virtual micro internship" WIL pilot with NSW State Government.* Paper presented at the WIL 2020: Pushing the boundaries, 2016 Australian Collaborative Education Network National Conference, Sydney, Australia.

Jenkins, M., Browne, T., Walker, R., & Hewitt, R. (2011). The development of technology enhanced learning: Findings from a 2008 survey of UK higher education institutions. *Interactive Learning Environments*, *19*(5), 447–465. doi:10.1080/10494820903484429

Johnson, L. (2014). *NMC Horizon Report 2014 Higher Education Edition*. Retrieved from https://www.nmc.org/pdf/2014-nmc-horizon-report-he-EN.pdf

Johnson, L., Adams Becker, S., Cummins, M., Estrada, V., Freeman, A., & Hall, C. (2016). *NMC horizon report: 2016 higher education edition*. Austin, TX: The New Media Consortium.

Johnston, J., & Baker, L. T. (2002). *Assessing the impact of technology in teaching and learning: A source book for evaluators*. Ann Arbor, MI: University of Michigan.

Jones, D. (2016, September 11). Which comes first? Pedagogy or technology? [Blog post]. Retrieved from http://djon.es/blog/2016/09/11/which-comes-first-pedagogy-or-technology/

Jones, H. M., & Warnock, L. (2014). *Towards a Competency Framework for Student Work Based Learning*. Higher Education Academy. Retrieved 13 April, 2017, from https://www.heacademy.ac.uk/sites/default/files/resources/towards_a_competency _framework_for_student_work-based_learning.pdf

Joyce, P. (2005). A framework for portfolio development in postgraduate nursing practice. *Journal of Clinical Nursing*, *14*(4), 456–463. doi:10.1111/j.1365-2702.2004.01075.x PMID:15807752

Joyce, S. P. (2013). Be visible on LinkedIn. *Career Planning and Adult Development Journal*, *29*(3), 88–90.

Junco, R. (2012). Too much face and not enough books: The relationship between multiple indices of Facebook use and academic performance. *Computers in Human Behavior*, *28*(1), 187–198. doi:10.1016/j.chb.2011.08.026

Kaider, F., Henschke, K., Richardson, J., & Kelly, M. P. (2009). *Designing blended spaces to maximise student learning in work integrated learning programs*. Paper presented at the ASCILITE 2009 - The Australasian Society for Computers in Learning in Tertiary Education.

Kallio, P., Kolehmainen, M., Laaksonen, D. E., Kekalainen, J., Salopuro, T., Sivenius, K., & Poutanen, K. S. et al. (2007). Dietary carbohydrate modification induces alterations in gene expression in abdominal subcutaneous adipose tissue in persons with the metabolic syndrome: The FUNGENUT Study. *The American Journal of Clinical Nutrition*, *85*(5), 1417–1427. PMID:17490981

Kalow, W., & Tang, B. K. (1993). The use of caffeine for enzyme assays: A critical appraisal. *Clinical Pharmacology and Therapeutics*, *53*(5), 503–514. doi:10.1038/clpt.1993.63 PMID:8491061

Karaksha, A., Grant, G., Anoopkumar-Dukie, S., Nirthanan, S. N., & Davey, A. K. (2013). Student engagement in pharmacology courses using online learning tools. *American Journal of Pharmaceutical Education*, *77*(6), 125. doi:10.5688/ajpe776125 PMID:23966728

Karaksha, A., Grant, G., Davey, A. K., & Anoopkumar-Dukie, S. (2011). Development and evaluation of computer-assisted learning (CAL) teaching tools compared to the conventional didactic lecture in pharmacology education. *Proceedings of EDULEARN11 Conference.*

Karaksha, A., Grant, G., Davey, A., Anoopkumar-Dukie, S., & Nirthanan, S. (2013). Educational benefit of an embedded animation used as supplement to didactic lectures in nursing pharmacology courses. *Proceedings of the 7th International Technology, Education and Development Conference (INTED'13).*

Karaksha, A., Grant, G., Nirthanan, S. N., Davey, A. K., & Anoopkumar-Dukie, S. (2014). A Comparative Study to Evaluate the Educational Impact of E-Learning Tools on Griffith University Pharmacy Students' Level of Understanding Using Bloom's and SOLO Taxonomies. *Education Research International.*

Karlowicz, K. A. (2000). The value of student portfolios to evaluate undergraduate nursing programs. *Nurse Educator*, *25*(2), 82–87. doi:10.1097/00006223-200003000-00010 PMID:11052006

Karpati, A. (2011). *Digital literacy in education*. Moscow, Russia: UNESCO Institute for Information Technologies in Education.

Karthikeyana, P., & Ramalingamb, K. P. (2017). E-learning initiatives in delivering the undergraduate physiotherapy education program in Papua New Guinea. *Asia Pacific Journal of Contemporary Education and Communication Technology (APJCECT), 3*(1).

Kasemsap, K. (2017). *Mastering educational computer games, educational video games, and serious games in the digital age*. IGI Global. doi:10.4018/978-1-5225-1034-5.ch003

Kazemi, H., Rappel, J. K., Poston, T., Lim, B. H., Burdet, E., & Teo, C. L. (2010). Assessing suturing techniques using a virtual reality surgical simulator. *Microsurgery*, *30*(6), 479–486. doi:10.1002/micr.20766 PMID:20201052

Keedy, A. W., Durack, J. C., Sandhu, P., Chen, E. M., O'Sullivan, P. S., & Breiman, R. S. (2011). Comparison of traditional methods with 3D computer models in the instruction of hepatobiliary anatomy. *Anatomical Sciences Education*, *4*(2), 84–91. doi:10.1002/ase.212 PMID:21412990

Kemp, J., & Livingstone, D. (2006). Putting a Second Life "metaverse" skin on learning management systems. *Proceedings of the Second Life education workshop at the Second Life community convention.*

Kerby, J., Shukur, Z. N., & Shalhoub, J. (2011). The relationships between learning outcomes and methods of teaching anatomy as perceived by medical students. *Clinical Anatomy (New York, N.Y.), 24*(4), 489–497. doi:10.1002/ca.21059 PMID:20949485

Khemaja, M. (2016). Using a knapsack model to optimize continuous building of a hybrid intelligent tutoring system: Application to information technology professionals. *International Journal of Human Capital and Information Technology Professionals*, *7*(2), 1–18. doi:10.4018/IJHCITP.2016040101

Khot, Z., Quinlan, K., Norman, G. R., & Wainman, B. (2013). The relative effectiveness of computer-based and traditional resources for education in anatomy. *Anatomical Sciences Education*, *6*(4), 211–215. doi:10.1002/ase.1355 PMID:23509000

Kicklighter, J. R., Dorner, B., Hunter, A. M., Kyle, M., Pflugh Prescott, M., Roberts, S., & Byrne, C. et al. (2017). Visioning Report 2017: A Preferred Path Forward for the Nutrition and Dietetics Profession. *Journal of the Academy of Nutrition and Dietetics*, *117*(1), 110–127. doi:10.1016/j.jand.2016.09.027 PMID:28010848

Kim, Y., Kim, H., & Kim, Y. O. (2017). Virtual reality and augmented reality in plastic surgery: A review. *Archives of Plastic Surgery*, *44*(3), 179–187. doi:10.5999/aps.2017.44.3.179 PMID:28573091

Kinash, S., Crane, L., Judd, M. M., Mitchell, K., McLean, M., Knight, C., & Schulz, M. et al. (2015). *Supporting graduate employability from generalist disciplines through employer and private institution collaboration*. Sydney: Australian Government Office for Learning and Teaching.

Kinnison, T., Forrest, N. D., Frean, S. P., & Baillie, S. (2009). Teaching Bovine Abdominal Anatomy: Use of a Haptic Simulator. *Anatomical Sciences Education*, *2*(6), 280–285. doi:10.1002/ase.109 PMID:19780149

Kirschner, P. A., & Karpinski, A. C. (2010). Facebook® and academic performance. *Computers in Human Behavior*, *26*(6), 1237–1245. doi:10.1016/j.chb.2010.03.024

Knight, J. (2008). The internationalization of higher education: Are we on the right track? *Academic Matters: The Journal of Higher Education*, *52*, 5–9.

Knight, J. (2015). Updated internationalisation definition. *Industry and Higher Education*, *33*, 2–3.

Knight, P. T., & York, M. (2010). Employability and Good Learning in Higher Education. *Teaching in Higher Education*, *8*(1), 3–18. doi:10.1080/1356251032000052294

Knight, P., & Yorke, M. (2004). *Learning, curriculum and employability in higher education*. London: Routledge.

Koch, L. H., Lampros, J. N., Delong, L. K., Chen, S. C., Woosley, J. T., & Hood, A. F. (2009). Randomized comparison of virtual microscopy and traditional glass microscopy in diagnostic accuracy among dermatology and pathology residents. *Human Pathology*, *40*(5), 662–667. doi:10.1016/j.humpath.2008.10.009 PMID:19144382

Kohlmeier, M., De Caterina, R., Ferguson, L. R., Gorman, U., Allayee, H., Prasad, C., & Martinez, J. A. et al. (2016). Guide and Position of the International Society of Nutrigenetics/Nutrigenomics on Personalized Nutrition: Part 2 - Ethics, Challenges and Endeavors of Precision Nutrition. *Journal of Nutrigenetics and Nutrigenomics*, *9*(1), 28–46. doi:10.1159/000446347 PMID:27286972

Kontaxis, G., Polychronakis, M., & Markatos, E. P. (2012). Minimizing information disclosure to third parties in social login platforms. *International Journal of Information Security*, *11*(5), 321–332. doi:10.1007/s10207-012-0173-6

Kostic, A. D., Xavier, R. J., & Gevers, D. (2014). The microbiome in inflammatory bowel disease: Current status and the future ahead. *Gastroenterology*, *146*(6), 1489–1499. doi:10.1053/j.gastro.2014.02.009 PMID:24560869

Krathwohl, D. R. (2002). A Revision of Bloom's Taxonomy: An Overview. *Theory into Practice*, *41*(4), 212–218. doi:10.1207/s15430421tip4104_2

Krause, K.-L. (2009). *GIHE Good Practice Guide on Blended Learning*. Retrieved from http://www.griffith.edu.au/gihe/pdf/gihe_tipsheet_web_bl.pdf

Kukulska-Hulme, A. (2012). How should the higher education workforce adapt to advancements in technology for teaching and learning? *The Internet and Higher Education*, *15*(4), 247–254. doi:10.1016/j.iheduc.2011.12.002

Kumar, R. K., Freeman, B., Velan, G. M., & De Permentier, P. J. (2006). Integrating histology and histopathology teaching in practical classes using virtual slides. *Anatomical Record. Part B, New Anatomist*, *289*(4), 128–133. doi:10.1002/ar.b.20105 PMID:16865702

Kutz, G. (2006). *Nutrigenetic Testing Tests Purchased from Four Web Sites Mislead Consumers. Statement of Gregory Kutz, Managing Director Forensic Audits and Special Investigations.* Retrieved from http://www.gao.gov/assets/120/114612.pdf

Kwon, S. R., Hernández, M., Blanchette, D. R., Lam, M. T., Gratton, D. G., & Aquilino, S. A. (2015). Effect of computer-assisted learning on students' dental anatomy waxing performance. *Journal of Dental Education*, *79*(9), 1093–1100. PMID:26329034

Lahaie, U. (2007). Web-Based Instruction: Getting Faculty Onboard. *Journal of Professional Nursing*, *26*(6), 335–342. doi:10.1016/j.profnurs.2007.01.024 PMID:18053959

Lam, A. K., Veitch, J., & Hays, R. (2005). Resuscitating the teaching of anatomical pathology in undergraduate medical education: Web-based innovative clinicopathological cases. *Pathology*, *37*(5), 360–363. doi:10.1080/00313020500253331 PMID:16194846

Lamrani, R., Chraibi, S., Qassimi, S., Hafidi, M., & El Amrani, A. (2017). *Serious Game to Enhance and Promote Youth Entrepreneurship. In Europe and MENA Cooperation Advances in Information and Communication Technologies* (pp. 77–85). Springer. doi:10.1007/978-3-319-46568-5_8

Lane, A., Caird, S., & Weller, M. (2014). The potential social, economic and environmental benefits of MOOCs: Operational and historical comparisons with a massive 'closed online' course. *Open Praxis*, *6*(2), 115–123. doi:10.5944/openpraxis.6.2.113

Langenberg, C., Sharp, S. J., Franks, P. W., Scott, R. A., Deloukas, P., Forouhi, N. G., & Wareham, N. J. et al. (2014). Gene-lifestyle interaction and type 2 diabetes: The EPIC interact case-cohort study. *PLoS Medicine*, *11*(5), e1001647. doi:10.1371/journal.pmed.1001647 PMID:24845081

Lanning, S. K., Wetzel, A. P., Baines, M., & Byrne, B. E. (2012). Evaluation of a revised curriculum: A four year qualitative study of student perceptions. *Journal of Dental Education, 76*(10), 1323–1333. PMID:23066131

Larue, C., Pepin, J., & Allard, É. (2015). Simulation in preparation or substitution for clinical placement: A systematic review of the literature. *Journal of Nursing Education and Practice, 5*(9), 132. doi:10.5430/jnep.v5n9p132

Lateef, F. (2010). Simulation-based learning: Just like the real thing. *Journal of Emergencies, Trauma and Shock, 3*(4), 348. doi:10.4103/0974-2700.70743 PMID:21063557

Lau, A., & Pang, M. (2000). Career strategies to strengthen graduate employees' employment position in the Hong Kong labour market. *Education + Training, 42*(3), 135–149. doi:10.1108/00400910010372689

Lauby, S. (2011). 9 Dynamic Digital Resumes That Stand Out From The Crowd. *Mashable.* Retrieved from http://mashable.com/2011/02/21/dynamic-digital-resumes/#oK_r3LwnIGq7

Le Beux, P., & Fieschi, M. (2007). *Virtual biomedical universities and e-learning*. Elsevier.

Leask, B. (2009). Using formal and informal curricula to improve interactions between home and international students. *Journal of Studies in International Education, 13*(2), 205–221. doi:10.1177/1028315308329786

Lee, M., & Pohio, L. (2012). An ePortfolio theoretical approach for provisionally registered teachers. In M. Brown, M. Hartwell, & T. Stewart (Eds.), Proceedings of ascilite Wellington 2012: Future challenges, sustainable futures (pp. 550–559). Academic Press.

Lee, N. (2013). *Learning to fly: Capstones and the transformation of student experience*. Paper presented at the Griffith University Learning and Teaching Conference: Capstones: The time is now! Brisbane, Australia.

Lee, E. A.-L., & Wong, K. W. (2014). Learning with desktop virtual reality: Low spatial ability learners are more positively affected. *Computers & Education, 79*, 49–58. doi:10.1016/j.compedu.2014.07.010

Lee, S. H. (2005). Virtual microscopy: Applications to hematology education and training. *Hematology, 10*(sup1), 151–153. doi:10.1080/10245330512331390249 PMID:16188659

Leifer, Z. (2015). The use of virtual microscopy and a wiki in pathology education: Tracking student use, involvement, and response. *Journal of Pathology Informatics, 6*(1), 30. doi:10.4103/2153-3539.158063 PMID:26110097

Lempicke, T. (2011, February 12). History of the Resume. *Business Insider*. Retrieved from https://www.businessinsider.com.au/how-resumes-have-evolved-since-their-first-creation-in-1482-2011-2?r=US&IR=T#the-first-resumes-1

Levinson, A. J., Weaver, B., Garside, S., McGinn, H., & Norman, G. R. (2007). Virtual reality and brain anatomy: A randomised trial of e-learning instructional designs. *Medical Education, 41*(5), 495–501. doi:10.1111/j.1365-2929.2006.02694.x PMID:17470079

Lewis, M. J., Davies, R., Jenkins, D., & Tait, M. I. (2005). A review of evaluative studies of computer-based learning in nursing education. *Nurse Education Today, 25*(8), 586–597. doi:10.1016/j.nedt.2005.09.006 PMID:16289489

Lim, J. S., Singh, O., Ramasamy, R. D., Ramasamy, S., Subramanian, K., Lee, E. J., & Chowbay, B. (2010). Pharmacogenetics of CYP1A2, novel polymorphisms and haplotypes in three distinct Asian populations. *Drug Metabolism and Pharmacokinetics, 25*(6), 616–623. doi:10.2133/dmpk.DMPK-10-SC-051 PMID:20930417

Lin, J., Yang, R., Tarr, P. T., Wu, P. H., Handschin, C., Li, S., & Spiegelman, B. M. et al. (2005). Hyperlipidemic effects of dietary saturated fats mediated through PGC-1beta coactivation of SREBP. *Cell, 120*(2), 261–273. doi:10.1016/j.cell.2004.11.043 PMID:15680331

Li, S. X., Collins, J., Lawson, S., Thomas, J., Truby, H., Whelan, K., & Palermo, C. (2014). A preliminary qualitative exploration of dietitians' engagement with genetics and nutritional genomics: Perspectives from international leaders. *Journal of Allied Health, 43*(4), 221–228. PMID:25433186

Li, S. X., Ye, Z., Whelan, K., & Truby, H. (2016). The effect of communicating the genetic risk of cardiometabolic disorders on motivation and actual engagement in preventative lifestyle modification and clinical outcome: A systematic review and meta-analysis of randomised controlled trials. *British Journal of Nutrition, 116*(5), 924–934. doi:10.1017/S0007114516002488 PMID:27405704

Lisk, K., McKee, P., Baskwill, A., & Agur, A. M. R. (2015). Student perceptions and effectiveness of an innovative learning tool: Anatomy Glove Learning System. *Anatomical Sciences Education, 8*(2), 140–148. doi:10.1002/ase.1459 PMID:24757171

Locatis, C., Vega, A., Bhagwat, M., Liu, W.-L., & Conde, J. (2008). A virtual computer lab for distance biomedical technology education. *BMC Medical Education, 8*(1), 12. doi:10.1186/1472-6920-8-12 PMID:18366629

Long, J. D., Gannaway, P., Ford, C., Doumit, R., Zeeni, N., Sukkarieh-Haraty, O., & Song, H. et al. (2016). Effectiveness of a Technology-Based Intervention to Teach Evidence-Based Practice: The EBR Tool. *Worldviews on Evidence-Based Nursing, 13*(1), 59–65. doi:10.1111/wvn.12132 PMID:26773417

Losco, C. D., Grant, W. D., Armson, A., Meyer, A. J., & Walker, B. F. (2017). Effective methods of teaching and learning in anatomy as a basic science: A BEME systematic review: BEME guide no. 44. *Medical Teacher, 39*(3), 234–243. doi:10.1080/0142159X.2016.1271944 PMID:28129720

Lowden, K., Hall, S., Elliot, D., & Lewin, J. (2011). *Employers' perceptions of the employability skills of new graduates*. London: Edge Foundation.

Lowe, S., Adams, R., & O'Kane, A. (2007). *A framework for the categorization of the Australian health professional workforce - discussion paper.* Retrieved from https://sarrah.org.au/sites/default/files/docs/framework_for_the_categorization_of_the_australian_health_workforce_summary_statement_august_2007.pdf

Lynn, V. A., Yenser, A., & Harman, R. (2015). Body apps: iPads for undergrad Anatomy and Physiology students. *College & Research Libraries News*, *76*(3), 149–152. doi:10.5860/crln.76.3.9281

MacLean, J., Scott, K., Marshall, T., & Asperen, P. (2011). Evaluation of an e-learning teaching resource: What is the medical student perspective? *Focus on Health Professional Education: A Multi-Disciplinary Journal, 13*(2), 53-63.

MacManaway, L. A. (1970). Teaching methods in higher educaion - innovation and research. *Higher Education Quarterly*, *24*(3), 321–329. doi:10.1111/j.1468-2273.1970.tb00346.x

Mącznik, A. K., Ribeiro, D. C., & Baxter, G. D. (2015). Online technology use in physiotherapy teaching and learning: A systematic review of effectiveness and users' perceptions. *BMC Medical Education*, *15*(1), 160. doi:10.1186/s12909-015-0429-8 PMID:26415677

Maggio, M. P., Hariton-Gross, K., & Gluch, J. (2012). The Use of Independent, Interactive Media for Education in Dental Morphology. *Journal of Dental Education*, *76*(11), 1497–1511. PMID:23144486

Magro, M., Sharp, J., Ryan, K., & Ryan, S. (2013). Investigating Ways to Use Facebook at the University Level: A Delphi Study. *Proceedings of the Informing Science and Information Technology Education Conference 2013*. https://www.learntechlib.org/p/114656

Magro, M., Sharp, J., Ryan, K., & Ryan, S. (2013). Investigating Ways to Use Facebook at the University Level: A Delphi Study. *Proceedings of the Informing Science and Information Technology Education Conference.*

Manogue, M., McLoughlin, J., Christensen, C., Delap, E., Lindh, C., Schoonheim-Klein, M., & Plasschaert, A. (2011). Curriculum structure, content, learning and assessment in Euorpean undergraduate dental education - update 2010. *European Journal of Dental Education*, *15*(3), 133–141. doi:10.1111/j.1600-0579.2011.00699.x PMID:21762317

Mantovani, F., Castelnuovo, G., Gaggioli, A., & Riva, G. (2003). Virtual reality training for health-care professionals. *Cyberpsychology & Behavior*, *6*(4), 389–395. doi:10.1089/109493103322278772 PMID:14511451

Marchevsky, A. M., Relan, A., & Baillie, S. (2003). Self-instructional "virtual pathology" laboratories using web-based technology enhance medical school teaching of pathology. *Human Pathology*, *34*(5), 423–429. doi:10.1016/S0046-8177(03)00089-3 PMID:12792914

Marsaux, C. F., Celis-Morales, C., Livingstone, K. M., Fallaize, R., Kolossa, S., Hallmann, J., & Saris, W. H. et al. (2016). Changes in Physical Activity Following a Genetic-Based Internet-Delivered Personalized Intervention: Randomized Controlled Trial (Food4Me). *Journal of Medical Internet Research*, *18*(2), e30. doi:10.2196/jmir.5198 PMID:26851191

Marsh, K. R., Giffin, B. F., & Lowrie, D. J. Jr. (2008). Medical student retention of embryonic development: Impact of the dimensions added by multimedia tutorials. *Anatomical Sciences Education*, *1*(6), 252–257. doi:10.1002/ase.56 PMID:19109854

Martin, A. J., & Marsh, H. W. (2003). Fear of failure: Friend or foe? *Australian Psychologist*, *38*(1), 31–38. doi:10.1080/00050060310001706997

Martin, E., Prosser, M., Trigwell, K., Ramsden, P., & Benjamin, J. (2000). What university teachers teach and how they teach it. *Instructional Science*, *28*(5), 387–412. doi:10.1023/A:1026559912774

Martin, F. (2008). Blackboard as the learning management system of a computer literacy course. *Journal of Online Learning and Teaching / MERLOT*, *4*(2), 138–145.

Martin, F., & Parker, M. A. (2014). Use of Synchronous Virtual Classrooms: Why, Who, and How? *Journal of Online Learning and Teaching / MERLOT*, *10*(2), 192.

Masters, K., & Ellaway, R. (2008). e-Learning in medical education Guide 32 Part 2: Technology, management and design. *Medical Teacher*, *30*(5), 474–489. doi:10.1080/01421590802108349 PMID:18576186

Mathur, A. S. (2015). *Low cost virtual reality for medical training*. Paper presented at the Virtual Reality (VR). doi:10.1109/VR.2015.7223437

Mattheos, N., Stefanovic, N., Apse, P., Attstrom, R., Buchanan, J., Brown, P., & Walmsley, A. D. et al. (2008). Potential of information technology in dental education. *European Journal of Dental Education*, *12*(s1S1), 85–91. doi:10.1111/j.1600-0579.2007.00483.x PMID:18289271

Maxmen, A. (2017). 23andMe given green-light to sell DNA tests for 10 diseases. *Nature news*. Retrieved from http://www.nature.com/news/23andme-given-green-light-to-sell-dna-tests-for-10-diseases-1.21802

Maxwell, S. R. J. (2012). An agenda for UK clinical pharmacology: How should teaching of undergraduates in clinical pharmacology and therapeutics be delivered and assessed? *British Journal of Clinical Pharmacology*, *73*(6), 893–899. doi:10.1111/j.1365-2125.2012.04232.x PMID:22360965

Mayer, R. E. (2001). *Multimedia Learning*. Cambridge, UK: Cambridge University Press. doi:10.1017/CBO9781139164603

Mayer, R. E., & Anderson, R. B. (1992). The Instructive Animation: Helping Students Build Connections Between Words and Pictures in Multimedia Learning. *J Educ Psychol*, *84*(4), 444–452. doi:10.1037/0022-0663.84.4.444

Mayer, R. E., & Moreno, R. (1998). A Split-Attention Effect in Multimedia Learning: Evidence for Dual Processing Systems in Working Memory. *J Educ Psychol*, *90*(2), 312–320. doi:10.1037/0022-0663.90.2.312

Mayer, R. E., & Moreno, R. (2003). Nine Ways to Reduce Cognitive Load in Multimedia Learning. *Educational Psychologist*, *38*(1), 43–52. doi:10.1207/S15326985EP3801_6

Mayo, P. H., Hackney, J. E., Mueck, J. T., Ribaudo, V., & Schneider, R. F. (2004). Achieving house staff competence in emergency airway management: Results of a teaching program using a computerized patient simulator. *Critical Care Medicine*, *32*(12), 2422–2427. doi:10.1097/01.CCM.0000147768.42813.A2 PMID:15599146

Mayrath, M., Clarke-Midura, J., & Robinson, D. (Eds.). (2012). *Technology-Based Assessments for 21st Century Skills: Theoretical and Practical Implications from Modern Research*. Charlotte, NC: Information Age Publishing.

McAllister, L., & Hauville, K. (2017). Striving for Sustainability: ePortfolio Pedagogy in Australian Higher Education. In ePortfolios in Australian Universities (pp. 13-32). Springer Singapore.

McAllister, L., & Nagarajan, S. V. (2016). Accreditation requirements in allied health education: Strengths, weaknesses and missed opportunities. *Journal of Teaching and Learning for Graduate Employability*, *6*(1), 2–24. doi:10.21153/jtlge2015vol6no1art570

McAlpine, A., Thomson, A., Ridler, G., White, J., & Plaisted, T. (2009). *Designing career development modules into the first year curriculum*. Paper presented at ALTC First Year Experience Curriculum Design Symposium. Retrieved from http://www.fyecd2009.qut.edu.au/resources/FYE_showcaseabstracts_4Feb09_FIN_SJ.pdf

McCorkle, D. E., Alexander, J. F., Reardon, J., & Kling, N. D. (2003, December). Developing self-marketing skills: Are marketing students prepared for the job search? *Journal of Marketing Education*, *25*, 196–207. doi:10.1177/0273475303257517

McGil, L. (2011). *Curriculum innovation: Pragmatic approaches to transforming learning and teaching through technologies*. Bristol, UK: JISC.

McNulty, H., Strain, J. J., Hughes, C. F., & Ward, M. (2017). Riboflavin, MTHFR genotype and blood pressure: A personalized approach to prevention and treatment of hypertension. *Molecular Aspects of Medicine*, *53*, 2–9. doi:10.1016/j.mam.2016.10.002 PMID:27720779

Mehta, N. B., Hull, A. L., Young, J. B., & Stoller, J. K. (2013). Just imagine: New paradigms for medical education. *Academic Medicine*, *88*(10), 1418–1423. doi:10.1097/ACM.0b013e3182a36a07 PMID:23969368

Meredith, S., & Burkle, M. (2008). Building bridges between university and industry: Theory and practice. *Education + Training*, *50*(3), 199–215. doi:10.1108/00400910810873982

Merriam-Webster On-line Dictionary. (2017). *Globalization*. Retrieved from https://www.merriam-webster.com/dictionary/globalization

Metzler, R., Stein, D., Tetzlaff, R., Bruckner, T., Meinzer, H.-P., Büchler, M. W., & Fischer, L. et al. (2012). Teaching on Three-Dimensional Presentation Does Not Improve the Understanding of According CT Images: A Randomized Controlled Study. *Teaching and Learning in Medicine*, *24*(2), 140–148. doi:10.1080/10401334.2012.664963 PMID:22490095

Meyer, E., Abrami, P. C., Wade, C. A., Aslan, O., & Deault, L. (2010). Improving literacy and metacognition with electronic portfolios: Teaching and learning with ePEARL. *Computers & Education*, *55*(1), 84–91. doi:10.1016/j.compedu.2009.12.005

Michel, M. C., Bischoff, A., & Jakobs, K. H. (2002). Comparison of problem-and lecture-based pharmacology teaching. *Trends in Pharmacological Sciences*, *23*(4), 168–170. doi:10.1016/S0165-6147(00)01940-4 PMID:11931991

Miclea, M., Miclea, S., & Ciuca, A. (2008). *Computer-Supported Psychotherapy Should Pay Attention To E-Learning*. Paper presented at the Cognitie, Creier, Comportament / Cognition, Brain, Behavior, Romanian Association for Cognitive Science.

Milkins, L., Moore, C., & Spiteri, J. (2014). *Simulation based education: Professional entry student education and training*. Retrieved from http://www.heti.nsw.gov.au/Global/NSS%20Simulation/SimulationBasedEducation_HETI.pdf

Miller, A. (2009). E-portfolios – Managing learner information in the vocational education and training sector. *Learning Communities: International Journal of Learning in Social Contexts*, (2), 16–30.

Miller, A. (2017). Professional Learning Ecosystem Support for ePortfolio Use in Australian Higher Education: An Historical Perspective. In ePortfolios in Australian Universities (pp. 1-11). Springer Singapore.

Miller, G. E. (1990). The assessment of clinical skills/competence/performance. *Journal of Academic Medicine*, *65*(9), S63–S67. doi:10.1097/00001888-199009000-00045 PMID:2400509

Mitchell, M. (1994). The views of students and teachers on the use of portfolios as a learning and assessment tool in midwifery education. *Nurse Education Today*, *14*(1), 38–43. doi:10.1016/0260-6917(94)90056-6 PMID:8159148

Miyazaki, T., Hotta, Y., Kunii, J., Kuriyama, S., & Tamaki, Y. (2009). A review of dental CAD/CAM: Current status and future perspectives from 20 years ofexperience. *Dental Materials Journal*, *28*(1), 44–56. doi:10.4012/dmj.28.44 PMID:19280967

Molnar, A. (1997). Computers in education: A brief history. *The Journal, 24*(11), 63-68.

Moore, M. G. (1973). *Speculations on a Definition of Independent Study*. Paper presented at the The Kellogg Invitational Conference (2nd), Vancouver, Canada.

Moran, M., & Jackson, L. (2012). The guide to everlasting employability. 10eightylimited.

Moreno, R., & Mayer, R. E. (1999). Cognitive Principles of Multimedia Learning: The Role of Modality and Contiguity. *J Educ Psychol*, *91*(2), 358–368. doi:10.1037/0022-0663.91.2.358

Mori, B., Carnahan, H., & Herold, J. (2015). Use of simulation learning experiences in physical therapy entry-to-practice curricula: A systematic review. *Physiotherapy Canada. Physiotherapie Canada*, *67*(2), 194–202. doi:10.3138/ptc.2014-40E PMID:25931672

Morley, L. (2001). Producing new workers: Quality, equality and employability in higher education. *Quality in Higher Education*, *7*(2), 131–138. doi:10.1080/13538320120060024

Moro, C., Stromberga, Z., Raikos, A., & Stirling, A. (2017). The Effectiveness of Virtual and Augmented Reality in Health Sciences and Medical Anatomy. *Anatomical Sciences Education*. doi:10.1002/ase.1696 PMID:28419750

Moyer, A. C., Young, W. A. II, Weckman, G. R., & Cutright, K. (2015). Rubrics on the Fly: Improving Efficiency and Consistency with a Rapid Grading and Feedback System. *Journal of Teaching and Learning with Technology*, *4*(2), 6–29. doi:10.14434/jotlt.v4n2.13473

Muller, M., & Kersten, S. (2003). Nutrigenomics: Goals and strategies. *Nature Reviews. Genetics*, *4*(4), 315–322. doi:10.1038/nrg1047 PMID:12671662

Mundkur, A., & Ellickson, C. (2012). Bringing the real world in: Reflection on building a virtual learning environment. *Journal of Geography in Higher Education*, *36*(3), 369–384. doi:10.1080/03098265.2012.692073

Murakami, T., Tajika, Y., Ueno, H., Awata, S., Hirasawa, S., Sugimoto, M., & Yorifuji, H. et al. (2014). An integrated teaching method of gross anatomy and computed tomography radiology. *Anatomical Sciences Education*, *7*(6), 438–449. doi:10.1002/ase.1430 PMID:24443310

Murphy, G., & Calway, B. (2008). Professional development for professional: Beyond sufficiency learning. *Australian Journal of Adult Learning*, *48*(3), 424–444.

Murray, J. (2016). *Technology in the classroom: What happens when it fails?* Retrieved 15 February, 2017, from http://www.teachhub.com/technology-classroom-what-happens-when-it-fails

Mustea, A., Naaji, A., & Herman, C. (2014). *Using Moodle for the development of Massive Open Online Courses*. Paper presented at the The International Scientific Conference eLearning and Software for Education.

Mwalumbwe, I., & Mtebe, J. S. (2017). Using Learning Analytics to Predict Students' Performance in Moodle Learning Management Systems: A case of Mbeya University of Science and Technology. *The Electronic Journal on Information Systems in Developing Countries*.

Myhrer, T., Evans, J. L., Haugen, H., Gorman, C., Kavanagh, Y., & Cameron, A. (2015). Exploring the consistency, transparency and portability of dental technology education: Benchmarking across Norway, Ireland and Australia. *European Journal of Dental Education*. doi:10.1111/eje.12160 PMID:26147858

Nagarajan, S. V., & McAllister, L. (2015). Integration of practice experiences into the allied health curriculum: Curriculum and pedagogic considerations before, during and after work-integrated learning experiences. *Asia Pacific Journal of Cooperative Education*, *16*(4), 279–290.

National Center for Biotechnology Information (NCBI). (1988). Retrieved from National Library of Medicine (US): https://www.ncbi.nlm.nih.gov/

National Health and Medical Research Council (NHMRC). (2010). *Medical Genetic Testing Information for Health Professionals*. Retrieved from https://www.nhmrc.gov.au/_files_nhmrc/publications/attachments/e99.pdf

National Health and Medical Research Council (NHMRC). (2013). *Discussing Direct-to-Consumer Genetic DNA Testing with Patients: A Short Guide for Health Professionals*. Retrieved from https://www.nhmrc.gov.au/_files_nhmrc/publications/attachments/g7_discussing_direct_to_consumer_genetic_testing_patients.pdf

National Health and Medical Research Council (NHMRC). (2015). *NHMRC additional levels of evidence and grades for recommendations for developers of guidelines*. Retrieved from https://www.nhmrc.gov.au/_files_nhmrc/file/guidelines/developers/nhmrc_levels_grades_evidence_120423.pdf

Naumann, F., Yang, J. L., Thai, T., Ford, C., & Polly, P. (2016). Virtual patient consultations and the use of an ePortfolio assessment to support student learning of integrated professional skills. *Focus on Health Professional Education: A Multi-Disciplinary Journal, 17*(3), 69.

Nelson, D., Ziv, A., & Bandali, K. S. (2012). Going glass to digital: Virtual microscopy as a simulation-based revolution in pathology and laboratory science. *Journal of Clinical Pathology, 65*(10), 877–881. doi:10.1136/jclinpath-2012-200665 PMID:22791768

Nestel, D., & Bearman, M. (2014). 0122 The Nhet-sim Program: A National Investment In Faculty Development. *BMJ Simulation and Technology Enhanced Learning, 1*(Suppl 1), A3–A3. doi:10.1136/bmjstel-2014-000002.6

Newble, D. I., & Jaeger, K. (1983). The effect of assessments and examinations on the learning of medical students. *Medical Education, 17*(3), 165–171. doi:10.1111/j.1365-2923.1983.tb00657.x PMID:6865814

Newton, R. (2003). Staff attitudes to the development and delivery of e-learning. *New Library World, 104*(10), 412–425. doi:10.1108/03074800310504357

Nguyen, L. T. C., & Gu, Y. (2013). Strategy-based instruction: A learner-focused approach to developing learner autonomy. *Language Teaching Research, 17*(1), 9–30. doi:10.1177/1362168812457528

Nguyen, N., Mulla, A., Nelson, A. J., & Wilson, T. D. (2014). Visuospatial anatomy comprehension: The role of spatial visualization ability and problem-solving strategies. *Anatomical Sciences Education, 7*(4), 280–288. doi:10.1002/ase.1415 PMID:24124041

Nguyen, N., Nelson, A. J., & Wilson, T. D. (2012). Computer visualizations: Factors that influence spatial anatomy comprehension. *Anatomical Sciences Education, 5*(2), 98–108. doi:10.1002/ase.1258 PMID:22232125

Nicholson, D. T., Chalk, C., Funnell, W. R. J., & Daniel, S. J. (2006). Can virtual reality improve anatomy education? A randomised controlled study of a computer-generated three-dimensional anatomical ear model. *Medical Education*, *40*(11), 1081–1087. doi:10.1111/j.1365-2929.2006.02611.x PMID:17054617

Nicol, D. (2010). Improving written feedback processes in mass higher education. *Assessment in Higher Education*, *35*(5), 501–517. doi:10.1080/02602931003786559

Nieder, G. L., Borges, N. J., & Pearson, J. C. (2011). Medical student use of online lectures: Exam performance, learning styles, achievement motivation and gender. *The Journal of the International Association of Medical Science Educators: JIAMSE*, *21*(3), 222–228. doi:10.1007/BF03341711

Nielsen, D. E., Shih, S., & El-Sohemy, A. (2014). Perceptions of genetic testing for personalized nutrition: A randomized trial of DNA-based dietary advice. *Journal of Nutrigenetics and Nutrigenomics*, *7*(2), 94–104. doi:10.1159/000365508 PMID:25170902

Nisbet, G., O'Keefe, M., & Henderson, A. (2016). Twelve tips for structuring student placements to achieve interprofessional learning outcomes. *MedEdPublish*, *5*(3), 23. doi:10.15694/mep.2016.000109

Nordstrom, K., Juth, N., Kjellstrom, S., Meijboom, F. L., & Gorman, U. (2013). Values at stake: Autonomy, responsibility, and trustworthiness in relation to genetic testing and personalized nutrition advice. *Genes & Nutrition*, *8*(4), 365–372. doi:10.1007/s12263-013-0337-7 PMID:23504640

NSW Government Health Centre for Genetics Education. (2016). *Ethical Issues in Human Genetics and Genomics*. Retrieved from http://www.genetics.edu.au/Publications-and-Resources/Genetics-Fact-Sheets/FactSheetELSI

NSW Health Centre for Genetics Education. (n.d.). *About MTHFR - Information for GPs*. Retrieved from http://www.genetics.edu.au/health-professionals/mthfr-dna-test

Nuzhat, A., Salem, R. O., Al Shehri, F. N., & Al Hamdan, N. (2014). Role and challenges of simulation in undergraduate curriculum. *Medical Teacher*, *36*(Suppl 1), S69–S73. doi:10.3109/0142159X.2014.886017 PMID:24617788

O'Connor, E., Obst, P., Furlong, M., & Hansen, J. (2015). Using the TARL model in psychology: Supporting first and final year students to compose reflections. In *Teaching Reflective Learning in Higher Education* (pp. 77–91). Springer International Publishing. doi:10.1007/978-3-319-09271-3_6

O'Donovan, C. B., Walsh, M. C., Forster, H., Woolhead, C., Celis-Morales, C., Fallaize, R., & Gibney, E. R. et al. (2016). The impact of MTHFR 677C --> T risk knowledge on changes in folate intake: Findings from the Food4Me study. *Genes & Nutrition*, *11*(1), 25. doi:10.1186/s12263-016-0539-x PMID:27708721

O'Flaherty, J., & Phillips, C. (2015). The use of flipped classrooms in higher education: A scoping review. *Internet and Higher Education*, *25*, 85–95. doi:10.1016/j.iheduc.2015.02.002

O'Shaughnessy, L., Haq, I., Maxwell, S., & Llewelyn, M. (2010). Teaching of clinical pharmacology and therapeutics in UK medical schools: Current status in 2009. *British Journal of Clinical Pharmacology*, *70*(1), 143–148. doi:10.1111/j.1365-2125.2010.03665.x PMID:20642558

Oh, C.-S., Kim, J.-Y., & Choe, Y. H. (2009). Learning of cross-sectional anatomy using clay models. *Anatomical Sciences Education*, *2*(4), 156–159. doi:10.1002/ase.92 PMID:19588481

Ohtake, P. J., Lazarus, M., Schillo, R., & Rosen, M. (2013). Simulation experience enhances physical therapist student confidence in managing a patient in the critical care environment. *Physical Therapy*, *93*(2), 216–228. doi:10.2522/ptj.20110463 PMID:23329555

Oliveira, T., & Martins, M. F. (2011). Literature review of information technology adoption models at firm level. *The Electronic Journal Information Systems Evaluation*, *14*(1), 110–121.

Oliver, B. (2013). Graduate Attributes as a focus for institution-wide curriculum renewal: Innovations and challenges. *Higher Education Research & Development*, *32*(3), 450–463. doi:10.1080/07294360.2012.682052

Oliver, B., von Konsky, B. R., Nikoletatos, P., Wilsinson, H., Ng, J., Quirke, T., & Moore, R. (2010). *Iportfolio, ITunesU, iPhone app: Capturing, tagging and sharing evidence of learning*. Presented at the *Association or Authentic Experiential and Evidence-Based Learning Conference*, Boston, MA.

Olson, P. W. (2005). Significant success factors in distance education. *International Journal of Case Method Research & Application*, *17*(2), 235–245.

Onah, D. F., Sinclair, J., Pang, E. L., & Jantjies, M. (2016). Exploring the multi-dimensional attainment of self-regulatory learning skills in educational contexts: A comparative study. *EDULEARN16 Proceedings*, 1-10.

Orr, D., Baram-Tsabari, A., & Landsman, K. (2016). Social media as a platform for health-related public debates and discussions: The Polio vaccine on Facebook. *Israel Journal of Health Policy Research*, *5*(1), 34. doi:10.1186/s13584-016-0093-4 PMID:27843544

Owen, J. (2016). *Renewing Australia's Promise Report Card 2016*. Foundation of Young Australians. Retrieved from http://www.fya.org.au

Owen, J. (2016). *Renewing Australia's promise Report Card*. Foundation of Australians. Retrieved from http://www.fya.org.au/report/renewing-australias-promise-report-card-2016/

Pahinis, K., Stokes, C. W., Walsh, T. F., & Cannavina, G. (2007). Evaluating a Blended-Learning Course Taught to Different Groups of Learners in a Dental School. *Journal of Dental Education*, *71*(2), 269–278. PMID:17314389

Palermo, C., Capra, S., Beck, E. J., Ash, S., Jolly, B., & Truby, H. (2016). Are dietetics educators' attitudes to assessment a barrier to expanding placement opportunities? Results of a Delphi study. *Nutrition & Dietetics: the Journal of the Dietitians Association of Australia*, *73*(3), 254–259. doi:10.1111/1747-0080.12205

Palermo, C., Chung, A., Beck, E. J., Ash, S., Capra, S., Truby, H., & Jolly, B. (2015). Evaluation of assessment in the context of work-based learning: Qualitative perspectives of new graduates. *Nutrition & Dietetics: the Journal of the Dietitians Association of Australia, 72*(2), 143–149. doi:10.1111/1747-0080.12126

Pani, J. R., Chariker, J. H., & Naaz, F. (2013). Computer-Based Learning: Interleaving Whole and Sectional Representation of Neuroanatomy. *Anatomical Sciences Education, 6*(1), 11–18. doi:10.1002/ase.1297 PMID:22761001

Pani, J. R., Chariker, J. H., Naaz, F., Mattingly, W., Roberts, J., & Sephton, S. E. (2014). Learning with interactive computer graphics in the undergraduate neuroscience classroom. *Advances in Health Sciences Education: Theory and Practice, 19*(4), 507–528. doi:10.1007/s10459-013-9483-3 PMID:24449123

Pan, Z., Cheok, A. D., Yang, H., Zhu, J., & Shi, J. (2006). Virtual reality and mixed reality for virtual learning environments. *Computers & Graphics, 30*(1), 8. doi:10.1016/j.cag.2005.10.004

Park, S. E., & Howell, T. H. (2015). Implemenation of a flipped classroom educational model in a predoctoral dental course. *Journal of Dental Education, 79*(5), 563–570. PMID:25941150

Pasek, J., More, E., & Hargittai, E. (2009). Facebook and Academic Performance: Reconciling a Media Sensation with Data. *First Monday Peer-Reviewed Journal on the Internet, 14*(5).

Patel, F., & Lynch, H. (2013). Glocalisation as an alternative to internationalisation in higher education: Embedding positive glocal learning perspectives. *International Journal on Teaching and Learning in Higher Education, 25*(2), 223–230.

Patrick, C.-j., Peach, D., Pocknee, C., Webb, F., Fletcher, M., & Pretto, G. (2008 December). *The WIL (work integrated learning) report: A national scoping study* [Australian Learning and Teaching Council (ALTC) Final Report]. Brisbane, Australia: Queensland University of Technology.

Pavlidis, C., Lanara, Z., Balasopoulou, A., Nebel, J. C., Katsila, T., & Patrinos, G. P. (2015). Meta-Analysis of Genes in Commercially Available Nutrigenomic Tests Denotes Lack of Association with Dietary Intake and Nutrient-Related Pathologies. *OMICS: A Journal of Integrative Biology, 19*(9), 512–520. doi:10.1089/omi.2015.0109 PMID:26348710

Pavlidis, C., Nebel, J. C., Katsila, T., & Patrinos, G. P. (2016). Nutrigenomics 2.0: The Need for Ongoing and Independent Evaluation and Synthesis of Commercial Nutrigenomics Tests' Scientific Knowledge Base for Responsible Innovation. *OMICS: A Journal of Integrative Biology, 20*(2), 65–68. doi:10.1089/omi.2015.0170 PMID:26689492

Peacock, S., Gordon, L., Murray, S., Morss, K., & Dunlop, G. (2010). Tutor response to implementing an ePortfolio to support learning and personal development in further and higher education institutions in Scotland. *British Journal of Educational Technology, 41*(5), 827–851. doi:10.1111/j.1467-8535.2009.00986.x

Pearson, A., & the Centre for Learning Futures. (2017). *ePortfolios to promote employability in Health students.* Retrieved from https://app.griffith.edu.au/explore/entry/3125/view

Pebble Learning Ltd. (2012). *Pebble+ Help: Pebble Pocket.* Retrieved from http://www.pebblepad.co.uk/pp3help/helpfile.aspx?t=1&vn=9.0&v=10&tg=3bf540bf-f5a7-4714-a00e-bca93111676b&f=193&v3k=d2a5149c-1595-4e4e-a02a-494a9f52d7c5

Pegg, A., Waldock, J., Hendy-Isaac, S., & Lawton, R. (2012). *Pedagogy for employability.* Higher Education Academy. Retrieved from: http://oro.open.ac.uk/30792/1/Pedagogy_for_employability_170212_1724.pdf

Perren, L. (2003). The role of e-mentoring in entrepreneurial education and support: A meta- review of academic literature. *Education + Training, 45*(8), 517–525. doi:10.1108/00400910310508900

Phillips, K. P. A. (2008). *Review of career development services in Australian tertiary institutions.* Canberra, Australia: Department of Education, Employment and Workplace Relations.

Podolskiy, O. (2012). Audio-visual (AV) learning. In N. Seel (Ed.), *Encyclopedia of the Sciences of Learning* (pp. 384–386). New York: Springer.

Polly, P., Marcus, N., Maguire, D., Belinson, Z., & Velan, G. M. (2014). Evaluation of an adaptive virtual laboratory environment using Western Blotting for diagnosis of disease. *BMC Medical Education, 14*(1), 222. doi:10.1186/1472-6920-14-222 PMID:25331335

Posey, L., Plack, M. M., & Snyder, R. (2015). Developing a Pathway for an Institution Wide ePortfolio Program. *International Journal of ePortfolio, 5*(1), 75-92.

Posey, L., Plack, M. M., Snyder, R., Dinneen, P. L., Feuer, M., & Wiss, A. (2015). Developing a pathway for an institution wide eportfolio program. *International Journal of ePortfolio, 5*(1), 75–92.

Preast, V., Danielson, J., Bender, H., & Bousson, M. (2007). Effectiveness of a computer-based tutorial for teaching how to make a blood smear. *Veterinary Clinical Pathology, 36*(3), 245–252. doi:10.1111/j.1939-165X.2007.tb00219.x PMID:17806072

Prensky, M. (2001). Digital Natives, Digital Immigrants Part 1. *On the Horizon, 9*(5), 1–6. doi:10.1108/10748120110424816

Prensky, M. (2009). H. sapiens digital: From digital immigrants and digital natives to digital wisdom. *Innovate: Journal of Online Education, 5*(3), 1–9.

Prensky, M. (2009). H. Sapiens digital: From immigrants and digitalnatives to digital wisdom. *Innovate: Journal of Online Education, 5*(3), 1–9.

Prince, K. J. A. H., Scherpbier, A. J. A. A., Van Mameren, H., Drukker, J., & Van Der Vleuten, C. P. M. (2005). Do students have sufficient knowledge of clinical anatomy? *Medical Education, 39*(3), 326–332. doi:10.1111/j.1365-2929.2005.02096.x PMID:15733169

Psotka, J. (1995). Immersive training systems: Virtual reality and education and training. *Instructional Science, 23*(5), 405–431. doi:10.1007/BF00896880

Puentedura, R. (2010). *SAMR and TPCK: Intro to advanced practice.* Retrieved August 16, 2017, from http://hippasus.com/resources/sweden2010/SAMR_TPCK_IntroToAdvancedPractice.pdf

Pytlikzilling, L. M., Bodvarsson, M., & Bruning, R. (2005). Technology-Based Education. Information Age Publishing.

Qi, Q., Wang, X., Strizich, G., & Wang, T. (2015). Genetic Determinants of Type 2 Diabetes in Asians. *International Journal of Diabetology & Vascular Disease Research*, (Suppl 1). doi:10.19070/2328-353X-SI01001 PMID:27583258

Quail, M., Brundage, S. B., Spitalnick, J., Allen, P. J., & Beilby, A. J. (2016). Student self-reported communication skills, knowledge and confidence across standardised patient, virtual and traditional clinical learning environments. *BMC Medical Education*, *16*(1), 73. doi:10.1186/s12909-016-0577-5 PMID:26919838

Quinton, S., & Smallbone, T. (2008). PDP implementation at English universities: What are the issues? *Journal of Further and Higher Education*, *32*(2), 99–109. doi:10.1080/03098770701851839

Radloff, A., & Coates, H. (2009). *Australasian Student Engagement Survey 2009 institution report*. Academic Press.

Radloff, A., & Coates, H. (2010). *Doing more for learning: enhancing engagement and outcomes: Australasian Survey of Student Engagement: Australasian Student Engagement Report*. Academic Press.

Rajanbabu, A., Drudi, L., Lau, S., Press, J. Z., & Gotlieb, W. H. (2014). Virtual reality surgical simulators: A prerequisite for robotic surgery. *Indian Journal of Surgical Oncology*, *5*(2), 125–127. doi:10.1007/s13193-014-0314-7 PMID:25114465

Ramsden, P. (2003). Learning to teach in higher education: Approaches to learning (2nd ed.). London: Routledge Falmer.

Ramsden, P. (1992). *Learning to teach in higher education*. London: Routledge. doi:10.4324/9780203413937

Ramsden, P. (2003). *Learning to teach in higher education; approaches to learning* (2nd ed.). London: Routledge.

Reardon, R. C., Lumsden, J. A., & Meyer, K. E. (2005). Developing an e-portfolio program: Providing a comprehensive tool for student development, reflection, and integration. *Journal of Student Affairs Research and Practice*, *42*(3), 630–642. doi:10.2202/1949-6605.1513

Reddan, G. (2008). The benefits of job-search seminars and mock interviews in a work experience course. *Asia Pacific Journal of Cooperative Education*, *9*(2), 113–127.

Reese, M., & Levy, R. (2009). *Assessing the future: E-portfolio trends, uses, and options in higher education*. Academic Press.

Reese, M., & Levy, R. (2009). Assessing the future: E-portfolio trends, uses, and options in higher education. *Research Bulletin*, *4*, 1–12.

Reifeis, P. E., Kirkup, M. L., Willis, L. H., & Browning, W. D. (2014). Introducing CAD/CAM into a predoctoral dental curriculum: A case study. *Journal of Dental Education*, *78*(10), 1432–1441. PMID:25281677

Reilly, P. R., & Debusk, R. M. (2008). Ethical and legal issues in nutritional genomics. *Journal of the American Dietetic Association*, *108*(1), 36–40. doi:10.1016/j.jada.2007.10.016 PMID:18155987

Rennie, F., & Morrison, T. (2012). *E-learning and social networking handbook: Resources for higher education*. Routledge.

Rice, S., & McKendree, J. (2014). e-learning. In T. Swantick (Ed.), Understanding medical education (pp. 161-173). Oxford, UK: Wiley and Sons.

Rice, S., & McKendree, J. (2014). e-learning. In T. Swanwick (Ed.), Understanding medical education: Evidence, theory and practice (2nd ed.; pp. 161-173). Oxford, UK: Wiley & Sons.

Rich, J. (2015). *Employability: Degrees of value*. HEPI Occasional Paper 12. Retrieved 20 April, 2017, from www.hepi.ac.uk

Roach, V. A., Brandt, M. G., Moore, C. C., & Wilson, T. D. (2012). Is three-dimensional videography the cutting edge of surgical skill acquisition? *Anatomical Sciences Education*, *5*(3), 138–145. doi:10.1002/ase.1262 PMID:22278856

Roblyer, M. D., & Doering, A. H. (2010). *Integrating Educational Technology Into Teaching* (5th ed.). Allyn & Bacon.

Rodger, S., Rodger, J., & Hoffman, S. (2010). Where in the world is interprofessional education? A global environmental scan. *Journal of Interprofessional Care*, *24*(5), 479–491. doi:10.3109/13561821003721329 PMID:20718594

Rogers, P. L., Jacob, H., Rashwan, A. S., & Pinsky, M. R. (2001). Quantifying learning in medical students during a critical care medicine elective: A comparison of three evaluation instruments. *Critical Care Medicine*, *29*(6), 1268–1273. doi:10.1097/00003246-200106000-00039 PMID:11395619

Rook, L. (2016). *Challenges implementing WIL in human resource management*. Paper presented at the WIL 2020: Pushing the boundaries, 2016 Australian Collaborative Education Network National Conference, Sydney, Australia.

Ross, J., & Collier, A. (2016). Complexity, mess, and not-yetness: Teaching online with emerging technologies. In G. Veletsianos (Ed.), *Emergence and innovation in digital learning: foundations and applications* (pp. 17–33). Edmonton, Canada: AU Press. doi:10.15215/aupress/9781771991490.01

Roswall, N., Angquist, L., Ahluwalia, T. S., Romaguera, D., Larsen, S. C., Ostergaard, J. N., & Tjonneland, A. et al. (2014). Association between Mediterranean and Nordic diet scores and changes in weight and waist circumference: Influence of FTO and TCF7L2 loci. *The American Journal of Clinical Nutrition*, *100*(4), 1188–1197. doi:10.3945/ajcn.114.089706 PMID:25099543

Roulin, N., & Bangerter, A. (2013). Students' use of extra-curricular activities for positional advantage in competitive job markets. *Journal of Education and Work*, *26*(1), 21–47. doi:10.1080/13639080.2011.623122

Rountree, M. L., & Davis, L. (2011). A dimensional qualitative research approach to understanding medically unnecessary aesthetic surgery. *Psychology and Marketing*, *28*(10), 1027–1043. doi:10.1002/mar.20426

Rowley, L. (2008). *How to Market and Sell Your Art, Music, Photographs, and Handmade Crafts Online: Turn Your Hobby Into a Cash Machine*. Atlantic Publishing Company.

Royal College of Pathologists of Australasia, & the Genetic Advisory Committee. (n.d.). *Position Statement MTHFR Genetic Tests*. Retrieved from https://www.rcpa.edu.au/Library/College-Policies/Position-Statements/MTHFR-Genetic-Tests

Rudolph, J. W., Raemer, D. B., & Simon, R. (2014). Establishing a safe container for learning in simulation: The role of the presimulation briefing. *Simulation in Healthcare*, *9*(6), 339–349. doi:10.1097/SIH.0000000000000047 PMID:25188485

Rudolph, J. W., Simon, R., Raemer, D. B., & Eppich, W. J. (2008). Debriefing as formative assessment: Closing performance gaps in medical education. *Academic Emergency Medicine*, *15*(11), 1010–1016. doi:10.1111/j.1553-2712.2008.00248.x PMID:18945231

Rudolph, J. W., Simon, R., Rivard, P., Dufresne, R. L., & Raemer, D. B. (2007). Debriefing with good judgment: Combining rigorous feedback with genuine inquiry. *Anesthesiology Clinics*, *25*(2), 361–376. doi:10.1016/j.anclin.2007.03.007 PMID:17574196

Rust, C., & Froud, L. (2011). 'Personal literacy': The vital, yet often overlooked, graduate attribute. *Journal of Teaching and Learning for Graduate Employability*, *2*(1), 28–40. doi:10.21153/jtlge2011vol2no1art551

Sabus, C., Sabata, D., & Antonacci, D. (2011). Use of a virtual environment to facilitate instruction of an interprofessional home assessment. *Journal of Allied Health*, *40*(4), 199–205. PMID:22138875

Sanderson, G. (2008). A foundation for the Internationalization of the academic self. *Journal of Studies in International Education*, *12*(3), 276–307. doi:10.1177/1028315307299420

Sankey, M., & Hill, R. S. (2005). *Multimodal design for hybrid learning materials in a second level economics course*. Paper presented at the the Eleventh Australasian Teaching Economics Conference: Innovation for Student Engagement in Economics, Sydney, Australia.

Sari, A. (2012). Impact of Determinants on Student Performance towards Information Communication Technology in Higher Education. *International Journal of Learning and Development*, *2*(2), 18–30. doi:10.5296/ijld.v2i2.1371

Scalese, R. J., Obeso, V. T., & Issenberg, S. B. (2008). Simulation technology for skills training and competency assessment in medical education. *Journal of General Internal Medicine*, *23*(1), 46–49. doi:10.1007/s11606-007-0283-4 PMID:18095044

Schaub-de Jong, M., Schönrock-Adema, J., Dekker, H., Verkerk, M., & Cohen-Schotanus, J. (2011). Development of a student rating scale to evaluate teachers' competencies for facilitating reflective learning. *Medical Education, 45*(2), 155–165. doi:10.1111/j.1365-2923.2010.03774.x PMID:21208261

Scoville, S. A., & Trent, D. B. (2007). Traditional and virtual microscopy compared experimentally in a classroom setting. *Clinical Anatomy (New York, N.Y.), 20*(5), 565–570. doi:10.1002/ca.20440 PMID:17109440

Sealey, R., Raymond, J., Groeller, H., Rooney, K., Crabb, M., & Watt, K. (2013). *Current practice of clinical exercise physiology placement supervision in Australia.* 2013 Report.

Sédille-Mostafaie, N., Engler, H., Lutz, S., & Korte, W. (2013). Advancing haemostasis automation–successful implementation of robotic centrifugation and sample processing in a tertiary service hospital. *Clinical Chemistry and Laboratory Medicine, 51*(6), 1273–1278. doi:10.1515/cclm-2012-0625 PMID:23241682

Seel, N. M. (Ed.). (2011). *Encyclopedia of the Sciences of Learning*. New York: Springer.

Seery, M. K., Agustian, H. Y., Doidge, E. D., Kucharski, M. M., O'Connor, H. M., & Price, A. (2017). Developing laboratory skills by incorporating peer-review and digital badges. *Chemistry Education Research and Practice, 18*(3), 403–419. doi:10.1039/C7RP00003K

Severt, N. (2016, October 26). 14 best online resume builders reviewed [Blog post]. Retrieved from https://uptowork.com/blog/best-online-resume-builders

Seybert, A. L., Kobulinsky, L. R., & McKaveney, T. P. (2008). Human Patient Simulation in a Pharmacotherapy Course. *American Journal of Pharmaceutical Education, 72*(2), 37. doi:10.5688/aj720237 PMID:18483603

Shaffer, K. (2004). Teaching anatomy in the digital world. *The New England Journal of Medicine, 351*(13), 1279–1281. doi:10.1056/NEJMp048100 PMID:15385652

Shakroum, M. A., Wong, K. W., & Fung, C. (2016). The effectiveness of the Gesture-Based learning system (GBLS) and its impact on learning experience. *Journal of Information Technology Education: Research, 15*, 191–210.

Shavinina, L., & Loarer, E. (1999). Psychological Evaluation of Educational Multimedia Applications. *European Psychologist, 4*(1), 33–44. doi:10.1027//1016-9040.4.1.33

Shead, D., Roos, R., Olivier, B., & Ihunwo, A. O. (2016). Gross anatomy curricula and pedagogical approaches for undergraduate physiotherapy students: A scoping review protocol. *JBI Database of Systematic Reviews and Implementation Reports, 14*(10), 98–104. doi:10.11124/JBISRIR-2016-003164 PMID:27846120

Sheppard, L., & Mackintosh, S. (1998). Technology in education: What is appropriate for rural and remote allied health professionals? *The Australian Journal of Rural Health, 6*(4), 189–193. doi:10.1111/j.1440-1584.1998.tb00311.x PMID:9919075

Siemens, G. (2005). Connectivism: Learning as network-creation. *ASTD Learning News, 10*(1).

Silage, D. A., & Gil, J. (1985). Digital image tiles: A method for the processing of large sections. *Journal of Microscopy, 138*(2), 221–227. doi:10.1111/j.1365-2818.1985.tb02615.x PMID:3894672

Simcock, D. C., Chua, W. H., Hekman, M., Levin, M. T., & Brown, S. (2017). A survey of first-year biology student opinions regarding live lectures and recorded lectures as learning tools. *Advances in Physiology Education, 41*(1), 69–76. doi:10.1152/advan.00117.2016 PMID:28143825

Simms, M. H., Mendis-Handagama, C., & Moore, R. N. (2007). Virtual microscopy in a veterinary curriculum. *Journal of Veterinary Medical Education, 34*(4), 416–422. doi:10.3138/jvme.34.4.416 PMID:18287467

Simpson, P., & Thyer, L. (2016). *Fitting together the pieces: Using the jigsaw classroom to facilitate paramedic WIL.* Paper presented at the WIL 2020: Pushing the boundaries, 2016 Australian Collaborative Education Network National Conference, Sydney, Australia.

Sinclair, N. (2015). How should our pedagogy keep up with rapidly changing technology? *Journal of Initial Teacher Inquiry, 1*, 31–33.

Singer, N. (2015, March 11). Privacy pitfalls as education apps spread haphazardly. *The New York Times*. Retrieved from https://www.nytimes.com/2015/03/12/technology/learning-apps-outstrip-school-oversight-and-student-privacy-is-among-the-risks.html?_r=0

Singh, J. (2017). *Moodle Stats – Moodle surpasses the 100 million users mark and India rises in the top 10 Moodle countries list #moodlestats*. Retrieved 06/04, 2017, from http://www.moodleworld.com/moodle-stats-moodle-surpasses-the-100-million-users-mark-and-india-rises-in-the-top-10-moodle-countries-list-moodlestats/

Sirhan, G. (2007). Learning difficulties in chemistry: An overview. *Journal of Turkish science education, 4*(2), 2.

Siu, F. K. P. (2013). The incorporation of eportolios into EFL courses: Barriers encountered in the diffusion of technology. *Journal of Interactive Learning Research, 24*(2), 211–231.

Skills Australia. (2010). *Australian workforce futures: A national workforce development strategy*. Canberra, Australia: Commonwealth of Australia.

Skills Australia. (2010). *Australian workforce futures: A national workforce development strategy.* Retrieved from https://docs.education.gov.au/system/files/doc/other/wwf_strategy-2010.pdf

Slade, C., Murfin, K., & Readman, K. (2013). Evaluating processes and platforms for potential eportfolio use: The role of the middle agent. *International Journal of ePortfolio, 3*(2), 177–188.

Slade, C., Murfin, K., & Readman, K. (2013). Evaluating Processes and Platforms for Potential ePortfolio Use: The Role of the Middle Agent. *International Journal of ePortfolio, 3*(2), 177-188.

Sloman, M. (2009). Learning and technology - What have we learnt? *Impact: Journal of Applied Research in Workplace E-learning, 1*(1), 12–26.

Smith, M., Brooks, S., Lichtenberg, A., McIlveen, P., Torjul, P., & Tyler, J. (2009). *Career development learning: Maximising the contribution of work-integrated learning to the student experience*. Final Project Report. University of Wollongong. Careers Central. Academic services Division.

Smither, R., Houston, J., & McIntire, S. (2016). *Organization development: Strategies for changing environments*. New York, NY: Routledge.

Smythe, G., & Hughes, D. (2008). Self-directed learning in gross human anatomy: Assessment outcomes and student perceptions. *Anatomical Sciences Education*, *1*(4), 145–153. doi:10.1002/ase.33 PMID:19177401

Soumya, B. G., & Ramachandra, S. S. (2011). Haptics Application in Dentistry: Is the Time Poised Yet? *Dental Hypotheses*, *19*. doi:10.5436/j.dehy.2011.2.00019

Stanciu, A., Mihai, F., & Aleca, O. (2012). Social Networking as an Alternative Environment for Education. *Accounting and Information Management Systems*, *11*(1), 56–75.

Stankov, S., Glavinic, V., & Rosic, M. (2011). *Intelligent tutoring systems in e-learning environments: Design, implementation and evaluation*. IGI Global. doi:10.4018/978-1-61692-008-1

Stark, C. M., & Pope, J. (2014). Massive open online courses: How registered dietitians use MOOCs for nutrition education. *Journal of the Academy of Nutrition and Dietetics*, *114*(8), 1147–1155. doi:10.1016/j.jand.2014.04.001 PMID:24842306

Steadman, R. H., Coates, W. C., Huang, Y. M., Matevosian, R., Larmon, B. R., McCullough, L., & Ariel, D. (2006). Simulation-based training is superior to problem-based learning for the acquisition of critical assessment and management skills. *Critical Care Medicine*, *34*(1), 151–157. doi:10.1097/01.CCM.0000190619.42013.94 PMID:16374169

Stein, C. D., Eisenberg, E. S., O'Donnell, J. A., & Spallek, H. (2014). What dental educators need to understand about emerging technologies to incorporate them effectively into the educational process. *Journal of Dental Education*, *78*(4), 520–529. PMID:24706681

Stephenson, C. R., Wang, A. T., Szostek, J. H., Bonnes, S. L., Ratelle, J. T., Mahapatra, S., & Wittich, C. M. et al. (2016). Flipping the continuing medical education classroom: Validating a measure of attendees' perceptions. *The Journal of Continuing Education in the Health Professions*, *36*(4), 256–262. doi:10.1097/CEH.0000000000000113 PMID:28350306

Sterling, R. (2008). The on-line promotion and sale of nutrigenomic services. *Genetics in Medicine*, *10*(11), 784–796. doi:10.1097/GIM.0b013e31818c0441 PMID:18941418

Stewart, J., Bevans-Williams, K., Bhattacharya, A., Ye, C., Miyazaki, K., & Kurtycz, D. (2008). Virtual microscopy: An educator's tool for the enhancement of cytotechnology student's locator skills. *Diagnostic Cytopathology*, *36*(6), 363–368. doi:10.1002/dc.20821 PMID:18478604

Stewart, J., & Knowles, V. (2001). Graduate recruitment: Implications for business and management courses in HE. *Journal of European Industrial Training*, *25*(2), 98–108. doi:10.1108/03090590110395771

Stewart-Knox, B. J., Bunting, B. P., Gilpin, S., Parr, H. J., Pinhao, S., Strain, J. J., & Gibney, M. et al. (2009). Attitudes toward genetic testing and personalised nutrition in a representative sample of European consumers. *British Journal of Nutrition*, *101*(7), 982–989. doi:10.1017/S0007114508055657 PMID:18775102

Stillman, P. L., Burpeau-Di Gregorio, M. Y., Nicholson, G. I., Sabers, D. L., & Stillman, A. E. (1983). Six years of experience using patient instructors to teach interviewing skills. *Academic Medicine*, *58*(12), 941–946. doi:10.1097/00001888-198312000-00004 PMID:6644777

Stirling, A., & Birt, J. (2014). An enriched multimedia eBook application to facilitate learning of anatomy. *Anatomical Sciences Education*, *7*(1), 19–27. doi:10.1002/ase.1373 PMID:23650104

Stokes, S. (2002). Visual Literacy in Teaching and Learning: A Literature Perspective. *Electronic Journal for the Integration of Technology in Education*, *1*(1), 10–19.

Storrs, M. J., Alexander, H. G. I., Sun, J., Kroon, J., & Evans, J. L. (2015). Measuring teams-based interprofessional education outcomes in cinical dentistry: Psychometric evaluation of a new scale at an Australian dental school. *Journal of Dental Education*, *79*(3), 249–258. PMID:25729018

Storrs, M. J., Alexander, H. G. I., Sun, J., Kroon, J., & Evans, J. L. (2015). Measuring teams-based interprofessional education outcomes in clinical dentistry: Psychometric evaluation of a new scale at an Australian dental school. *Journal of Dental Education*, *79*(3), 249–258. PMID:25729018

Strampel, K., Sibson, R., & Main, S. (2017). Professional Development to Support the Embedding of ePortfolios in Higher Education Programs. In ePortfolios in Australian Universities (pp. 33-46). Springer Singapore. doi:10.1007/978-981-10-1732-2_3

Strauss, W., & Howe, N. (1991). *Generations: The History of America's Future, 1584 to 2069*. HarperCollins.

Stwine, E. E., & Alves, M. G. (2010). Higher education and the employability of graduates. *European Educational Research Journal*, *9*(1), 32–44. doi:10.2304/eerj.2010.9.1.32

Su, C. H., & Cheng, C. H. (2015). A mobile gamification learning system for improving the learning motivation and achievements. *Journal of Computer Assisted Learning*, *31*(3), 268–286. doi:10.1111/jcal.12088

Sugand, K., Abrahams, P., & Khurana, A. (2010). The anatomy of anatomy: A review for its modernization. *Anatomical Sciences Education*, *3*(2), 83–93. doi:10.1002/ase.139 PMID:20205265

Sung, Y. H., Kwon, I. G., & Ryu, E. (2008). Blended learning on medication administration for new nurses: Integration of e-learning and face-to-face instruction in the classroom. *Nurse Education Today*, *28*(8), 943–952. doi:10.1016/j.nedt.2008.05.007 PMID:18599162

Sun, P.-C., Tsai, R. J., Finger, G., Chen, Y.-Y., & Yeh, D. (2008). What drives a successful e-Learning? An empirical investigation of the critical factors influencing learner satisfaction. *Computers & Education*, *50*(4), 1183–1202. doi:10.1016/j.compedu.2006.11.007

Sutherland, K., & Symmons, R. (2012). *Development of processes and assessment to facilitate a broad multidisciplinary Work Integrated Learning package*. Paper presented at the Australian Collaborative Education Network National Conference.

Svirko, E., & Mellanby, J. (2017). Teaching Neuroanatomy Using Computer-Aided Learning: What Makes for Successful Outcomes? *Anatomical Sciences Education*. doi:10.1002/ase.1694 PMID:28431201

Sweller, J. (1994). Cognitive load theory, learning difficulty, and instructional design. *Learning and Instruction*, *4*(4), 295–312. doi:10.1016/0959-4752(94)90003-5

Tam, M. D. B. S., Hart, A. R., Williams, S., Heylings, D., & Leinster, S. (2009). Is learning anatomy facilitated by computer-aided learning? A review of the literature. *Medical Teacher*, *31*(9), e393–e396. doi:10.1080/01421590802650092 PMID:19811174

Tanzawa, T., Futaki, K., Kurabayashi, H., Goto, K., Yoshihama, Y., Hasegawa, T., & Maki, K. et al. (2012). Medical Emergency Education Using a Robot Patient in a Dental Setting. *European Journal of Dental Education*. doi:10.1111/j.1600-0579.2012.00770.x PMID:23279398

Tanzawa, T., Futaki, K., Tani, C., Hasegawa, T., Yamamoto, M., Miyazaki, T., & Maki, K. (2011). Introduction of a Robot Patient into Dental Education. *European Journal of Dental Education*, *16*(1), e195–e199. doi:10.1111/j.1600-0579.2011.00697.x PMID:22251346

Taplin, R. H., Low, L. H., & Brown, A. M. (2011). Students' satisfaction and valuation of web-based lecture recording technologies. *Australasian Journal of Educational Technology*, *27*(2), 175–191. doi:10.14742/ajet.964

Taylor, B. (1999). The Darwinian shake-out in financial services. In Driving strategic change in financial services. Cambridge, UK: Woodhead Publishing Limited. doi:10.1016/B978-1-85573-431-9.50008-6

Taylor, N. (2015) The industrial revolution's next wave. In *CEDA Research Report, Australia's Future Workforce?* Retrieved 17 April, 2017, from http://www.ceda.com.au/research-and-policy/policy-priorities/workforce

ten Brinke, B., Klitsie, P. J., Timman, R., Busschbach, J. J. V., Lange, J. F., & Kleinrensink, G.-J. (2014). Anatomy Education and Classroom Versus Laparoscopic Dissection-Based Training: A Randomized Study at One Medical School. *Academic Medicine*, *89*(5), 806–810. doi:10.1097/ACM.0000000000000223 PMID:24667502

TEQSA. (n.d.). *Higher Education Standards Framework*. Canberra, Australia: Australian Government. Retrieved from http://www.teqsa.gov.au/teqsa-contextual-overview-hes-framework

Tess, P. A. (2013). The Role of Social Media in Higher Education Classes (Real and Virtual)—A Literature Review. *Computers in Human Behavior*, *29*, A60–A68.

Thomas, S. (2016). *Future Ready Learning: Reimagining the Role of Technology in Education. 2016 National Education Technology Plan*. Washington, DC: Office of Educational Technology, US Department of Education.

Thompson, C. J. (2016). Disruptive innovation: The rise of distance education. *Clinical Nurse Specialist CNS*, *30*(4), 238–241. doi:10.1097/NUR.0000000000000213 PMID:27309788

Thyer, L., & Simpson, M. D. (2016). *Wellness for health students during WIL*. Paper presented at the WIL 2020: Pushing the boundaries, 2016 Australian Collaborative Education Network National Conference, Sydney, Australia.

Tomlinson, M. (2006). 'The degree is not enough': Students' perceptions of the role of higher education credentials for graduate work and employability. *British Journal of Sociology of Education*, *29*(1), 49–61. doi:10.1080/01425690701737457

Tong, Y., Lin, Y., Zhang, Y., Yang, J., Zhang, Y., Liu, H., & Zhang, B. (2009). Association between TCF7L2 gene polymorphisms and susceptibility to type 2 diabetes mellitus: A large Human Genome Epidemiology (HuGE) review and meta-analysis. *BMC Medical Genetics*, *10*(1), 15. doi:10.1186/1471-2350-10-15 PMID:19228405

Townsend, G., & Winning, T. (2011). Research in PBL - where to from here for dentistry? *European Journal of Dental Education*, *15*(3), 193–198. doi:10.1111/j.1600-0579.2010.00655.x PMID:21762325

Towns, M., Harwood, C. J., Robertshaw, M. B., Fish, J., & O'Shea, K. (2015). The digital pipetting badge: A method to improve student hands-on laboratory skills. *Journal of Chemical Education*, *92*(12), 2038–2044. doi:10.1021/acs.jchemed.5b00464

Trent, R. (2014). Direct-to-consumer DNA testing and the general practitioner. *Australian Family Physician*, *43*(7), 436–439. PMID:25006602

Trigwell, K., & Prosser, M. (1996). Congruence Between Intention and Strategy in University Science Teachers' Approaches to Teaching. *Higher Education*, *32*(1), 77–87. doi:10.1007/BF00139219

Trigwell, K., Prosser, M., & Waterhouse, F. (1999). Relations between teachers' approaches to teaching and students' approaches to learning. *Higher Education*, *37*(1), 57–70. doi:10.1023/A:1003548313194

Turney, B. W. (2007). Anatomy in a Modern Medical Curriculum. *Annals of the Royal College of Surgeons of England*, *89*(2), 104–107. doi:10.1308/003588407X168244 PMID:17346399

Turnitin. (2012). *White paper: The Plagiarism Spectrum*. Retrieved from http://go.turnitin.com/paper/plagiarism-spectrum

Tuttle, N. A., & Bialocerkowski, A. (2014). *Finding a videoconferencing platform for simulated telemedicine is not a trivial pursuit*. Academic Press.

Tuttle, N. (2005). Do changes within a manual therapy treatment session predict between-session changes for patients with cervical spine pain? *The Australian Journal of Physiotherapy*, *51*(1), 43–48. doi:10.1016/S0004-9514(05)70052-0 PMID:15748124

Tuttle, N. (2009). Is It Reasonable to Use an Individual Patient's Progress After Treatment as a Guide to Ongoing Clinical Reasoning? *Journal of Manipulative and Physiological Therapeutics*, *32*(5), 396–403. doi:10.1016/j.jmpt.2009.04.002 PMID:19539124

Tuttle, N., Waite, M., & Bialocerkowksi, A. (2015). Increasing external clinical placement capacity and supplementing placement content through a centrally located telemedicine simulated learning environment. *Physiotherapy*, *101*, e1552. doi:10.1016/j.physio.2015.03.1548

Tworek, J. K., Jamniczky, H. A., Jacob, C., Hallgrímsson, B., & Wright, B. (2013). The LINDSAY Virtual Human Project: An immersive approach to anatomy and physiology. *Anatomical Sciences Education*, *6*(1), 19–28. doi:10.1002/ase.1301 PMID:22791664

Tymon, A. (2013). The student perspective on employability. *Studies in Higher Education*, *38*(6), 841–856. doi:10.1080/03075079.2011.604408

U.S. Food and Drug Administration. (2013). *Inspections, Compliance, Enforcement, and Criminal Investigations*. Retrieved from https://www.fda.gov/iceci/enforcementactions/warningletters/2013/ucm376296.htm

U.S. Food and Drug Administration. (2015). *FDA permits marketing of first direct-to-consumer genetic carrier test for Bloom syndrome*. Retrieved from https://www.fda.gov/NewsEvents/Newsroom/PressAnnouncements/ucm435003.htm

University of Minnesota. (2017). *Hype cycle for education: Emerging technologies in higher education*. Retrieved 2 February, 2017, from http://hypecycle.umn.edu/

University of Queensland. (n.d.). *Three Minute Thesis*. Retrieved 13 April, 2017, from http://threeminutethesis.org/

van der Zande, M. M., Gorter, R. C., & Wismeijer, D. (2013). Dental practioners and a digital future: An inital exploration of barriers and incentives to adopting digital technologies. *British Dental Journal*, *215*(11E21), 1–5. doi:10.1038/sj.bdj.2013.1146 PMID:24309814

Van Nuland, S. E., & Rogers, K. A. (2015). The anatomy of e-learning tools: Does software usability influence learning outcomes? *Anatomical Sciences Education*, *9*(4), 378–390. doi:10.1002/ase.1589 PMID:26671838

Vanderlelie, J. (2017). *Development of students professional identity through Me in a Minute presentations*. Retrieved from https://app.secure.griffith.edu.au/explore/entry/3765/view

Vanderlelie, J., & Dobinson, T. (2017). *Enhancing employability within curriculum using the Career Focus Module*. Retrieved from https://app.secure.griffith.edu.au/explore/entry/4625/view

vanNoort, R. (2012). The future of dental device is digital. *Dental Materials*, *28*(1), 3–12. doi:10.1016/j.dental.2011.10.014 PMID:22119539

Venkatiah, J. (2010). Computer-assisted modules to enhance the learning of anatomy by dissection. *Medical Education*, *44*(5), 523–524. doi:10.1111/j.1365-2923.2010.03657.x PMID:20519005

Vernick, S. H., Reardon, R. C., & Sampson, J. P. (2002). *Process and Evaluation of a Career Course: A Replication and Extension (Technical Report 31)*. Tallahassee, FL: Florida State University. Retrieved from http://career.fsu.edu/documents/technical%20reports/Technical%20Report%2031/Technical%20Report%2031.htm

Viswanathan, R. (2012). Teaching and Learning through MOOC. *Frontiers of Language and Teaching*, *3*(1), 32–40.

Vogel-Walcutt, J. J., Gebrim, J. B., & Nicholson, D. (2010). Animated versus static images of team processes to affect knowledge acquisition and learning efficiency. *Journal of Online Teaching and Learning*, *6*(1), 163–173.

Vuchkova, J., Maybury, T. S., & Farah, C. S. (2011). Testing the Educational Potential of 3D Visualization Software in Oral Radiographic Interpretation. *Journal of Dental Education*, *75*(11), 1417–1425. PMID:22058390

W3C. (2016). *Accessibility. Web design and applications*. Retrieved 1 April, 2017, from https://www.w3.org/standards/webdesign/accessibility

Walley, T., Bligh, J., Orme, M., & Breckenridge, A. (1994). Clinical pharmacology and therapeutics in undergraduate medical education in the UK: The future. *British Journal of Clinical Pharmacology*, *37*(2), 137–143. doi:10.1111/j.1365-2125.1994.tb04253.x PMID:8186060

Wang, J., Hu, X., & Xi, J. (2012). Cooperative learning with role play in Chinese pharmacology education. *Indian Journal of Pharmacology*, *44*(2), 253–256. doi:10.4103/0253-7613.93862 PMID:22529486

Ward, L. S., & Killian, P. (2011). Virtual Community Internships in the Classroom: Testing an Intervention. *Nurse Educator*, *36*(1), 40–44. doi:10.1097/NNE.0b013e3182001e6c PMID:21135684

Waters, J. R., Van Meter, P., Perrotti, W., Drogo, S., & Cyr, R. J. (2005). Cat dissection vs. sculpting human structures in clay: An analysis of two approaches to undergraduate human anatomy laboratory education. *Advances in Physiology Education*, *29*(1), 27–34. doi:10.1152/advan.00033.2004 PMID:15718380

Watson, D. M. (2001). Pedagogy before technology: Re-thinking the relationship between ICT and teaching. *Education and Information Technologies*, *6*(4), 251–266. doi:10.1023/A:1012976702296

Watson, K., Wright, A., Morris, N., McMeeken, J., Rivett, D., Blackstock, F., & Watson, G. et al. (2012). Can simulation replace part of clinical time? Two parallel randomised controlled trials. *Medical Education*, *46*(7), 657–667. doi:10.1111/j.1365-2923.2012.04295.x PMID:22646319

Watson, R. (2011). A rationale for the development of an extracurricular employability award at a British university. *Research in Post-Compulsory Education*, *16*(3), 371–384. doi:10.1080/13596748.2011.602248

Watts, A. G. (2006). *Career development learning and employability. Learning and Employability Series Two.* York, UK: ESECT and HEA. Retrieved April 12, 2017, from http://www.heacademy.ac.uk/assets/documents/resources/resourcedatabase/id592_career_development_learning_and_employability.pdf

Watts, A. G., Sweet, R., Haines, C., & McMahon, M. (2006). International symposium on career development and public policy: Synthesis of country papers. *Australian Journal of Career Development, 15*(3), 33–44. doi:10.1177/103841620601500308

WCPT. (2011). *WCPT guideline for the clinical education component of the physical therapist professional entry level programme.* Retrieved from London: www.wcpt.org/guidelines/clinical-education

Weber, A. S. (2013). *Cloud computing in education. In Ubiquitous and mobile learning in the digital age* (pp. 19–36). Springer. doi:10.1007/978-1-4614-3329-3_2

Weinstein, R. S., Descour, M. R., Liang, C., Barker, G., Scott, K. M., Richter, L., & Bartels, P. H. et al. (2004). An array microscope for ultrarapid virtual slide processing and telepathology. Design, fabrication, and validation study. *Human Pathology, 35*(11), 1303–1314. doi:10.1016/j.humpath.2004.09.002 PMID:15668886

Weitzel, K. W., McDonough, C. W., Elsey, A. R., Burkley, B., Cavallari, L. H., & Johnson, J. A. (2016). Effects of Using Personal Genotype Data on Student Learning and Attitudes in a Pharmacogenomics Course. *American Journal of Pharmaceutical Education, 80*(7), 122. doi:10.5688/ajpe807122 PMID:27756930

Wenger, E., Dermott, R. M., & Snyder, W. M. (2002). *Cultivating communities of practice: A guide to managing knowledge.* Boston: Harvard Business School.

Wen, R., Tay, W.-L., Nguyen, B. P., Chng, C.-B., & Chui, C.-K. (2014). Hand gesture guided robot-assisted surgery based on a direct augmented reality interface. *Computer Methods and Programs in Biomedicine, 116*(2), 68–80. doi:10.1016/j.cmpb.2013.12.018 PMID:24438993

Westerkamp, D., & Gahm, T. (1993). Non-distorted assemblage of the digital images of adjacent fields in histological sections. *Analytical Cellular Pathology, 5*, 235–247. PMID:8363984

Wheeler, A., Austin, S., & Glass, J. (2012). E-mentoring for employability. In Centre for Engineering and Design Education (Ed.), EE2012—Innovation, Practice and Research in Engineering Education (pp. 1–9). Loughborough University.

Wierinck, E., Puttamen, V., Swinnen, S., & van Steenberghe, D. (2005). Effect of Augmented Visual Feedback from a Virtual Reality Simulation System on Manual Dexterity Training. *European Journal of Dental Education, 9*(1), 10–16. doi:10.1111/j.1600-0579.2004.00351.x PMID:15642018

Williams, A., Birch, E., & Hancock, P. (2012). The impact of online lecture recordings on student performance. *Australasian Journal of Educational Technology, 28*(2), 199–213. doi:10.14742/ajet.869

Williams, A., Simmons, C., Levett-Jones, T., Sher, W., & Bowen, L. (2012). *Facilitating work integrated learning (WIL) through skills-enabled ePortfolios in construction and nursing final report*. Sydney: Office for Learning and Teaching, Department of Industry, Innovation, Science, Research and Tertiary Education. Retrieved from http://www.olt.gov.au/project-facilitating-wil-eportfolios-uon-2009

Williams, B., Boyle, M., Brightwell, R., McCall, M., McMullen, P., Munro, G., & Webb, V. et al. (2013). A cross-sectional study of paramedics' readiness for interprofessional learning and cooperation: Results from five universities. *Nurse Education Today*, *33*(11), 1369–1375. doi:10.1016/j.nedt.2012.06.021 PMID:22818954

Williams, S. L. (2006). The effectiveness of distance education in allied health science programs: A meta-analysis of outcomes. *American Journal of Distance Education*, *20*(3), 127–141. doi:10.1207/s15389286ajde2003_2

Willmarth-Stec, M., & Beery, T. (2015). Operationalizing the Student Electronic Portfolio for Doctoral Nursing Education. *Nurse Educator*, *40*(5), 263–265. doi:10.1097/NNE.0000000000000161 PMID:25783814

Wilson, C. P., McNulty, H., Ward, M., Strain, J. J., Trouton, T. G., Hoeft, B. A., & Scott, J. M. et al. (2013). Blood pressure in treated hypertensive individuals with the MTHFR 677TT genotype is responsive to intervention with riboflavin: Findings of a targeted randomized trial. *Hypertension*, *61*(6), 1302–1308. doi:10.1161/HYPERTENSIONAHA.111.01047 PMID:23608654

Wilson, C. P., Ward, M., McNulty, H., Strain, J. J., Trouton, T. G., Horigan, G., & Scott, J. M. et al. (2012). Riboflavin offers a targeted strategy for managing hypertension in patients with the MTHFR 677TT genotype: A 4-y follow-up. *The American Journal of Clinical Nutrition*, *95*(3), 766–772. doi:10.3945/ajcn.111.026245 PMID:22277556

Wilson, M., & Gerber, L. E. (2008). How Generational Theory can Improve Teaching: Strategies for Working with the "Millennials". *Currents in Teaching and Learning*, *1*(1).

Winchester-Seeto, T., Rowe, A., & Mackaway, J. (2016). Sharing the load: Understanding the roles of academics and host supervisors in work-integrated learning. *Asia Pacific Journal of Cooperative Education*, *17*(2), 101–118.

Wise, I., Skues, J., & Williams, B. (2011). *Facebook in Higher Education Promotes Social but not Academic Engagement.* Paper presented at the Annual Australasian Society of Computers in Learning in Tertiary Education (ASCILITE), Hobart, Australia.

Wise, L., Skues, J., & Williams, B. (2011). *Facebook in Higher Education Promotes Social but not Academic Engagement.* Paper presented at the Annual Australasian Society of Computers in Learning in Tertiary Education (ASCILITE) 2011, Hobart, Australia.

Woodley, C., & Sims, R. (2011). EPortfolios, professional development and employability: Some student perceptions. *Campus-Wide Information Systems, 28*(3), 164–174. doi:10.1108/10650741111145698

Wright, S., Mandrusiak, A., Ramsbotham, N., Hayles, E., & Kelly, K. (2014). The use of simulated learning to enhance cardiorespiratory acute paediatric physiotherapy across Queensland. *Pediatric Critical Care Medicine, 15*(4_suppl), 222.

Wright, A., Moss, P., Watson, K., Rue, S., Jull, G., Mandrusiak, A., & MacIntosh, S. et al. (2015). A profession-wide collaboration to embed role-play simulation into Australian entry-level physiotherapy clinical training. *Physiotherapy, 101*, e1047. doi:10.1016/j.physio.2015.03.1924

Wright, A., Moss, P., Watson, K., Rue, S., Jull, G., Mandrusiak, A., & Palmer, T. (2016). *Simulation in Physiotherapy Clinical Training*. Academic Press.

Wright, O. R. (2014). Systematic review of knowledge, confidence and education in nutritional genomics for students and professionals in nutrition and dietetics. *Journal of Human Nutrition and Dietetics, 27*(3), 298–307. doi:10.1111/jhn.12132 PMID:23781868

Xiannong, C. (2010). *Chinese acupuncture and moxibustion* (3rd ed.). Beijing: Foreign Languages Press.

Yamagata-Lynch, L. C. (2014). Blending online asynchronous and synchronous learning. *The International Review of Research in Open and Distributed Learning, 15*(2). doi:10.19173/irrodl.v15i2.1778

Yancey, K. B. (2001). Digitized student portfolios. *Electronic portfolios: Emerging practices in student, faculty, and institutional learning*, 15-30.

Yang, R. (2002). University internationalisation: Its meaning, rationales and implications. *Intercultural Education, 13*(1), 81–95. doi:10.1080/14675980120112968

Yelland, N., Tsembas, S., & Hall, L. (2008). E learning: Issues of pedagogy and practice for the information age. In P. Kell, W. Vialle, D. Konza, & G. Vogyl (Eds.), Introduction - learning and the learner: Exploring learning for new times (pp. 95-111). University of Wollongong.

Yen, K., & Gorelick, M. H. (2013). New Biomedical Devices That Use Near-Infrared Technology to Assist With Phlebotomy and Vascular Access. *Pediatric Emergency Care, 29*(3), 383–385. doi:10.1097/PEC.0b013e31828680f9 PMID:23462399

Yorke, M. (2006). Employability in higher education: What it is–what it is not. *Learning and Employability Series, 1*. Higher Education Academy. Retrieved from https://www.heacademy.ac.uk/knowledge-hub/employability-higher-education-what-it-what-it-not

Young, J. R. (2008). Blackboard customers consider alternatives. *The Chronicle of Higher Education*, *55*(3), A1.

Zaption. (2016, June 30). Zaption joins Workday [Blog post]. Retrieved from http://blog.zaption.com/post/146724427719/zaption-joins-workday

Zeichner, K., & Wray, S. (2001). The teaching portfolio in US teacher education programs: What we know and what we need to know. *Teaching and Teacher Education*, *17*(5), 613–621. doi:10.1016/S0742-051X(01)00017-8

Zgheib, N. K., Simaan, J. A., & Sabra, R. (2011). Using Team-based Learning to Teach Clinical Pharmacology in Medical School: Student Satisfaction and Improved Performance. *Journal of Clinical Pharmacology*, *51*(7), 1101–1111. doi:10.1177/0091270010375428 PMID:20671296

Zheng, L., Yue, L., Zhou, M., & Yu, H. (2013). Dental laboratory technology education in China: Current situation and challenges. *Journal of Dental Education*, *77*(3), 345–347. PMID:23486899

Zissis, D., & Lekkas, D. (2012). Addressing cloud computing security issues. *Future Generation Computer Systems*, *28*(3), 583–592. doi:10.1016/j.future.2010.12.006

Zitzelsberger, H., Campbell, K. A., Service, D., & Sanchez, O. (2015). Using wikis to stimulate collaborative learning in two online health sciences courses. *The Journal of Nursing Education*, *54*(6), 352–355. doi:10.3928/01484834-20150515-08 PMID:26057431

About the Contributors

Indu Singh has more than 30 years' experience practising laboratory medicine in Hong Kong and Australia with more than 15 years of teaching Haematology, Transfusion Science and Laboratory Medicine to undergraduate and postgraduate students. She obtained MSc in Histopathology from India, MSc in Laboratory Medicine from Charles Sturt University, New South Wales and PhD from RMIT University, Victoria, Australia. After 14 years' experience in Hong Kong Adventist Hospital Pathology she moved to Australia to work as a scientist at Melbourne Pathology and Cabrini Hospital in Melbourne while teaching and managing Haematology and transfusion at RMIT University. Currently she is an Associate Professor and Program Director of Medical Laboratory Science program at Griffith University, Queensland, Australia. Her research focus is haemostasis, antiplatelet therapy, and preventive role of antioxidants on life style induced oxidative stress related Metabolic Syndrome including Diabetes and Cardiovascular Diseases. In last 12 years, she has published more than 20 scientific journal articles, Change to 4 book chapters and 1 book and obtained funding to continue her research and support research of her more than 10 masters and PhD students.

* * *

Melissa Adamski, BSc, MND, APD, is an Accredited Practising Dietitian currently working at Monash University in Melbourne, in the area of nutritional genomics and the translation to nutrition practice. Melissa also works one on one with patients, providing practical experience in the implementation of the science of nutritional genomics into nutrition practice.

Mahmoud Bakr, BDS, MDS, Grad Cert High Ed, ADC, received his Bachelor Degree in Dental Medicine and Surgery from Cairo University in 2004. He completed his Masters Degree in Oral Biology from Cairo University in 2010. He was appointed as an academic within different departments in the Faculty of Dentistry (Cairo University) with a special focus on Oral Histopathology and Restorative

Dentistry in 2005, where he gained experience in Dental Education for five years. After moving to Australia in 2010, Dr. Bakr was appointed to teach within the School of Biomedical Sciences (University of Queensland). Dr. Bakr held different positions in Griffith University and in 2012, Dr. Bakr was appointed as a full-time Lecturer in General Dental Practice. In 2013, he completed a Graduate Certificate in Higher Education from Griffith University. Currently Dr. Bakr is the First Year Coordinator for dental science students within the School of Dentistry and Oral Health - Griffith University. Dr. Bakr has published over 25 peer reviewed articles in different fields including dental education, bone biology, periodontology, oral histopathology and preventative dentistry.

Natalie Colson, BHSc (Hons), Grad Cert Higher Ed, MND, PhD, is a Molecular Geneticist and Accredited Practising Dietitian. Natalie is currently a senior lecturer and program director at Griffith University Australia where she develops and delivers curricula to medical and allied health students, undertakes nutritional genomics research and supervises graduate students. Natalie has been formally recognized for her teaching approaches, including a National Citation for Outstanding Contribution to Student Learning. Natalie has authored over 30 publications in peer-reviewed scientific journals in the areas of genetics, nutrition, nutritional genomics and tertiary education.

Jane Evans is an Associate Professor in the School of Dentistry and Oral Health at Griffith University. She has researched, designed and developed the Bachelor of Oral Health in Dental Technology as the inaugural degree program for dental technology in Australia. Jane completed her doctoral studies on Interprofessional Education in Dental Technology Education. She writes and presents broadly on dental technology education. An earlier career as a successful dental technologist in the private and public sectors has resulted in an unconventional academic career path that provides an authentic context for academic work.

Vinod Gopalan is a Senior Lecturer in Medical Education in the School of Medicine at Griffith University, Gold Coast, Australia. Gopalan has over 15 years of experience in teaching/training medical students around the world and primarily focused on promoting self-directed learning and problem based learning among medical students. With a background in medicine and science, Gopalan has published multiple learning and teaching publications and grants in learning and teaching. His primary focuses in education include pathology/histology, pre-clinical, science and work integrated learning.

Brooke Harris-Reeves is a Senior Lecturer and Program Director in the School of Allied Health Sciences at Griffith University. Brooke's teaching and research interests are focused on making a difference in people's lives by focusing on Health & Education. She draws on her knowledge and experience in education to design curriculum and assessment 'for student learning', not 'of student learning' and is committed to ensuring students are 'work-ready' upon graduation.

Abdullah Karaksha is a Lecturer and the First Year Coordinator in the School of Medical Science at Griffith University. Abdullah's passion is teaching and helping students improve in their academic career. Abdullah's research interests include enhancing student engagement at higher education by designing online materials to supplement courses to increase student preference and performance. Abdullah collaborates with other academics to support students using his knowledge in online teaching.

Leanne Kenway completed her Bachelor of Physiotherapy, with Honours, at the University of Queensland in 1991, and her Doctor of Philosophy, at Griffith University in 2015. She is currently a Course Convenor for Anatomy and Physiology Systems delivered to Health students in their foundation year. Her 25-year background as a clinical physiotherapist enables her to bring real-world examples to the classroom, helping consolidate student knowledge and relevance of the basic sciences. She holds publications in the field of behavioural Neuroscience, and has a special interest in developing online tools to supplement her anatomy teaching.

Avinash Kundur completed his education and training in Bachelor of Pharmacy at JNTU University in 2008, Masters of Medical Science at RMIT University and Doctor Of Philosophy at Griffith University in 2017. He is currently a Course Convener for Cells, Tissues & Regulation and has many publications in the field of Haematology in association with Antioxidant Therapy, Anti-platelet Therapy and Cardiovascular Diseases.

E-Liisa Laakso is an Associate Professor of Physiotherapy, and former Head of Physiotherapy/Deputy Head of the School of Allied Health Sciences at Griffith University. Her research interests include physiotherapy education, and cancer care. Her teaching ranges across ethics, leadership and professional issues, to tissue healing and repair, cancer and palliative care, and electrophysical agents.

Robert Loudon is currently an educational designer at Griffith University (Australia) working with academics in the Health Faculty, particularly the School of Medicine, where he has overseen the development of extensive systems to support the delivery of learning and teaching resources to the MD program. Other recent activities include assisting an initiative at Griffith to roll out a new eportfolio and personal learning environment application to all courses, and the development of a bespoke assessment management system. Robert received a Master of Education in 2007; prior qualifications completed include a Grad. Cert. Learning Technology (2004), B.Multimedia (2001), B.Surveying (1980).

Lana Mitchell is a lecturer and First Year Coordinator in the Department of Nutrition & Dietetics at Griffith University. In addition to lecturing and research, Lana co-coordinates a variety of Learning & Teaching projects aimed at improving student learning and employability. As part of this, Lana has lead the implementation of the PebblePad ePortfolio tool within the Bachelor of Nutrition & Dietetics degree.

Sapha Mosawy is an academic within the School of Medical Science at Griffith University. Dr Mosawy has worked as a medical laboratory scientist in both public and private pathology departments. Currently, Dr Mosawy is an academic for Haematology and Transfusion Science.

Trude Myhrer is an Assistant Professor and a Certified Dental Technologist with a Master in Vocational Pedagogy. She is Head of studies for Radiography and Dental Technology, at Oslo and Akershus University College of Applied Sciences, and has participated in design and developing the Bachelor degree program for Dental Technology in Norway. Trude leads a digitalization project at the Faculty of Health science, and is developing digital educational resources for internal, national and international use. Her research focus is pedagogical themes, international collaboration, elderly and oral health, and use of digital resources in higher education. Trude has worked as a successful dental technologist as an owner and general manager in the private sectors for nearly 20 years prior to entering an academia in 1999, this background provides an authentic context for academic work.

Yun-Mi Nguy is a Medical Scientist graduate from the University of Technology, Sydney. Over the past 12 years, she has worked in various Haematology and Blood Bank laboratories and is currently working as a Haematology and Transfusion Science Scientific Officer at Griffith University Gold Coast Campus. While currently in this role, her main initiatives are to continually improve tertiary level practical laboratory techniques and processes in all areas of Haematology and simulate pathology laboratories found across the nation and globally around the world.

Andrew Pearson is a Senior Lecturer and the First Year Coordinator in the School of Medical Science at Griffith University. Andrew is dedicated to positively addressing the challenges of scaffolding the academic success of diverse groups of students with a demanding curriculum through the development diagnostic testing and supplementary academic support, academic recovery, innovative assessment, embedding employability into the curriculum, the creation of online resources, and enhancing student engagement and learning.

Ganeshan Rao is currently the Blended Learning Manager, Health Faculty at Griffith University (Australia). He received his Master in Library Science (1991) from University of British Columbia (Canada) and Post Graduate Diploma in Marine Studies (1999), Graduate Certificate in Education (1981) & BSc (Biology & Chemistry, 1981) from the University of the South Pacific (Fiji). He is responsible for blended learning and educational design services for the faculty enabling in the increased, enhanced, and appropriate use of technology including learning management system in the design of student-centered learning experiences informed by evidence-based strategies and resources. He develops, implements and oversees academic staff development initiatives that address the needs of academics and help them increase capabilities to meet the objective of increased uptake and appropriate use of educational technology to enhance student learning.

Roselyn Rose'Meyer has taught the discipline of pharmacology for 25 years to undergraduate students including pharmacy, biomedical science, medicine and nursing students. Her research background and expertise is in cardiovascular pharmacology. She has a history of research training with many PhD, Masters of Medical Research and Honours students completing research projects in pharmacology with most of the students completing research into hypertension, aging and diabetes. While pharmacological research has been the cornerstone of her postgraduate teaching and mentorship, she has also expanded the scope of research interests as an educator, investigating learning and teaching pedagogy that underpins current pharmacology education, research ethics and tacit knowledge skills in biomedical research.

Abishek Santhakumar completed his Doctor of Philosophy at Griffith University in 2014. His research investigates the role of natural dietary antioxidant compounds in reducing the risk factors of cardiovascular and metabolic diseases. Abishek started his academic career in Medical Laboratory Science (Pathology) at Griffith University in 2011. In 2014, he was appointed as a Lecturer in Haematology in the Pathology discipline at Central Queensland University. Abishek is currently a Lecturer and Researcher in Haematology and Blood Banking at the School of Biomedical Sciences, Charles Sturt University and a Chief Investigator at the ARC ITTC Centre for Functional Grains. During his research tenure, Abishek has led nationally registered human clinical trials investigating the feasibility and efficacy of natural antioxidant compounds as therapeutic alternatives in diverse pro-thrombotic populations. Abishek is a Fellow of the Institute of Biomedical Sciences (FIBMS) and a full professional member of the Australian Institute of Medical Scientists (MAIMS).

Mary-Ann Shuker is a Blended Learning Advisor in the Health Group at Griffith University (Australia). For the past 5 years she has supported academics to increase their capabilities across the 8 Health schools in planning, designing and implementing evidence-informed blended learning solutions in order to enhance their teaching to improve both student experience and outcomes. She has investigated many technologies to meet academic needs. She is currently assisting in Griffith initiatives to appropriately engage academics with new enterprise platforms in active learning (Echo360 ALP) and adaptive learning (SmartSparrow). She was previously involved in technology trials of online marking tools and the large scale migration from one Learning Management System to another. Mary-Ann received a Graduate Certificate in Higher Education in 2016. Prior qualifications completed include Master of Library and Information Management (2012), Graduate Diploma in Adult Education (1995) and B Applied Science (Computing) (1986). She continues her professional development with online courses including Applying the Quality Matters Rubric, Learning to Teach Online, Carpe Diem and Gamification.

Neil Tuttle (BSc, GradDipAdvManipTher, MPhil, PhD) is a Senior Lecturer in Physiotherapy at Grifith University. Hehas been a musculoskeletal physiotherapist for over 35 years with his time being divided between clinical practice and teaching for most of those years. He completed his PhD in 2008, He has received over $1.5 million in grants for simulated learning.

Jessica Vanderlelie, as the Innovative Research Universities Vice Chancellors' Fellow, leads a collaborative approach to research, design, innovate and disseminate scalable, practices to improve student outcomes across all demographics. Jessica is a passionate academic that has demonstrated sustained leadership in learning and teaching in Australian Higher Education with a key focus on supporting student and graduate success. At Griffith University Jessica led a significant program of activities to embed authentic employability based curriculum across the Faculty of Health. Jessica's achievements in the development and implementation of practice-based curriculum have been recognised nationally through a series of prestigious awards, including the Australian Award for Excellence in Teaching (early career) in 2012 and an OLT citation for her work in innovative assessment design in biochemistry. In 2015, Jessica was awarded an Australian Office of Learning and Teaching Fellowship for a project entitled 'Engaging alumni for graduate success'.

Index

P

R

S

T

V

W

www.ingramcontent.com/pod-product-compliance
Lightning Source LLC
LaVergne TN
LVHW080342011026
849161LV00009B/2159